Evaluating Climate Change Impacts

Evaluating Climate Change Impacts

Edited by
Vyacheslav Lyubchich
Yulia R. Gel
K. Halimeda Kilbourne
Thomas J. Miller
Nathaniel K. Newlands
Adam B. Smith

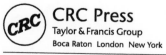

CRC Press
Taylor & Francis Group
Boca Raton London New York

CRC Press is an imprint of the
Taylor & Francis Group, an **informa** business

A CHAPMAN & HALL BOOK

First edition published 2021
by CRC Press
6000 Broken Sound Parkway NW, Suite 300, Boca Raton, FL 33487-2742

and by CRC Press
4 Park Square, Milton Park, Abingdon, Oxon OX14 4RN

First issued in paperback 2023

© 2021 Taylor & Francis Group, LLC
CRC Press is an imprint of Taylor & Francis Group, an Informa business

Reasonable efforts have been made to publish reliable data and information, but the author and publisher cannot assume responsibility for the validity of all materials or the consequences of their use. The authors and publishers have attempted to trace the copyright holders of all material reproduced in this publication and apologize to copyright holders if permission to publish in this form has not been obtained. If any copyright material has not been acknowledged please write and let us know so we may rectify in any future reprint.

Except as permitted under U.S. Copyright Law, no part of this book may be reprinted, reproduced, transmitted, or utilized in any form by any electronic, mechanical, or other means, now known or hereafter invented, including photocopying, microfilming, and recording, or in any information storage or retrieval system, without written permission from the publishers.

For permission to photocopy or use material electronically from this work, access www.copyright.com or contact the Copyright Clearance Center, Inc. (CCC), 222 Rosewood Drive, Danvers, MA 01923, 978-750-8400. For works that are not available on CCC please contact mpkbookspermissions@tandf.co.uk

Trademark Notice: Product or corporate names may be trademarks or registered trademarks, and are used only for identification and explanation without intent to infringe.

Publisher's Note
The publisher has gone to great lengths to ensure the quality of this reprint but points out that some imperfections in the original copies may be apparent.

ISBN-13: 978-0-8153-9237-8 (hbk)
ISBN-13: 978-0-367-55213-8 (pbk)
ISBN-13: 978-1-351-19083-1 (ebk)

DOI: 10.1201/9781351190831

Typeset in LMRoman
by Vyacheslav Lyubchich and Nova Techset Private Limited, Bengaluru & Chennai, India

Contents

Preface — xi

I Ecosystem Impacts — 1

1 On Evaluation of Climate Models — 3
Kaibo Gong and Snigdhansu Chatterjee
1.1 Introduction — 3
1.2 A brief tour of climate models — 4
1.3 Evaluation of climate model outputs: summary measures — 5
1.4 Ensemble-based approaches — 7
1.5 Probabilistic model evaluation techniques — 11
1.6 Ensemble using empirical likelihood — 15
1.7 Conclusions and future directions — 17
References — 18

2 A Statistical Analysis of North Atlantic Tropical Cyclone Changes — 25
Thomas J. Fisher, Robert Lund, and Michael W. Robbins
2.1 Introduction — 25
2.2 Data — 27
2.3 Statistical methods — 28
2.4 Results — 33
2.5 Comments and conclusions — 39
References — 41

3 Fire-Weather Index and Climate Change — 45
Zuzana Hubnerova, Sylvia Esterby, and Steve Taylor
3.1 Introduction — 45
3.2 Statistical modeling of the fire-weather index monthly maxima — 48
3.3 Summary and discussion — 56
References — 61

4 Probabilistic Projections of High-Tide Flooding for the State of Maryland in the Twenty-First Century — 65
Ming Li, Fan Zhang, Yijun Guo and Xiaohong Wang
4.1 Introduction — 65
4.2 Methods — 69

	4.3	Results	72
	4.4	Conclusions	80
		References	83

5 Response of Benthic Biodiversity to Climate-Sensitive Regional and Local Conditions in a Complex Estuarine System — 87
Ryan J. Woodland and Jeremy M. Testa

5.1	Introduction	87
5.2	Methods	89
5.3	Results	96
5.4	Discussion	104
5.5	Conclusions	115
	References	115

6 Using Structural Comparisons to Measure the Behavior of Complex Systems — 123
Ryan E. Langendorf

6.1	Introduction	123
6.2	Data	125
6.3	Network alignment	126
6.4	Visualization	127
6.5	Example: the Chesapeake Bay	128
6.6	Critical considerations	130
6.7	Recipe	132
6.8	Final thought	135
	References	135

7 Causality Analysis of Climate and Ecosystem Time Series — 139
Mohammad Gorji Sefidmazgi and Ali Gorji Sefidmazgi

7.1	Introduction	139
7.2	Methods of causality detection	141
7.3	Simulations	149
7.4	Conclusions	157
	References	159

II Socioeconomic Impacts — 163

8 Statistical Issues in Detection of Trends in Losses from Extreme Weather and Climate Events — 165
Richard W. Katz

8.1	Introduction	165
8.2	Loss distribution	170
8.3	Bias, uncertainty, and variability in losses	176
8.4	Detection and attribution of trends in losses	178
8.5	Summary and discussion	182
	References	185

9 Event Attribution: Linking Specific Extreme Events to Human-Caused Climate Change 187
Stephanie Herring
- 9.1 Why is this chapter in this book? 187
- 9.2 Background on event attribution 188
- 9.3 Event attribution methodologies 188
- 9.4 Impact attribution 192
- 9.5 FAR = 1 or "Not possible without climate change" ... 194
- 9.6 Communicating event attribution studies 195
- 9.7 Summary 197
- References 197

10 Financing Weather and Climate Risks in the United States 201
Roger S. Pulwarty, David R. Easterling, Jeffery Adkins, and Adam B. Smith
- 10.1 Disasters in the United States—the recent record ... 201
- 10.2 Climate and extremes 203
- 10.3 Assessing economic impacts 206
- 10.4 Insurance and risk financing 211
- 10.5 Data and analytical challenges 219
- 10.6 Implementation challenges 222
- 10.7 Financing mitigation and resilience 223
- 10.8 Pathways and conclusion 226
- References 229

11 Extreme Events, Population, and Risk: An Integrated Modeling Approach 235
Lelys Bravo de Guenni, Desireé Villalta, and Andrés Sajo-Castelli
- 11.1 Introduction 235
- 11.2 Conceptual framework for risk modeling 236
- 11.3 Applications of the conceptual framework 238
- 11.4 Discussion, conclusions, and future work 252
- References 255

12 Aspects of Climate-Induced Risk in Property Insurance 259
Ola Haug
- 12.1 Introduction 259
- 12.2 The role of statistics in assessing insurance climate risk ... 260
- 12.3 Water damage to properties in Norway 263
- 12.4 The Gjensidige case study 264
- 12.5 Climate change and property insurance interactions ... 271
- 12.6 Conclusions 274
- References 275

13 Climate Change Impacts on the Nation's Electricity Sector — 277
Craig D. Zamuda
- 13.1 Introduction ... 277
- 13.2 Climate impacts and implications for the electricity sector . 280
- 13.3 Resilience approaches and options ... 288
- 13.4 Analytical approaches for assessing costs and benefits of resilience investments ... 290
- 13.5 Gaps and opportunities for improvement in resilience planning ... 296
- References ... 301

14 Impacts of Inclement Weather on Traffic Accidents in Mexico City — 307
Sophie Bailey, S. Marcelo Olivera-Villarroel, and Vyacheslav Lyubchich
- 14.1 Introduction ... 307
- 14.2 Data description ... 310
- 14.3 Methods ... 313
- 14.4 Results ... 316
- 14.5 Conclusions ... 320
- References ... 321

15 Statistical Modeling of Dynamic Greenhouse Gas Emissions — 325
Nathaniel K. Newlands
- 15.1 Overview ... 325
- 15.2 Background ... 326
- 15.3 Introduction ... 326
- 15.4 Statistical framework ... 328
- 15.5 Ecosystem dynamical optimization ... 331
- 15.6 Numerical results ... 334
- 15.7 Summary ... 338
- 15.8 Appendix: model parameters and variables ... 339
- References ... 343

16 Agricultural Climate Risk Management and Global Food Security: Recent Progress in Southeast Asia — 347
Louis Kouadio and Eric Rahn
- 16.1 Climate risks management in agriculture—use of climate prediction in crop models ... 348
- 16.2 Current approaches integrating SCFs and crop simulation models applied in Southeast Asia ... 349
- 16.3 Examples of integrated SCF-crop modeling approach for climate risk management in Southeast Asia ... 350

16.4 Challenges for operationalizing seasonal climate-crop modeling frameworks in Southeast Asia 355
16.5 Improved climate risk management in Southeast Asia—the way forward 357
References 359

17 Poppy Cultivation and Eradication in Mexico, 2000–2018: The Effects of Climate 363
S. Marcelo Olivera-Villarroel and Maria del Pilar Fuerte Celis
17.1 Introduction 363
17.2 Context 365
17.3 Methodology 366
17.4 Results 370
17.5 Discussion 375
17.6 Conclusions 376
References 377

Index 381

Preface

We are delighted to introduce this book on *Evaluating Climate Change Impacts*. It presents the topic of assessing and quantifying climate change and its impacts from a multifaceted perspective of ecosystem, social, and infrastructure resilience, given through a lens of statistics and data science. Recall the group of men who tried to describe an elephant without seeing the animal: the conclusion of each man was "locally correct," but it was hard to comprehend the overall picture. Similarly, climate variability and the impact of climate change cannot be described sufficiently well solely with trends in temperature or in concentrations of greenhouse gases. Moreover, even if these trends are known for each area on the globe, the implications are usually unclear, leaving the elephant unrecognized and possibly mistreated. Thus, the book provides a multidisciplinary view on the implications of climate variability and shows how the new data science paradigm can help us to mitigate climate-induced risk and to enhance climate adaptation strategies.

While encompassing the frontier approaches of data science for climate variability and being quantitatively oriented, the book targets a broad audience, providing the background and overview of the current state of the knowledge and open interdisciplinary research directions. The book emphasizes the key role of uncertainty quantification and, more generally, of statistics and data science in assessing the climate change outcomes and associated risk management.

The book consists of chapters solicited from leading topical experts and presents their perspectives on climate change effects in two general areas: natural ecosystems (Part I) and socioeconomic impacts (Part II). No sole-author book can achieve a comparable interdisciplinary depth and rigor in describing the details of seemingly disparate but tightly interrelated problems. We put an effort to arrange the chapters in a cohesive story, unveiling from "distant" and general topics of atmospheric circulation, climate modeling, and long-term prediction, then approaching the problems of increasing frequency of particular extreme events, local sea-level rise, forest fires, and reaching closer and deeper into economic losses, analyses of climate impacts for insurance, agriculture, fisheries, and electric and transport infrastructures.

The book contributes to the body of knowledge in three major ways:

1. Provides an integrated view on the climate change processes, describing climate change effects not only in physical systems, but

also in biodiversity, national security, infrastructure resilience, and financial well-being.

2. Showcases the importance of data science in tackling the interconnected problems, including problems related to high frequency, high dimensions, large volume of data, and multisource multiresolution data sources.

3. Gathers an interdisciplinary group of experts and exposes the links between different areas and processes associated with climate change.

We are grateful to all the contributors for their collaboration. We also thank John Kimmel of Taylor & Francis for his patience and support during the preparation of this book.

Part I
Ecosystem Impacts

1
On Evaluation of Climate Models

Kaibo Gong and Snigdhansu Chatterjee
University of Minnesota, Minneapolis, MN, USA

CONTENTS

1.1	Introduction	3
1.2	A brief tour of climate models	4
1.3	Evaluation of climate model outputs: summary measures	5
	1.3.1 Simple summary measures	5
	1.3.2 Evaluation by process isolation, instrument simulators, and initial value techniques	6
1.4	Ensemble-based approaches	7
	1.4.1 Multimodel ensembles	8
	1.4.2 Perturbation-parameter ensembles	8
	1.4.3 Reliability ensemble averaging	8
	1.4.4 Bayesian ensembles	9
	1.4.5 Machine-learning ensemble approaches	10
1.5	Probabilistic model evaluation techniques	11
	1.5.1 Model comparison by moving-block bootstrap	11
	1.5.2 Evaluation using functional representations	12
1.6	Ensemble using empirical likelihood	15
1.7	Conclusions and future directions	17
References		18

1.1 Introduction

An excellent starting place for learning about climate models and about evaluation of climate models is Flato et al (2014). In particular, a comprehensive discussion on several aspects of climate model evaluation is present there and omitted here, to keep this chapter within reasonable length as well as cohesive in content. Such omitted topics include experimental strategies for climate model comparison, the details of the simulation processes for atmosphere, ocean, sea ice, and other spheres of study as well as simulations for variability and extremes, topics like regional climates, downscaling, climate feedbacks, and detailed data analysis results. A very recent discussion on the state-of-the-art in model evaluation, based primarily from a climate science perspective, can be found in Eyring et al (2019). The general pattern of how well climate models have performed in the past has been studied in Hausfather et al (2020).

In this chapter, we focus mostly on the *data science methodology, principles, and caveats* related to the science of evaluating the performance of climate models. We present a very brief, and necessarily incomplete, overview of climate models in Section 1.2. This is followed by a review of the statistical and machine learning techniques that have been used to assess the quality of climate models. In course of this review, we note interesting technical and methodological details, and important caveats noted by different teams of authors, and also include our own remarks.

We begin by discussing the first generation of climate model evaluation strategies in Section 1.3, which are typically simple summary measures of discrepancy between model outputs and observed data. A more sophisticated approach resulted from the efforts to construct ensembles of climate model outputs, which are discussed in Section 1.4. The current generation of probabilistic scoring and ranking of climate models is discussed in Section 1.5. A new approach, based on empirical likelihood, and combining some of the strengths of the probabilistic scoring as well as the ensemble-based approach, is very briefly discussed in Section 1.6. Owing to the scope of the problem, our review is necessarily limited in coverage and details.

1.2 A brief tour of climate models

Climate models are developed from the first principles of physics, like energy, mass, and momentum conservation. These principles translate to a complex system of mathematical formalizations under a variety of idealistic assumptions, for example, using numerous interrelated partial differential equations. Such complex systems of equations can only be solved using numeric methods, typically involving approximations over a discretized grid of space and time values. However, several natural processes are too complex and are not resolved by a discretized system of equations. Examples of such processes mentioned in Flato et al (2014) include biochemical processes in vegetation and cloud processes and turbulence. As a result, conceptual models or parameterizations of several physical, chemical, and biological processes are additionally required, further increasing complexity of the mathematical framework. In addition, some components of climate models are deterministic, while others are not (Gleckler et al, 2008).

A realistic solution system for such a framework requires a model resolution that represent compromises on assumptions on the physical processes and parameterizations, on assignment of relative importance of the different constituent processes including exclusion of some processes or components, based on available computational resources. There are several kinds of climate models, from basic energy balance models, complex Atmosphere–Ocean General Circulation Models (AOGCMs) that can include components for atmosphere, ocean, land and sea ice, greenhouse gases and aerosols, to full-scale Earth System Models (ESMs) that can further include the carbon cycle, the sulfur cycle, or ozone. Climate models may be global or regional in terms of their spatial coverage, and both these kinds have their own constraints and features. See Chapter 4 for an example of implementing a regional ocean model.

Owing to the scale and complexity of the entire system, generally major components like the atmosphere or oceans are individually modeled and then assembled together. A small number of model parameters are used to benchmark the model in a process called *model tuning*, that is, ensure that the model adheres to large-scale observational constraints like global averages.

1.3 Evaluation of climate model outputs: summary measures

Given the variety of modeling and numeric constraints that are necessary for obtaining simulation outputs from climate model runs, as well as the gaps in our knowledge of the Earth's climate, quality assessments are needed for these outputs. An evaluation of the quality of climate model outputs will help us understand the physics better and better design climate models. For example, the tasks of assigning relative importance to different Earth system components, or different parameterizations or model conditions, may be facilitated by better understanding of the quality of simulations from different model runs.

In essence, the various techniques for evaluating climate model performance approach the problem by making the technical assumption that the observed data and the simulation runs from different climate models are random fields. This assumption can be justified from a number of viewpoints: there are measurement errors, approximations, and inaccuracies in observations, and the models are subject to both aleatoric and epistemic uncertainties. Additionally note that, statistical models reflect usefulness and not exactness, and the fact that climate models contain intractable deterministic components should not hinder modeling such processes using stochastic terms.

1.3.1 Simple summary measures

The performance of a climate model may be assessed over different spatial regions and different time scales, and for multiple climate variables. In the

Fifth Assessment Report of the Intergovernmental Panel on Climate Change, multiple methodologies were adopted for evaluating the performance of various climate models (Flato et al, 2014). These included evaluating overall model results using scalar performance metrics, cluster analysis that collected together multiple kinds of scalar metrics, and visualization tools, based on Cadule et al (2010), Gleckler et al (2008), Nishii et al (2012), Pincus et al (2008), Sahany et al (2012), Waugh and Eyring (2008), Yokoi et al (2011).

As a scalar metric of performance, a popular tool is the *root mean squared error* (RMSE), defined as the square-root of the sum of squared differences between observed data and model simulated output. Other popular tools include bias (difference between averages of observed and model-generated data), correlation, variance. These tools have been used by Cadule et al (2010), Gleckler et al (2008), Pincus et al (2008), Sahany et al (2012), and Waugh and Eyring (2008) to study multiple variables including atmospheric temperature, wind, sea surface temperature, and ocean surface heat and momentum fluxes, clouds, precipitation, and radiation and so on. These evaluations have been done at several spatial and temporal scales and resolutions (for example, monthly means over the planet), and for multiple statistical characteristics (for example, median instead of mean, measures of variability, and so on). The multiple scalar metrics are generally statistically related to each other, but nevertheless may point to different strengths and weaknesses of the models, and may be hard to interpret, and cluster analysis was proposed as a summarization tool (Nishii et al, 2012, Yokoi et al, 2011). Caveats about interpreting such metrics are included in the literature, for example, Gleckler et al (2008) observe, " (...) *we expect metrics to provide symptoms of problems, but to be less informative than diagnostics for illuminating their causes.*" Recent open-source products to obtain summary metrics on climate models include Eyring et al (2016) and Gleckler et al (2016).

However, the capacity of any metric to indicate a problem with a climate model depends on the statistical properties of the metric, for example, its distribution under the hypothesis that there is no problem with the model. Additional caveats on interpretation of simple metrics like a bias or RMSE should be in place, based on statistical considerations. Such metrics, as well as off-the-shelf cluster analysis or other multivariate data analysis techniques, can yield meaningful results under statistical assumptions that may or may not hold for the observed data, or a simulated output from a climate model. In addition, robustness and sensitivity properties of the results with respect to both data quality and technical assumptions, and computational approximations used to arrive at the numeric values should be carefully studied.

1.3.2 Evaluation by process isolation, instrument simulators, and initial value techniques

As opposed to considering temporal or spatial averages of model outputs and comparing those to corresponding data averages, one may consider physically distinct regimes or processes instead. This approach may be more informative about the strengths and deficiencies of a climate model, since its components may not be similar in quality or fidelity. Among papers that use this approach are Bellucci et al (2010), Brient and Bony (2013), Brown et al (2010), Ichikawa et al (2012), Jiang et al (2012, 2015), Konsta et al (2012), Schneider et al (2017), Su et al (2013), Tsushima et al (2013), Wood et al (2011), and several others.

Instrument simulator approaches compute variants of observation-equivalents that a satellite might have recorded if it were observing a model, and provide alternative data sources for evaluating models; see Bodas-Salcedo et al (2008, 2011), Klein et al (2013), Pincus et al (2012), Stubenrauch et al (2013), Williams and Webb (2009), Yokohata et al (2010), and related studies.

Climate and weather modeling have similar atmospheric model components (Phillips et al, 2004). Consequently, the atmospheric component may be evaluated using weather prediction models with appropriate initialization. Research in this direction has been carried out by Klocke and Rodwell (2014), Ma et al (2014), Santer et al (2019), Suzuki et al (2015), Webb et al (2017), Xie et al (2012), Zhang et al (2010), and several others.

From a data science perspective, the studies discussed in this part involve machinery similar to those mentioned in Section 1.3.1, but there is scope for more deeper methodological research here, some of which is already underway (Dueben and Bauer, 2018, O'Gorman and Dwyer, 2018, Rasp et al, 2018, Scher and Messori, 2019).

1.4 Ensemble-based approaches

A different track on assessing the uncertainty in climate model simulations is to use *ensemble methods*, which primarily refer to either multimodel ensembles, or perturbed-parameter ensembles. Instead of ranking models or assigning a quality score to each climate model, trying to create an optimal ensemble of models can be of more practical value for future projections. Additionally, the weights assigned to the models in an optimal ensemble may be interpreted as quality scores. However, ensembles may not be reflective of physical reality, and the uncertainty, accuracy, precision, or probabilistic properties of ensembles may not be easy to obtain. In Section 1.4.1 and Section 1.4.2, we describe very briefly the two kinds of ensembles that have been considered in the literature, namely, multimodel and perturbed-parameter ensembles.

A statistical problem associated with constructing ensembles of climate models is how to define optimality, for both kinds of ensembles. Traditionally, optimality has been computed in terms of two criteria: (i) performance on historical data, and (ii) agreement with other climate models. The first criterion is based on an evaluation of how well a model performs with observed data, for example, with hindcasts. The second criterion, which can be more debatable, is an evaluation of how much a model is in agreement with other models. In Section 1.4.1 and following subsections in this section, we briefly discuss a few prominent ensemble construction methodology, that explicitly or implicitly define optimality in terms of weighted averages of historical performance and consensus.

1.4.1 Multimodel ensembles

Multimodel ensembles assemble simulated runs from different modeling centers, and are expected to be informative about structural uncertainty and internal variability. However, since the underlying physics for different models is often the same and there are even shared components (Masson and Knutti, 2011), the statistical properties of multimodel ensembles may not emulate the sample average of several independent and identical random variates. Details on multimodel ensembles, including caveats about interpreting results from this approach, are available in Abramowitz et al (2019), Herger et al (2018), Knutti (2010), Knutti et al (2010a,b, 2013, 2017), Lorenz et al (2018), Sanderson et al (2015, 2017), Sunyer et al (2014), Tebaldi and Knutti (2007), among other places.

1.4.2 Perturbation-parameter ensembles

Perturbed-parameter ensembles are based on a single model, but use simulations with different parameter values (Rougier et al, 2009). This allows for greater clarity on the roles of the different parameters in contributing to model uncertainty, however, the results naturally depend on the quality and features of the underlying climate model. Ensembles primarily using Bayesian statistical machinery, including those that may encompass both multimodel and perturbed-parameter ensembles have been proposed (Furrer et al, 2007a, Milliff et al, 2011, Sanderson, 2013, Sexton and Murphy, 2012, Sexton et al, 2012). However, it seems that systematic errors and effects due to components that are not explicitly controlled or parameterized may be unaccounted for in such ensemble-based approaches. In addition, the stochastic properties of either multimodel or perturbed-parameter ensembles are not transparent, so a Bayesian or non-Bayesian approach towards studying ensembles requires additional assumptions that may not be easy to verify.

1.4.3 Reliability ensemble averaging

The reliability ensemble averaging (REA) method obtains average, uncertainty range, and a measure of reliability of simulated atmosphere-ocean general circulation model (AOGCM) simulation (Giorgi and Mearns, 2002). Consider the case of temperature as an example, with L models and observed data, and the goal is to obtain an ensemble to model change in temperatures ΔT. Let R_i be the *model reliability factor*, whose definition is given later. The REA ensemble estimator of ΔT is a weighted average

$$\widetilde{\Delta T} = \left(\sum_{i=1}^{L} R_i\right)^{-1} \sum_{i=1}^{L} R_i \Delta T_i$$

of the ΔT_i's, the i-th model's estimate of ΔT, for $i = 1, \ldots, N$. The model reliability factor R_i's explicitly use model performance and the convergence as reliability criteria. Define the *model bias* $B_{T,i}$ as the difference between the i-th model simulated and observed mean temperature for the present-day period (taken to be 1961–1990 in Giorgi and Mearns, 2002). Also, let $D_{T,i}$ denote the distance between ΔT_i and $\widetilde{\Delta T}$. In terms of these, the model reliability factor R_i is defined as

$$R_i = \left((R_{B,i})^m (R_{D,i})^n\right)^{1/(m \times n)}, \text{ where}$$
$$R_{B,i} = \min\left(1, \frac{\epsilon_T}{|B_{T,i}|}\right), \text{ and}$$
$$R_{D,i} = \min\left(1, \frac{\epsilon_T}{|D_{T,i}|}\right),$$

where ϵ_T is a measure of natural variability calculated from data, and m, n are tuning constants, typically set to $m = n = 1$. Note that since $\widetilde{\Delta T}$ involved $D_{T,i}$ through the R_i's, an iterative scheme may be used for the numeric computations of the above.

The technical statistical assumptions that underlie this method are not explicit, and the choice of the relative weights assigned to model quality and model consensus, controlled through m and n, seems to be up to the user. The probabilistic properties of $\widetilde{\Delta T}$ or the R_i's is not clear, for example, it is not apparent that with an updated or slightly changed data set the R_i's would not drastically alter their relative rankings or values.

1.4.4 Bayesian ensembles

Following Giorgi and Mearns (2002), more sophisticated schemes for constructing ensembles were reported, primarily based on Bayesian statistical principles. We highlight two prominent works in this area, namely, Smith et al (2009) and Tebaldi et al (2005).

Suppose X_ℓ and Y_ℓ are the model outputs for present and future temperatures for the ℓ-th model, and X_0 is the current observed temperature. These are modeled as

$$X_\ell \sim N\left(\mu, \lambda_\ell^{-1}\right), \ell = 0, 1, \ldots, L, \text{ and}$$
$$Y_\ell \sim N\left(\nu, (\theta \lambda_\ell)^{-1}\right), \ell = 1, \ldots, L,$$

where $N(\mu, \lambda^{-1})$ is Gaussian distribution with mean μ and variance $1/\lambda$. Flat priors are set for μ and ν, and the λ_ℓ's for $\ell = 1, \ldots, L$ are assigned a gamma prior. A separate gamma prior is set for θ, and λ_0 is a fixed constant representing natural variability. A Markov Chain Monte Carlo (MCMC) scheme is used to approximate the posterior distribution. It can be computed that the posterior mean for λ_ℓ is inversely proportional to two terms, one represents model performance and the other is a measure of model convergence.

A variant of the above assumes that (X_ℓ, Y_ℓ) have a bivariate normal distribution, which alters the relative importance given to model performance and consensus. The paper by Smith et al (2009) strengthens the above framework, by introducing a hierarchical structure on the gamma priors, using cross-validation steps to validate the statistical assumptions, using a multivariate model and corresponding Gibbs-metropolis updating equations. Other variants are due to Greene et al (2006) and Furrer et al (2007b).

The relative importance given to model performance in terms of being able to replicate observed data, and consensus in terms of not being too unlike other models, is controlled by the parameter θ. In the event that λ_ℓ values are small, that is, the variance of model output for past and present times is high, the Bayesian ensemble tends to put a very high weight on consensus.

1.4.5 Machine-learning ensemble approaches

Modern machine-learning approaches for understanding the properties and predictions of climate models have been advocated in several places (Anderson and Lucas, 2018, Dijkstra et al, 2019, Ivatt and Evans, 2019, Scher, 2018). The primary focus of these studies has been on improving forecasts and predictions, but there has also been some effort at replicating climate model outputs using neural networks and other machines, with a view towards understanding their properties better.

We briefly mention a strategy of constructing ensembles based on *sequential* or *online learning*, which have been used with climate model outputs in McQuade and Monteleoni (2017), Monteleoni et al (2011), Strobach and Bel (2015) and several references therein. Unlike Bayesian modeling approaches described in Section 1.4.4, the online learning approach does not require probabilistic assumptions, but can still come up with some guarantees of prediction error in terms of performance relative to the best model in hindsight. The online learning algorithm starts typically with equal weight on each model, and then updates the weights based on the model's ability to replicate past observed data. This is done sequentially over time: the motivation being that over time models that have better performance will tend to have more weight. This sequential learning approach seems to value past performance of climate models, and consequently does not force consensus as an additional condition.

1.5 Probabilistic model evaluation techniques

The evaluation measures discussed above typically consider summary statistical measures quantifying the difference between observed data and simulated model runs, but do not associate probabilistic scores to such summary measures. Thus, they are not informative on whether the bias or mean squared error of a particular model is ignorable and insignificant variation, or a significant modeling deficiency. The summary statistics themselves are generally simple, standard metrics, and not motivated from the probabilistic principles of data science or statistics. Thus, there is no guarantee that the simple performance metrics have any optimality or robustness properties.

Sophisticated ensemble methods, like the Bayesian or machine learning methods, may be retooled for a proper probabilistic evaluation, but major data science challenges lie ahead. For example, the relative weights of an optimal ensemble do not inform about whether some, or all, the models are poor/excellent quality, or about the variability or distribution of the weights. Probabilistic model evaluation techniques, discussed in this section, provide reliable quality scores for each model, and associated uncertainty measures.

An additional matter of concern for the approaches described earlier is that those tend to compare a climate model output to an observation at a fixed time and location, thus performance is measured under the implicit assumption that the ideal model would produce exact numeric values as in observed data. However, climate models are based on first principles of physics, and in the best of cases they would be able to replicate the *patterns* of observed data, and not exact numeric values. Consequently, it is possible that the above evaluation techniques may undervalue model performance by requiring that a model simulated output exactly match a noisy observation, or in the case of machine learning approaches of Section 1.4.5, may overfit the data.

For the rest of this section, we assume that the observed and model generated data are time series, for simplicity. We denote observed data by $\mathbf{Y}_0 = (Y_{0,1}, \ldots, Y_{0,N_0})^\top \in \mathbb{R}^{N_0}$, and the ℓ-th model run by $\mathbf{Y}_\ell = (Y_{\ell,1}, \ldots, Y_{\ell,N_\ell})^\top \in \mathbb{R}^{N_\ell}$, for $\ell = 1, \ldots, L$. Much of the discussion below can be generalized to spatiotemporal data with little or no conceptual extension.

1.5.1 Model comparison by moving-block bootstrap

One of the first primarily data-driven approaches for evaluating climate model performance comes from Braverman et al (2011). They propose a non-parametric likelihood-based approach, using summary statistics to characterize important features of any model run, then approximating the distribution of such summary statistics using a moving-block bootstrap method, and finally evaluating the likelihood of the same summary statistics computed on the observed data. We briefly describe the methodology adopted by Braverman et al (2011) below.

Let $\{A = \ell\}$ be the event that model ℓ properly represents the physical process, or equivalently, with the same properties as the observed series, summarized by the statistic $g(\mathbf{Y}_0)$. Suppose $f(g(\mathbf{Y}_0)|A = \ell)$ is the probability mass/density function, under model ℓ, evaluated at the observed summary statistic value $g(\mathbf{Y}_0)$, which may thus be interpreted as the likelihood of model ℓ. In this framework an evaluation of a model is similar to comparing the posterior probabilities $\mathbb{P}[A = \ell | g(\mathbf{Y}_0)] \propto f(g(\mathbf{Y}_0)|A = \ell)\mathbb{P}[A = \ell]$. Setting $\mathbb{P}[A = \ell]$ to be equal for all $\ell = 1, \ldots, L$, this then reduces to comparing the likelihoods of the observed data, as summarized by $g(\mathbf{Y}_0)$, under each model.

The choice of summary statistics $g(\mathbf{Y}_0)$ was fixed at the first, second, and third empirical quartiles by Braverman et al (2011). Then, the authors use a moving block bootstrap method to obtain empirically the values of $f(g(\mathbf{Y}_0)|A = \ell)$. The moving block algorithm is implemented as follows: the original simulation run $\mathbf{Y}_\ell = (Y_{\ell,1}, \ldots, Y_{\ell,N_\ell})^T \in \mathbb{R}^{N_\ell}$ of the ℓ-th model is broken into overlapping, contiguous blocks of length k, say $\{\tilde{Y}_{\ell,i_1} = \{Y_{\ell,i_1}, \ldots, Y_{\ell,i_1+k}\}, i_1 = 1, \ldots, N_\ell - k + 1\}$. Then these $\tilde{Y}_{\ell,i_1}$ are sampled with replacement $h = [N_\ell/k]$ (the largest integer less than or equal to $[N_\ell/k]$) times, say these randomly drawn contiguous blocks are $\{\tilde{Y}_{\ell,i}^*, \ldots, \tilde{Y}_{\ell,h}^*\}$. These are then concatenated together to generate the resample $\mathbf{Y}_{\ell,b}^* = (Y_{\ell,1,b}, \ldots, Y_{\ell,hk,b})^T$ of approximately the same length as N_ℓ. The summary statistics are computed on this resample, thus obtaining $g(\mathbf{Y}_{\ell,b})$. The above steps are repeated a large B number of times to obtain the resampled summary values $\{g(\mathbf{Y}_{\ell,b}), b = 1, \ldots, B\}$, and then the function $f(\cdot)$ is estimated by density estimation techniques from these resampled summary values. The authors discuss a computational tractable method for choosing k. The moving block bootstrap assumes stationarity of the time series $\mathbf{Y}_\ell = (Y_{\ell,1}, \ldots, Y_{\ell,N_\ell})^T$.

1.5.2 Evaluation using functional representations

A different line of thinking motivated the series of research papers by Braverman et al (2017), Chatterjee (2019), and Gong et al (2018). These papers identified the observed data and simulation outputs from discretely observed instances of functions $\{\mathbf{Y}_\ell(t), t \in [0,1]\}$, $\ell = 0, 1, \ldots, L$, where t denotes time. These functions contain the deterministic or stochastic trend terms, multi-decadal, decadal, and shorter-term (like El Niño Southern Oscillation, ENSO) oscillations and fluctuations, very short-term components that essentially characterize weather (as opposed to climate), as well as noise terms: entirely as far as $\mathbf{Y}_0(\cdot)$ is concerned, and with varying degrees of fidelity for the different model runs $\mathbf{Y}_\ell(\cdot)$, $\ell = 1, \ldots, L$.

The issue of climate model performance evaluation then becomes one of isolating the climate-related components from the observed or simulated discretely-observed functions, and then comparing them. In the absence of a mathematically precise definition of *climate*, Chatterjee (2019) proposed that low-frequency components of the function $\mathbf{Y}_0(\cdot)$ be considered as climate, higher frequency components being more akin to associated weather and noise, such a definition was implicit in Braverman et al (2017). The formal approach taken by Braverman et al (2017), Chatterjee (2019), Gong et al (2018) is to use wavelets for decomposing the functions $\{\mathbf{Y}_\ell(t), t \in [0,1]\}$, $\ell = 0, 1, \ldots, L$, thus obtaining a multiscale time-frequency representation of each observed time series. The low-frequency components correspond to coarse wavelet scales in this representation. In Gong and Chatterjee (2020), a nonstationary Fourier functional representation is used instead. Other functional representations may also be used and may be equivalent to using frequency or time-scale representations in terms of the theoretical foundations, but wavelets and nonstationary spectral representations seem particularly useful in the present context in view of the oscillatory nature of many climate components.

Assume that the observed and the model-generated series have been detrended and de-seasonalized, which can be easily done using the scaling (father wavelet) function in the wavelet representations. Then, we may write $\mathbf{Y}_\ell(t) = \mu_\ell(t) + E_\ell(t)$ for $\ell = 0, 1, \ldots, L$, where $\mu_\ell(t)$ stands for the climate components and $E_\ell(t)$ gather the weather and noise terms.

Then, the problem of whether the ℓ-th climate model accurately depicts this planet's climate is reduced to the hypothesis-testing problem $H_0 : \mu_\ell(\cdot) = \mu_0(\cdot)$. Readers will recognize this approach as the *two-sample testing* problems, extended to the case of functional parameters with the observations being random fields! A comparison of trends can be easily worked into this framework by including the trends in $\mu_\ell(\cdot)$. Different scales may be separately analyzed, for example, to study whether a model represents the ENSO or some multi-decadal oscillation adequately. The alternative to the above null hypothesis can vary according to the context and use-case, and can be either a simple negation of the null, or that $\mu_\ell(\cdot)$ is a location-scale shifted version of $\mu_0(\cdot)$, and so on. This framework extends very easily to spatial and spatiotemporal data, the only change needed for such cases is to define the domain of the data and parameter functions appropriately, which is just $t \in [0,1]$ in the current time series comparison context. Multiple climate variables can also be considered simultaneously, and interesting tests involving co-integrating or other relations between the variables is feasible.

Extremely importantly, this approach can adequately address the fact that simulated runs from climate models are supposed to be representative numeric outputs, and are neither designed to be nor expected to be exact matches for the observed numeric values of a climate variable, say temperature, at different times and locations. In statistical terms, both the climate model output and observed data are *samples* from their respective populations, and it is of interest to test if the *climate components* of these populations match. Some of the *ad hoc* summary metrics or ensemble-based techniques may fail to take this factor into account.

Naturally, there are several challenges in this functional statistics approach as well. First, there are numeric problems to overcome: standard implementation of Mallat's algorithm for wavelet decomposition is available for evenly spaced data, with sample size or length of time series being a power of 2. This limitation was overcome in Gong et al (2018) by using a data interpolation technique. Another practical issue is that in much software, wavelet decomposition packages may not exist for two or higher dimensions, thus limiting current usage for spatial or spatiotemporal climate data. The present framework models the periodicities or frequencies of the climate and weather-related oscillations in a way that is algorithmically convenient, rather than adapting to their natural patterns. The choice of wavelet basis functions has some influence on the results of the hypothesis test.

More serious challenges are tied to the theoretical framework assumptions and methodological steps needed to construct an appropriate test statistic, and to get the distribution of the test statistic under the null and alternative hypotheses. For test statistics, Braverman et al (2017) and Chatterjee (2019) consider functions of the vector of wavelet coefficients from the coarse levels, while Gong et al (2018) reconstruct the climate signal using such coarse-level wavelets and construct a statistic from the amplitude of the oscillations. Resampling has been the main tool to obtain the test statistic distribution in Braverman et al (2017) and Chatterjee (2019), while Gong et al (2018) used a more traditional testing approach. We now present a brief description of the resampling-based approaches used in Braverman et al (2017) and Chatterjee (2019).

Fix $\ell = 1$ and assume that $N_0 = N_1 = 2^J$ for some $J > 0$. We further assume that linear trends and seasonality have been removed from $\mathbf{Y}_0$ and $\mathbf{Y}_1$, leaving us with the residuals $\tilde{\mathbf{Y}}_0$ and $\tilde{\mathbf{Y}}_1$, which are then represented as $\tilde{\mathbf{Y}}_\ell(t) = \mu_\ell(t) + E_\ell(t)$, $\ell = 0, 1$.

Let $\{V(t), W_{jk}(t), j = 0, 1, \ldots, k = 0, 1, \ldots, 2^j - 1\}$ be a family of wavelet basis functions. Suppose $J_N < J$ is some predefined fixed positive integer, which may be determined by the underlying physics of climate, or by data-driven techniques as in Heyman and Chatterjee (2020). We define

$$\mu_\ell(t) = \sum_{j=0}^{J_N - 1} \sum_{k=0}^{2^j - 1} \gamma_{\ell jk} W_{jk}(t). \tag{1.1}$$

Linear trends can be included here using the scaling function $V(\cdot)$; we ignore that for simplicity.

Define $p_n = 2^{J_N} - 1$ and the p_n-dimensional vector γ_ℓ consisting of the $\gamma_{\ell jk}$'s, for $\ell = 0, 1$. Matching the climate signals from the observations and the model simulations amounts to the test

$$H_0: \gamma_1 = \gamma_0, \quad H_1: \gamma_1 \neq \gamma_0, \tag{1.2}$$

and a T^2-type test statistic, with a matrix of weights carrying relative weights of coefficients at different wavelet scales, may be used as a test statistic. This was the approach used by Braverman et al (2017). In Chatterjee (2019), a slightly different test was used. Projecting γ_1 on the space spanned by γ_0 results in the relation

$$\gamma_\ell = \beta\gamma_0 + \delta, \quad \text{where} \quad \beta = \left[||\gamma_0||^2\right]^{-1} \langle \gamma_0, \gamma_1 \rangle, \quad \text{and} \quad \langle \gamma_0, \delta \rangle = 0. \tag{1.3}$$

Thus, the testing problem of whether or not a climate model accurately emulates Earth's climate can be formulated as Chatterjee (2019)

$$H_0: \beta = 1, \quad H_1: \beta \neq \beta_*. \tag{1.4}$$

To simulate the distribution of test statistics under null hypotheses, in Braverman et al (2017) an ARIMA model was used on the residual series $R_\ell(t) = \tilde{Y}_\ell(t) - \hat{\mu}_\ell(t)$, and resampling using this ARIMA model was proposed. In Chatterjee (2019), a wild bootstrap scheme was used.

1.6 Ensemble using empirical likelihood

In this section, we present a new technique, that simultaneously attains three goals: (*i*) it obtains a multimodel ensemble of climate models, that is constrained to satisfy desirable restrictions on the output; (*ii*) uncertainty quantification on the entire ensemble, the weights assigned to individual models, on properties of the ensemble output, including obtaining confidence sets and conducting hypothesis tests are viable; and (*iii*) the weights may be used for relative ranking of models and hence reflective of model quality. We use empirical likelihood (Owen, 1990, 1991, 2001, Qin and Lawless, 1994) in this section and present only a sketch of the main ideas owing to space limitations. The constraints may be based on observed data, or on known physics, thus, the properties of the *empirical likelihood ensemble* are interpretable and physically meaningful.

The framework we adopt is similar to that of Section 1.5. That is, we consider the observed series $\{Y_{0,t}, \ t = 1, \ldots, T\}$, and the ℓ-th model time series $\{Y_{\ell,t}, \ t = 1, \ldots, T\}$ for $\ell = 1, \ldots, L$. The goal is to construct a new time series

$$Y_{\boldsymbol{w},t} = \sum_{\ell=1}^{L} w_\ell Y_{\ell,t},$$

by finding weights $\boldsymbol{w} = \{w_1, \ldots, w_L\}$ such that the series $\{Y_{\boldsymbol{w},t}\}$ satisfies all imposed constraints. In this section, we impose constraints to ensure that several properties of $\{Y_{\boldsymbol{w},t}\}$ and $\{Y_{0,t}\}$ match, but external constraints could have been used as well.

This is achieved by maximizing the *empirical likelihood* $\prod_{\ell=1}^{L} w_\ell$, subject to the constraints $w_\ell \geqslant 0$, $\sum_{\ell=1}^{L} w_\ell = 1$ and additional restrictions of the form

$G(\boldsymbol{w}) = 0$. The last component captures any condition we would like to impose on the ensemble. Uncertainty quantification, confidence sets, and hypothesis tests are based on the empirical likelihood paradigm that closely imitates traditional parametric likelihood framework, and innovations like Bartlett corrections, and Bayesian and high-dimensional formulations are available; we omit the details here.

Instead, we provide methodological details for using empirical likelihood for generating interpretable and both physically and statistically meaningful ensembles. First, we obtained a number of subsamples of the different times series. In each of these subsamples $b = 1, \ldots, B$, we use a curve-smoothing technique to obtain climate signals $Y_{\ell,b}^{(c)}$, $\ell = 0, 1, \ldots, L$. We use Tukey's biweight smoothing in the present work, but other curve-smoothing techniques like splines, kernel smoothers, or basis expansions may be used as well. Suppose $\hat{\rho}_{\ell,b,j}$ is the j-th autocorrelation from the b-th resample of the time series $\ell = 0, 1, \ldots, L$, and let $f(\hat{\rho}_{0,b,j})$ be its Fisher transformation. We fix J, the number of autocorrelations of the smoothed ensemble we wish to constrain to be equal to observed autocorrelations, and define

$$p_{0,j} = median_{1 \leqslant b \leqslant B}\{f(\hat{\rho}_{0,b,j})\}, \quad j = 1, \ldots, J.$$

We set the j-th constraint to be

$$G_j(\boldsymbol{w}) = \sum_{\ell=1}^{L} w_\ell (p_{\ell,j} - p_{0,j}) = 0, \quad j = 1, \ldots, J.$$

Based on calculations largely following from Qin and Lawless (1994), it can be determined that

$$w_\ell = \frac{1}{L} \frac{1}{1 + \boldsymbol{t}^\tau \tilde{\boldsymbol{p}}_\ell},$$

where $\tilde{\boldsymbol{p}}_\ell$ is $\left\{(p_{\ell,1} - p_{0,1}), \ldots, (p_{\ell,J} - p_{0,J})\right\}^\top$, and $\boldsymbol{t}^\tau$ can be obtained by solving

$$\sum_{\ell=1}^{L} w_\ell (p_{\ell,j} - p_{0,j}) = 0, \quad j = 1, \ldots, J.$$

We use the multivariate Newton method to solve the above numerically.

We applied the above empirical likelihood scheme to the monthly global average near-surface temperature anomaly data used in Braverman et al (2017), with the parameters $J = 11$ and $B = 60$. The ensemble series is based on 139 models, and the simple averages series is the average of all models with 1/139 as weight. The observed monthly global average near-surface temperature anomaly time series, the simple average over all model outputs, and the ensemble based on empirical likelihood is presented in Figure 1.1. Notice that the empirical likelihood ensemble, denoted by the black curve, captures the properties of the observed data (green curve) better than the simple average (blue curve). However, much more detailed study is needed on this approach, which we will conduct in future.

Conclusions and future directions

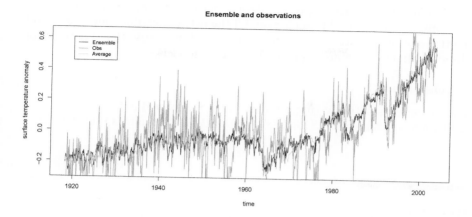

FIGURE 1.1: Monthly global average near-surface temperature anomaly time sequence, comparing with the average of 139 model series, and the ensemble based on empirical likelihood method with $J = 11$ and $B = 60$.

1.7 Conclusions and future directions

The brief review we presented in this chapter is primarily to help data science experts appreciate some of the challenges of evaluating climate models. Since the scope of this problem is vast, we had to pick and choose a selection of topics and references. One challenging aspect that remains to be addressed is the spatial and spatiotemporal patterns of climate data and model outputs: parts of the different methodologies briefly described above extend to such cases, but much more detailed studies are needed. A similar comment also holds for the case where multiple climate variables like temperature and precipitation, are considered simultaneously. A similar comment is also valid when the data on climate is gathered using multiple instruments and devices, each with its own source of bias and variability.

In a data science framework, internal variability of climate patterns is essentially considered to be colored noise. This aspect requires further investigation. Non-stationarity is a challenging aspect in the current context, and more studies are needed there. In this review, we have concentrated on only comparing model outputs to observed data, essentially treating the models themselves as impenetrable black boxes. A newer generation of data science models is in development on evaluation of the quality of such black boxes, for example, deep learning models in other contexts. However, much more progress on such procedures is needed before they are ready for use with climate models.

Considerable further progress in data science methodology and theoretical developments are needed to understand if the network aspects, multiscale and multiresolution patterns, or extreme values and tail distributional patterns of observed climate data are captured by climate models.

Acknowledgments

This research is partially supported by the US National Science Foundation (NSF) under grants #DMS-1622483, #DMS-1737918, and #OAC-1939916.

References

Abramowitz G, Herger N, Gutmann E, Hammerling D, Knutti R, Leduc M, Lorenz R, Pincus R, Schmidt GA (2019) Model dependence in multi-model climate ensembles: weighting, sub-selection and out-of-sample testing. Earth Syst Dynam 10:91–105

Anderson GJ, Lucas DD (2018) Machine learning predictions of a multiresolution climate model ensemble. Geophysical Research Letters 45(9):4273–4280

Bellucci A, Gualdi S, Navarra A (2010) The double-ITCZ syndrome in coupled general circulation models: the role of large-scale vertical circulation regimes. Journal of Climate 23(5):1127–1145

Bodas-Salcedo A, Webb M, Brooks M, Ringer M, Williams K, Milton S, Wilson D (2008) Evaluating cloud systems in the met office global forecast model using simulated CloudSat radar reflectivities. Journal of Geophysical Research: Atmospheres 113: D00A13

Bodas-Salcedo A, Webb MJ, Bony S, Chepfer H, Dufresne JL, Klein SA, Zhang Y, Marchand R, Haynes JM, Pincus R, et al (2011) Cosp: Satellite simulation software for model assessment. Bulletin of the American Meteorological Society 92(8):1023–1043

Braverman A, Cressie N, Teixeira J (2011) A likelihood-based comparison of temporal models for physical processes. Statistical Analysis and Data Mining: The ASA Data Science Journal 4(3):247–258

Braverman A, Chatterjee S, Heyman M, Cressie N (2017) Probabilistic evaluation of competing climate models. Advances in Statistical Climatology, Meteorology and Oceanography 3(2):93–105

Brient F, Bony S (2013) Interpretation of the positive low-cloud feedback predicted by a climate model under global warming. Climate Dynamics 40(9-10):2415–2431

Brown JR, Jakob C, Haynes JM (2010) An evaluation of rainfall frequency and intensity over the Australian region in a global climate model. Journal of Climate 23(24):6504–6525

References

Cadule P, Friedlingstein P, Bopp L, Sitch S, Jones CD, Ciais P, Piao SL, Peylin P (2010) Benchmarking coupled climate-carbon models against long-term atmospheric CO_2 measurements. Global Biogeochemical Cycles 24: GB2016

Chatterjee S (2019) The scale enhanced wild bootstrap method for evaluating climate models using wavelets. Statistics & Probability Letters 144:69–73

Dijkstra H, Hernandez-Garcia E, Lopez C, et al (2019) The application of machine learning techniques to improve El Nino prediction skill. Frontiers in Physics 7:153

Dueben PD, Bauer P (2018) Challenges and design choices for global weather and climate models based on machine learning. Geoscientific Model Development 11(10):3999–4009

Eyring V, Righi M, Lauer A, Evaldsson M, Wenzel S, Jones C, Anav A, Andrews O, Cionni I, Davin EL, et al (2016) Esmvaltool (v1.0)—a community diagnostic and performance metrics tool for routine evaluation of earth system models in CMIP. Geoscientific Model Development 9:1747–1802

Eyring V, Cox PM, Flato GM, Gleckler PJ, Abramowitz G, Caldwell P, Collins WD, Gier BK, Hall AD, Hoffman FM, et al (2019) Taking climate model evaluation to the next level. Nature Climate Change 9(2):102–110

Flato G, Marotzke J, Abiodun B, Braconnot P, Chou SC, Collins W, Cox P, Driouech F, Emori S, Eyring V, et al (2014) Evaluation of climate models. In: Climate change 2013: the physical science basis. Contribution of Working Group I to the Fifth Assessment Report of the Intergovernmental Panel on Climate Change, Cambridge University Press, 741–866

Furrer R, Knutti R, Sain SR, Nychka DW, Meehl GA (2007a) Spatial patterns of probabilistic temperature change projections from a multivariate Bayesian analysis. Geophysical Research Letters 34(6):L06711

Furrer R, Sain SR, Nychka D, Meehl GA (2007b) Multivariate Bayesian analysis of atmosphere–ocean general circulation models. Environmental and ecological statistics 14(3):249–266

Giorgi F, Mearns LO (2002) Calculation of average, uncertainty range, and reliability of regional climate changes from AOGCM simulations via the "reliability ensemble averaging" (REA) method. Journal of Climate 15(10):1141–1158

Gleckler P, Doutriaux C, Durack PJ, Taylor KE, Zhang Y, Williams DN, Mason E, Servonnat J (2016) A more powerful reality test for climate models. Eos 97

Gleckler PJ, Taylor KE, Doutriaux C (2008) Performance metrics for climate models. Journal of Geophysical Research: Atmospheres 113:D06104

Gong K, Chatterjee S (2020) Comparing non-stationary time series using spectral methods: a study on climate model quality assessment. preprint

Gong K, Chatterjee S, Braveman A (2018) On a technique for evaluating the quality of earth system models. In: Chen C, Cooley D, Runge J, Szekely E (eds) Proceedings of the 8th International Workshop on Climate Informatics (CI2018), NCAR Technical Note NCAR/TN-550+PROC, 93–96

Greene AM, Goddard L, Lall U (2006) Probabilistic multimodel regional temperature change projections. Journal of Climate 19(17):4326–4343

Hausfather Z, Drake HF, Abbott T, Schmidt GA (2020) Evaluating the performance of past climate model projections. Geophysical Research Letters 47:e2019GL085378

Herger N, Abramowitz G, Knutti R, Angélil O, Lehmann K, Sanderson BM (2018) Selecting a climate model subset to optimise key ensemble properties. Earth System Dynamics 9(1):135–151

Heyman M, Chatterjee S (2020) Partial linear model selection. preprint

Ichikawa H, Masunaga H, Tsushima Y, Kanzawa H (2012) Reproducibility by climate models of cloud radiative forcing associated with tropical convection. Journal of Climate 25(4):1247–1262

Ivatt PD, Evans MJ (2019) Improving the prediction of an atmospheric chemistry transport model using gradient boosted regression trees. Atmospheric Chemistry and Physics Discussions, 1–33

Jiang JH, Su H, Zhai C, Perun VS, Del Genio A, Nazarenko LS, Donner LJ, Horowitz L, Seman C, Cole J, et al (2012) Evaluation of cloud and water vapor simulations in CMIP5 climate models using NASA "A-Train" satellite observations. Journal of Geophysical Research: Atmospheres 117(D14)

Jiang X, Waliser DE, Xavier PK, Petch J, Klingaman NP, Woolnough SJ, Guan B, Bellon G, Crueger T, DeMott C, et al (2015) Vertical structure and physical processes of the Madden-Julian oscillation: Exploring key model physics in climate simulations. Journal of Geophysical Research: Atmospheres 120(10):4718–4748

Klein SA, Zhang Y, Zelinka MD, Pincus R, Boyle J, Gleckler PJ (2013) Are climate model simulations of clouds improving? An evaluation using the ISCCP simulator. Journal of Geophysical Research: Atmospheres 118(3):1329–1342

Klocke D, Rodwell M (2014) A comparison of two numerical weather prediction methods for diagnosing fast-physics errors in climate models. Quarterly Journal of the Royal Meteorological Society 140(679):517–524

Knutti R (2010) The end of model democracy? Climatic Change 102:395–404

Knutti R, Abramowitz G, Collins M, Eyring V, Gleckler PJ, Hewitson B, Mearns L (2010a) Good practice guidance paper on assessing and combining multi model climate projections. In: IPCC Expert Meeting on Assessing and Combining Multi Model Climate Projections: National Center for Atmospheric Research: Boulder, Colorado, USA: 25-27 January 2010: Meeting Report, IPCC Working Group I Technical Support Unit, University of Bern

Knutti R, Furrer R, Tebaldi C, Cermak J, Meehl GA (2010b) Challenges in combining projections from multiple climate models. Journal of Climate 23(10):2739–2758

Knutti R, Masson D, Gettelman A (2013) Climate model genealogy: Generation CMIP5 and how we got there. Geophysical Research Letters 40(6):1194–1199

References

Knutti R, Sedláček J, Sanderson BM, Lorenz R, Fischer EM, Eyring V (2017) A climate model projection weighting scheme accounting for performance and interdependence. Geophysical Research Letters 44(4):1909–1918

Konsta D, Chepfer H, Dufresne JL (2012) A process oriented characterization of tropical oceanic clouds for climate model evaluation, based on a statistical analysis of daytime A-train observations. Climate Dynamics 39(9-10):2091–2108

Lorenz R, Herger N, Sedláček J, Eyring V, Fischer EM, Knutti R (2018) Prospects and caveats of weighting climate models for summer maximum temperature projections over North America. Journal of Geophysical Research: Atmospheres 123(9):4509–4526

Ma HY, Xie S, Klein S, Williams K, Boyle J, Bony S, Douville H, Fermepin S, Medeiros B, Tyteca S, et al (2014) On the correspondence between mean forecast errors and climate errors in cmip5 models. Journal of Climate 27(4):1781–1798

Masson D, Knutti R (2011) Climate model genealogy. Geophysical Research Letters 38:L08703

McQuade S, Monteleoni C (2017) Spatiotemporal global climate model tracking. In: Large-Scale Machine Learning in the Earth Sciences, Chapman & Hall/CRC, 33–54

Milliff RF, Bonazzi A, Wikle CK, Pinardi N, Berliner LM (2011) Ocean ensemble forecasting. Part I: Ensemble Mediterranean winds from a Bayesian hierarchical model. Quarterly Journal of the Royal Meteorological Society 137(657):858–878

Monteleoni C, Schmidt GA, Saroha S, Asplund E (2011) Tracking climate models. Statistical Analysis and Data Mining: The ASA Data Science Journal 4(4):372–392

Nishii K, Miyasaka T, Nakamura H, Kosaka Y, Yokoi S, Takayabu YN, Endo H, Ichikawa H, Inoue T, Oshima K, et al (2012) Relationship of the reproducibility of multiple variables among global climate models. Journal of the Meteorological Society of Japan Ser II 90:87–100

O'Gorman PA, Dwyer JG (2018) Using machine learning to parameterize moist convection: Potential for modeling of climate, climate change, and extreme events. Journal of Advances in Modeling Earth Systems 10(10):2548–2563

Owen A (1990) Empirical likelihood ratio confidence regions. The Annals of Statistics 18(1):90–120

Owen A (1991) Empirical likelihood for linear models. The Annals of Statistics 19(4):1725–1747

Owen AB (2001) Empirical Likelihood. Chapman & Hall/CRC

Phillips TJ, Potter GL, Williamson DL, Cederwall RT, Boyle JS, Fiorino M, Hnilo JJ, Olson JG, Xie S, Yio JJ (2004) Evaluating parameterizations in general circulation models: Climate simulation meets weather prediction. Bulletin of the American Meteorological Society 85(12):1903–1916

Pincus R, Batstone CP, Hofmann RJP, Taylor KE, Glecker PJ (2008) Evaluating the present-day simulation of clouds, precipitation, and radiation in climate models. Journal of Geophysical Research: Atmospheres 113:D14209

Pincus R, Platnick S, Ackerman SA, Hemler RS, Patrick Hofmann RJ (2012) Reconciling simulated and observed views of clouds: MODIS, ISCCP, and the limits of instrument simulators. Journal of Climate 25(13):4699–4720

Qin J, Lawless J (1994) Empirical likelihood and general estimating equations. The Annals of Statistics 22(1):300–325

Rasp S, Pritchard MS, Gentine P (2018) Deep learning to represent subgrid processes in climate models. Proceedings of the National Academy of Sciences 115(39):9684–9689

Rougier J, Sexton DM, Murphy JM, Stainforth D (2009) Analyzing the climate sensitivity of the HadSM3 climate model using ensembles from different but related experiments. Journal of Climate 22(13):3540–3557

Sahany S, Neelin JD, Hales K, Neale RB (2012) Temperature–moisture dependence of the deep convective transition as a constraint on entrainment in climate models. Journal of the Atmospheric Sciences 69(4):1340–1358

Sanderson BM (2013) On the estimation of systematic error in regression-based predictions of climate sensitivity. Climatic Change 118(3-4):757–770

Sanderson BM, Knutti R, Caldwell P (2015) Addressing interdependency in a multimodel ensemble by interpolation of model properties. Journal of Climate 28(13):5150–5170

Sanderson BM, Wehner M, Knutti R (2017) Skill and independence weighting for multi-model assessments. Geoscientific Model Development 10(6):2379–2395

Santer BD, Fyfe JC, Solomon S, Painter JF, Bonfils C, Pallotta G, Zelinka MD (2019) Quantifying stochastic uncertainty in detection time of human-caused climate signals. Proceedings of the National Academy of Sciences 116(40):19821–19827

Scher S (2018) Toward data-driven weather and climate forecasting: Approximating a simple general circulation model with deep learning. Geophysical Research Letters 45(22):12–616

Scher S, Messori G (2019) Weather and climate forecasting with neural networks: using general circulation models (GCMs) with different complexity as a study ground. Geoscientific Model Development 12(7):2797–2809

Schneider T, Lan S, Stuart A, Teixeira J (2017) Earth system modeling 2.0: A blueprint for models that learn from observations and targeted high-resolution simulations. Geophysical Research Letters 44(24):12–396

Sexton DMH, Murphy JM (2012) Multivariate probabilistic projections using imperfect climate models. Part II: robustness of methodological choices and consequences for climate sensitivity. Climate Dynamics 38(11-12):2543–2558

Sexton DMH, Murphy JM, Collins M, Webb MJ (2012) Multivariate probabilistic projections using imperfect climate models. Part I: outline of methodology. Climate Dynamics 38(11-12):2513–2542

References

Smith RL, Tebaldi C, Nychka D, Mearns LO (2009) Bayesian modeling of uncertainty in ensembles of climate models. Journal of the American Statistical Association 104(485):97–116

Strobach E, Bel G (2015) Improvement of climate predictions and reduction of their uncertainties using learning algorithms. Atmospheric Chemistry and Physics 15(15):8631–8641

Stubenrauch C, Rossow W, Kinne S, Ackerman S, Cesana G, Chepfer H, Di Girolamo L, Getzewich B, Guignard A, Heidinger A, et al (2013) Assessment of global cloud datasets from satellites: project and database initiated by the GEWEX radiation panel. Bulletin of the American Meteorological Society 94(7):1031–1049

Su H, Jiang JH, Zhai C, Perun VS, Shen JT, Del Genio A, Nazarenko LS, Donner LJ, Horowitz L, Seman C, et al (2013) Diagnosis of regime-dependent cloud simulation errors in CMIP5 models using "A-Train" satellite observations and reanalysis data. Journal of Geophysical Research: Atmospheres 118(7):2762–2780

Sunyer MA, Madsen H, Rosbjerg D, Arnbjerg-Nielsen K (2014) A Bayesian approach for uncertainty quantification of extreme precipitation projections including climate model interdependency and nonstationary bias. Journal of Climate 27(18):7113–7132

Suzuki K, Stephens G, Bodas-Salcedo A, Wang M, Golaz JC, Yokohata T, Koshiro T (2015) Evaluation of the warm rain formation process in global models with satellite observations. Journal of the Atmospheric Sciences 72(10):3996–4014

Tebaldi C, Knutti R (2007) The use of the multi-model ensemble in probabilistic climate projections. Philosophical transactions of the royal society A: mathematical, physical and engineering sciences 365(1857):2053–2075

Tebaldi C, Smith RL, Nychka D, Mearns LO (2005) Quantifying uncertainty in projections of regional climate change: a Bayesian approach to the analysis of multimodel ensembles. Journal of Climate 18(10):1524–1540

Tsushima Y, Ringer MA, Webb MJ, Williams KD (2013) Quantitative evaluation of the seasonal variations in climate model cloud regimes. Climate dynamics 41(9-10):2679–2696

Waugh DW, Eyring V (2008) Quantitative performance metrics for stratospheric-resolving chemistry-climate models. Atmospheric Chemistry and Physics 8(18):5699–5713

Webb MJ, Andrews T, Bodas-Salcedo A, Bony S, Bretherton CS, Chadwick R, Chepfer H, Douville H, Good P, Kay JE, et al (2017) The cloud feedback model intercomparison project (CFMIP) contribution to CMIP6. Geoscientific Model Development 2017:359–384

Williams KD, Webb MJ (2009) A quantitative performance assessment of cloud regimes in climate models. Climate Dynamics 33(1):141–157

Wood R, Mechoso C, Bretherton C, Weller R, Huebert B, Straneo F, Albrecht BA, Coe H, Allen G, Vaughan G, et al (2011) The VAMOS ocean-cloud-atmosphere-land study regional experiment (VOCALS-REx): goals, platforms, and field operations. Atmospheric Chemistry and Physics 11(2):627–654

Xie S, Ma HY, Boyle JS, Klein SA, Zhang Y (2012) On the correspondence between short-and long-time-scale systematic errors in CAM4/CAM5 for the year of tropical convection. Journal of Climate 25(22):7937–7955

Yokohata T, Webb MJ, Collins M, Williams KD, Yoshimori M, Hargreaves JC, Annan JD (2010) Structural similarities and differences in climate responses to CO_2 increase between two perturbed physics ensembles. Journal of Climate 23(6):1392–1410

Yokoi S, Takayabu YN, Nishii K, Nakamura H, Endo H, Ichikawa H, Inoue T, Kimoto M, Kosaka Y, Miyasaka T, et al (2011) Application of cluster analysis to climate model performance metrics. Journal of Applied Meteorology and Climatology 50(8):1666–1675

Zhang Y, Klein SA, Boyle J, Mace GG (2010) Evaluation of tropical cloud and precipitation statistics of community atmosphere model version 3 using CloudSat and CALIPSO data. Journal of Geophysical Research: Atmospheres 115:D12205

2

A Statistical Analysis of North Atlantic Tropical Cyclone Changes

Thomas J. Fisher
Miami University, Oxford, OH, USA

Robert Lund
Clemson University, Clemson, SC, USA

Michael W. Robbins
RAND Corporation, Pittsburgh, PA, USA

CONTENTS

2.1	Introduction	25
2.2	Data	27
2.3	Statistical methods	28
	2.3.1 Penalized likelihood changepoint methods	29
	2.3.2 Poisson counts	31
	2.3.3 Correlated Gaussian data	32
2.4	Results	33
	2.4.1 Total cyclone counts	34
	2.4.2 Hurricanes and major storms	35
	2.4.3 Analyses with segment-length restrictions	36
	2.4.4 Accumulated cyclone energy	38
2.5	Comments and conclusions	39
References	....	41

2.1 Introduction

Climate change is one of the most important issues facing mankind today (Wanner et al, 2008). Many researchers have studied recent changes in the Earth's temperature record (Lu et al, 2005, Mann et al, 2008, Trenberth, 1990), with the issue becoming highly politicized in recent years (Giddens, 2009). A secondary issue pertains to frequency and strength changes in storms, particularly those involving hurricanes. Here, the issue is whether a warming planet will see more or stronger storms, or some combination of both. This chapter delves into this question, statistically examining the North Atlantic Basin's tropical cyclone record since 1851.

Hurricanes can be viewed as the Earth's way of sweating, moving heat from the topics to the poles in an attempt to equalize planet surface temperatures (Emanuel, 2005). In the Northern Hemisphere, sea surface temperatures have warmed in recent years, leading scientists to speculate that additional energy will need to be dissipated from the tropics. The prominent conjecture is that warming seas will inject more energy into the climate system, inducing more tropical cyclones, stronger cyclones, or some combination thereof. This issue has led to the formation of two antipodal camps. The first camp claims that the warming seas will give rise to stronger storms, but that their numbers should not increase greatly (Knutson et al, 2008, 2010). This camp largely justifies its position from climate model simulations. The other camp believes that more storms will form, but that the individual storms will not get much stronger (Mooney, 2007). This opinion is generally supported by the hurricane record itself. The popular book (Mooney, 2007) narrates the controversies and political mudslinging on the issue.

It is the intent of this chapter to present the statistical opinion on the topic. Here, the Atlantic Basin's tropical cyclone record since 1851 is statistically scrutinized for changes via multiple changepoint analysis techniques. Loosely speaking, a changepoint is a time of shift in the statistical properties that govern a time series. Multiple changepoint techniques estimate when and where such shifts have taken place, and how the changes have impacted the numbers and/or strengths of the storms. When changepoints are found, homogeneity of the series is rejected. Some of the changes identified here are attributable to changes in data collection procedures, but others do not lend themselves to such innocuous interpretations. In particular, we find that the North Atlantic Basin transitioned to an era of more frequent storms circa 1995, and that this era has yet to subside.

Before proceeding, it is worth acknowledging others who have analyzed the North Atlantic tropical cyclone record for changes: Elsner and Jagger (2006), Elsner et al (2000, 2008), Robbins et al (2011b). This list is incomplete; the edited compilation (Elsner and Jagger, 2009) contains many articles on this topic. To date, a multiple changepoint analysis of the North Atlantic Basin's record has not been run, which is our purpose here. This said, Robbins et al (2011b) presents a single changepoint analysis of this record.

The rest of this chapter proceeds as follows. The next section describes the North Atlantic Basin's tropical cyclone data. Section 2.3 moves to a statistical overview of multiple changepoint techniques. Section 2.4 describes what changes are found, and Section 2.5 concludes with comments and remarks.

2.2 Data

The data used here is the Atlantic Hurricane Database best tracking data, known as the Atlantic HURDAT2 data (Landsea and Franklin, 2013), which is a record spanning 1851–2018. There is significant uncertainty in the reliability of the first one-hundred years of this data. In particular, it is believed that many storms went undetected in the earlier years of this record, living their entire lives over open ocean waters and evading detection. This is believed to be especially problematic before the onset of aircraft reconnaissance. This concern is generally alleviated since the launch of the GOES satellites circa the mid-1960s. Since the early 2000s, a concerted effort has been made to reanalyze the HURDAT data to address inaccuracies and biases; for references, see Hodges et al (2017), Landsea (2007), Landsea et al (2008), Truchelut et al (2013). To our knowledge, the HURDAT2 record is the most comprehensive and complete data set on tropical cyclones in the North Atlantic Basin.

The HURDAT2 data contains measurements on cyclone location (latitude and longitude), wind speed, and barometric pressure, typically recorded every 6 hours. More recent storms include additional information on the size of a storm and other classifications (e.g., tropical depression or extra-tropical cyclone). Using the HURDAT2 data, we will study all storms that achieve tropical cyclone status at some time in their lives, which is a wind speed of 35 knots or higher. The storms are classified based on their maximum attained wind speed. Figure 2.1 displays an annual record of the storms

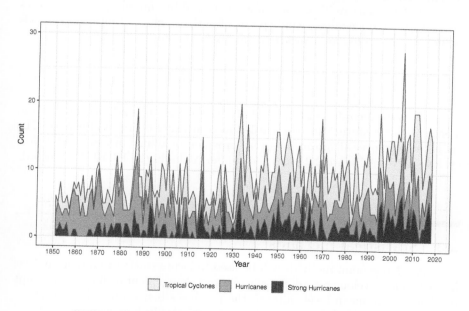

FIGURE 2.1: Time series plot of storm counts by year.

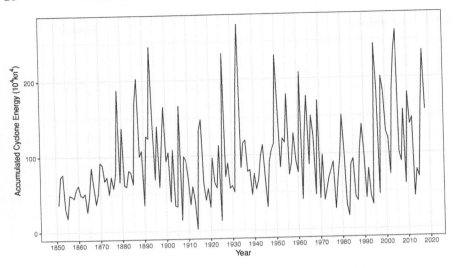

FIGURE 2.2: Time series plot of accumulated cyclone energy per year.

counts. Displayed separately are the counts of all tropical cyclones, those achieving hurricane status (wind speeds of 64 knots or higher), and strong storms (Saffir–Simpson category 3, 4, or 5 hurricanes, which have peak wind speeds of 96 knots or higher).

Another measure of the hurricane season is the accumulated cyclone energy (ACE). The ACE of a storm is calculated by summing up the squares of the estimated sustained wind speeds of active cyclones (only wind speeds of 35 knots or higher are considered) at six-hour intervals:

$$\text{ACE} = \frac{1}{10{,}000} \sum_{i=1}^{d} w_i^2, \qquad (2.1)$$

where w_i is the recorded sustained wind speed at the i-th six-hour observation. The ACE for a storm can be regarded as a measure of its total energy. The ACE summed over all storms in a year provides an annual measure of tropical cyclone activity. Figure 2.2 plots the annual ACEs in the HURDAT2 record.

2.3 Statistical methods

Multiple changepoint methods will be used to locate statistical discontinuities in the tropical cyclone record. Specifically, our changepoint techniques attempt to identify any mean level shifts in the processes being studied. If no shifts are found, the record is concluded to be statistically homogeneous in time.

Statistical methods

Multiple changepoint techniques (as opposed to single changepoint methods) are preferable if multiple shifts could have occurred over the study period.

If the record, in truth, had a linear increasing trend and no mean shifts, a multiple changepoint technique would signal one or more changepoints, each shifting the processes' mean levels higher in an attempt to match the series' pattern. In this manner, multiple changepoint analyses serve as a rudimentary check for data homogeneity. Tests for single changepoints in data that exhibit linear trends have been previously considered (Gallagher et al, 2013, Robbins et al, 2016); however, these methods have not been extended to the multiple changepoint setting. Also, mean shift models are known to model cyclone data well (see the single changepoint techniques for the North Atlantic tropical cyclone record in Robbins et al, 2011b). That study only considers data through 2008. Since this study analyzes both cyclone counts and ACE values and updates results through 2018, it provides a more complete statistical analysis of hurricane climatology changes in the North Atlantic Basin.

2.3.1 Penalized likelihood changepoint methods

Penalized likelihood methods will be used to estimate the number of changepoints and where they occur. We do not assume *a priori* that the number of changepoints is known. Suppose that a time series $\{X_t\}$ is observed for the times $t \in \{1,\ldots,N\}$. The likelihood of the observed data is typically taken as the joint probability density function of the model parameters given the observed data $X_1,\ldots,X_N$; see Casella and Berger (2002). The method of maximum likelihood estimates the model parameters as those that make the observed data the most likely; a penalty term is included to prevent overfitting (having a model with too many parameters).

Consider a model with m changepoints occurring at the times $\tau_1,\ldots,\tau_m$. We order the changepoint times via $1 < \tau_1 < \cdots < \tau_m$ (time 1 is not allowed to be a changepoint time for model identifiability). The m changepoints partition the data record into $m+1$ distinct regimes, the i-th regime containing the time indices $\tau_{i-1}+1,\ldots,\tau_i$. Here, the boundary conventions $\tau_0 = 1$ and $\tau_{m+1} = N+1$ are made. The likelihood, in general, is expressed as L, and is a function of the model parameters. The model parameters contain the changepoint configuration parameters $(m;\tau_1,\ldots,\tau_m)$ and any other model parameters, the latter of which is denoted by $\boldsymbol{\Theta}$. The notation

$$L(m;\tau_1,\ldots,\tau_m;\boldsymbol{\Theta}|X_1,\ldots,X_N)$$

denotes the model's likelihood, and the conditional bar | indicates that the data $X_1,\ldots,X_N$ is fixed. The maximum likelihood estimates are the arguments that maximize the likelihood

$$(\hat{m},\hat{\tau}_1,\ldots,\hat{\tau}_m;\widehat{\boldsymbol{\Theta}})' = \arg\sup L(m;\tau_1,\ldots,\tau_m;\boldsymbol{\Theta}|X_1,\ldots,X_N).$$

(In the above, $\prime$ indicates matrix transpose). These estimators are equivalent to those that minimize -2 times the log likelihood:

$$(\hat{m}, \hat{\tau}_1, \ldots, \hat{\tau}_m; \widehat{\boldsymbol{\Theta}})' = \arg\inf -2\log(L(m; \tau_1, \ldots, \tau_m; \boldsymbol{\Theta} | X_1, \ldots, X_N)).$$

As the number of changepoints increases in the model, the model fit becomes better and better. To prevent overfitting, a penalty is added to the likelihood to make sure that a parsimonious fit is achieved. Adding additional parameters into the model beyond what is optimal tends to increase the penalty more than reducing -2 times the log likelihood. Let $P(m; \tau_1, \ldots, \tau_m, \boldsymbol{\Theta})$ be the penalty for the model parameters. Our penalized likelihood estimates the model and its parameters as those that minimize the objective function

$$-2\log(L(m; \tau_1, \ldots, \tau_m; \boldsymbol{\Theta} | X_1, \ldots, X_N)) + P(m; \tau_1, \ldots, \tau_m, \boldsymbol{\Theta}).$$

Many different penalties have been proposed by statisticians over the years, two classic ones being the AIC and BIC (Akaike and Bayesian information criteria) penalties (Casella and Berger, 2002) given by $AIC = 2m$ and $BIC = m\log(N)$. These two penalties are proportional to the number of changepoints; changepoint locations are not accounted for in the penalty. Recently, minimum description length (MDL) penalties were developed from information theory and tailored to the changepoint problem in Davis et al (2006) and Lu et al (2010). MDL penalties take into account where the changepoints lie, penalizing changepoints that are close together more heavily than those that lie far away from each other. The MDL penalty has form

$$\text{MDL}(m; \tau_1, \ldots, \tau_m; \boldsymbol{\Theta}) = \log(m) + \sum_{i=1}^{m+1} \frac{\log(\tau_i - \tau_{i-1})}{2} + \sum_{i=2}^{m} \log(\tau_i) \quad (2.2)$$

when $m > 0$, and $\text{MDL} = 0$ when $m = 0$. Because of its superior performance in simulations and applications, MDL penalties will be used here.

Our future notation drops the condition $X_1, \ldots, X_N$ as the fact that the data are fixed is implied. Given a changepoint configuration $(m; \tau_1, \ldots, \tau_m)$, it is usually a standard statistical problem to estimate the parameters in $\boldsymbol{\Theta}$; examples are given below. Let

$$L_{\text{opt}}(m; \tau_1, \ldots, \tau_m) = \sup_{\theta \in \Theta} L(m; \tau_1, \ldots, \tau_m; \boldsymbol{\Theta})$$

be the optimal likelihood evaluated at the best estimates of $\boldsymbol{\Theta}$ when m and $\tau_1, \ldots, \tau_m$ are known and fixed. As seen below, L_{opt} can usually be computed explicitly or numerically. Hence, to find the best changepoint configuration, we must find the m and $\tau_1, \ldots, \tau_m$ that minimize the penalized likelihood (objective function)

$$O(m; \tau_1, \ldots, \tau_m) := -2\log(L_{\text{opt}}(m; \tau_1, \ldots, \tau_m)) + \text{MDL}(m; \tau_1, \ldots, \tau_m). \quad (2.3)$$

Statistical methods

2.3.2 Poisson counts

As a first task, consider a multiple changepoint analysis of the tropical cyclone counts. Such counts are often modeled by a Poisson statistical distribution (McDonnell and Holbrook, 2004, Mooley, 1981), which for a random count C has probability mass distribution

$$P(C = k) = \frac{e^{-\lambda}\lambda^k}{k!}, \quad k \in \{0, 1, \ldots\}, \qquad (2.4)$$

where $\lambda > 0$ is an unknown parameter that is the count mean: $\mathbb{E}[C] = \lambda$.

The maximum likelihood estimate of λ from the count observations $C_1, \ldots, C_N$, which are sampled from this distribution and assumed independent, is the sample mean: $\hat{\lambda} = N^{-1}\sum_{t=1}^{N} C_t$. The optimal likelihood L_{opt} with this value of λ is hence

$$-2\log(L_{\text{opt}}) = 2N\hat{\lambda}[1 - \log(\hat{\lambda})] + 2\sum_{t=1}^{N}\log(C_t!).$$

Our multiple changepoint model for Poisson data will allow the mean parameter λ to shift at each changepoint time. This is done by assuming that C_t has mean parameter λ_t for $t \in \{1, \ldots, N\}$ and imposing

$$\lambda_t = \begin{cases} \mu_1 & \tau_0 \leq t < \tau_1 \\ \mu_2 & \tau_1 \leq t < \tau_2 \\ \vdots & \vdots \\ \mu_{m+1} & \tau_m \leq t < \tau_{m+1} \end{cases}.$$

Here, the boundary conditions $\tau_0 = 1$ and $\tau_{m+1} = N + 1$ are imposed. Although the end issue is far from settled, the year-to-year counts do not seem to exhibit much temporal correlation (Livsey et al, 2018, Robbins et al, 2011b). Because of this, our likelihood is obtained by multiplying the probabilities in (2.4) in a time-varying form:

$$L(m; \tau_1, \ldots, \tau_m; \mu_1, \ldots, \mu_m) = \prod_{t=1}^{N}\frac{e^{-\lambda_t}\lambda_t^{C_t}}{C_t!}. \qquad (2.5)$$

Maximizing this over $\mu_1, \ldots, \mu_{m+1}$, which can be done by simple calculus, identifies the μ_i estimates as

$$\hat{\mu}_i = \frac{1}{\#(R_i)}\sum_{t \in R_i} C_t, \qquad (2.6)$$

which is the sample mean number of tropical cyclones during the i-th regime. Here, R_i is the set of times during which the data obeyed the i-th regime and $\#(R_i) = \tau_i - \tau_{i-1}$ is the number of years in the i-th regime. In this setting,

$\Theta = (\mu_1, \ldots, \mu_m)'$ is m-dimensional. Plugging these estimators back into (2.5) gives

$$L_{\text{opt}}(m; \hat{\mu}_1, \ldots, \hat{\mu}_m) = 2 \sum_{i=1}^{m+1} (\tau_i - \tau_{i-1}) \hat{\mu}_i [1 - \log(\hat{\mu}_i)] + 2 \sum_{t=1}^{N} \log(C_i!).$$

Since the C_t are fixed in this optimization, they can be ignored. Hence, our objective function can be reduced to

$$O(m; \tau_1, \ldots, \tau_m) = 2 \sum_{i=1}^{m+1} (\tau_i - \tau_{i-1}) \hat{\mu}_i [1 - \log(\hat{\mu}_i)] + \log(m)$$

$$+ \sum_{i=1}^{m+1} \frac{\log(\tau_i - \tau_{i-1})}{2} + \sum_{i=2}^{m} \log(\tau_i)$$

when $m > 0$; when $m = 0$, the objective function is $2N\hat{\mu}_1[1 - \log(\hat{\mu}_1)]$. Optimizing over all m and changepoint times yields an estimate of the best segmentation.

2.3.3 Correlated Gaussian data

Now consider a multiple changepoint analysis of the ACE series. The data here are continuous, but are allowed to exhibit year-to-year correlations. To accommodate this scenario, we will devise a model that has Gaussian marginal distributions, autocorrelation in its model errors, and mean shifts at each changepoint time. Lund et al (2007) and Robbins et al (2011a) show what can go wrong in a changepoint analysis when the correlations are ignored. While the ACE data are in truth somewhat non-Gaussian (foremost, ACE values must be non-negative), it is an unsettled statistical issue on how to construct an MDL matching a general non-Gaussian continuous distribution. More will be said about this mismatch later.

Our general model is
$$X_t = \alpha_t + \epsilon_t,$$
where $\alpha_t = \mathbb{E}[X_t]$ for each year t. To allow for a mean shift at each changepoint time, we impose the piecewise mean structure

$$\alpha_t = \begin{cases} \mu_1 & \tau_0 \leq t < \tau_1 \\ \mu_2 & \tau_1 \leq t < \tau_2 \\ \vdots & \vdots \\ \mu_{m+1} & \tau_m \leq t < \tau_{m+1} \end{cases}.$$

The time series errors $\{\epsilon_t\}$ are assumed to be a causal and invertible autoregressive moving-average (ARMA) model of orders p and q that satisfies the difference equation

$$\epsilon_t = \phi_1 \epsilon_{t-1} + \ldots + \phi_p \epsilon_{t-p} + Z_t + \eta_1 Z_{t-1} + \ldots + \eta_q Z_{t-q}.$$

Here, $\{Z_t\}$ is zero mean Gaussian white noise (independent and identically distributed variables) with variance $\text{Var}(Z_t) = \sigma_Z^2$, $\phi_1, \ldots, \phi_p$ are the autoregressive coefficients, and $\eta_1, \ldots, \eta_q$ are the moving-average coefficients. The autoregressive order p and the moving-average order q are assumed known; this is of little consequence in practice. For more on ARMA time series, see Brockwell and Davis (1991).

As in the last subsection, expressions for $L_{\text{opt}}(m; \mu_1, \ldots, \mu_m)$ and the penalty are needed. The penalty in this case is exactly as in (2.2); however, $L_{\text{opt}}(m; \mu_1, \ldots, \mu_m)$, the optimal likelihood given the changepoint configuration, will take additional work.

The Gaussian likelihood given the changepoint configuration is

$$L(\Theta|m; \tau_1, \ldots, \tau_m) = (2\pi)^{-N/2} \left(\prod_{t=1}^{N} v_{t-1} \right) \exp\left[-\frac{1}{2} \sum_{t=1}^{N} \frac{(X_t - \hat{X}_t)^2}{v_{t-1}} \right], \quad (2.7)$$

where Θ contains the parameters $\mu_1, \ldots, \mu_{m+1}, \phi_1, \ldots, \phi_p; \eta_1, \ldots, \eta_q$, and σ_Z^2. The other quantities here are as follows: $\hat{X}_t = P(X_t|1, X_1, \ldots, X_{t-1})$ is the best linear one-step-ahead forecast (minimal mean squared error) of X_t from a linear combination of a constant and all previous observations of the $\{X_t\}$ process; also, $v_t = \mathbb{E}[(X_t - \hat{X}_t)^2]$ is the mean squared prediction error of this forecast.

Identifying estimators of the time series and other parameters given that there are m changepoints occurring at the times $\tau_1, \ldots, \tau_m$ is a relatively standard problem, done as in Li and Lund (2012). First, the estimator of the mean μ_i is taken as the sample mean of the data in the i-th regime:

$$\hat{\mu}_i = \frac{1}{\#(R_i)} \sum_{t \in R_i} X_t, \quad (2.8)$$

This is simply (2.6). While these estimates are not the true likelihood estimators, they are very close to them and are used because their computation is so simple.

The ARMA parameters, which entail the autoregressive parameters $\phi_1, \ldots, \phi_p$, the moving-average parameters $\eta_1, \ldots, \eta_q$, and the white noise variance σ_Z^2 are estimated from the mean adjusted series defined by $X_t - \hat{\alpha}_t, 1 \leq t \leq N$. Here, $\hat{\alpha}_t$ is taken as $\hat{\mu}_i$ if time t is in regime i. Estimates of ARMA parameters and the associated best likelihood are computed using the `arima` function in base R (R Core Team, 2019).

2.4 Results

Optimizing the MDL over all m and $\tau_1, \ldots, \tau_m$ can be very challenging. The objective function has few convenient features, and exhaustive optimization over all admissible changepoint configurations would require fitting 2^{N-1} different models, an impossible task even on the world's fastest computers. To combat this, an exhaustive search over all possible changepoint configurations with $m \leqslant 5$ changepoints was conducted. Even this contains over one billion possible configurations for $N = 168$ years of data. This search was done in a parallel fashion utilizing the Ohio Supercomputer Center (Ohio Supercomputer Center, 1987). To also consider changepoint configurations with $m > 5$, a genetic algorithm (GA) in R (Scrucca, 2013, 2017) was used; GA findings are denoted with a * in the results below. In general, a GA has no bound on the total number of changepoints other than $m \leqslant N - 1$; the drawback is that GAs may fail to locate the true MDL minimum configuration. To combat this random aspect of GAs, multiple runs of the algorithm were done to give credence to the reported results.

2.4.1 Total cyclone counts

Table 2.1 provides results for the tropical cyclone counts in the North Atlantic Basin. MDL estimates $m = 7$ changepoints in the optimal segmentation, resulting in eight regimes. This model is graphically displayed in Figure 2.3 and appears to describe the data well. One implication is immediately clear: there have been significant changes over the years. Numeric information by regime is provided in Table 2.2.

The MDL approach has several small-length regimes, one having the two years 1886 and 1887 and one containing the single year 1914, wherein only one tropical cyclone was recorded. These can be interpreted as outlying periods. For those who do not want to consider such small segment lengths, we will refit the model imposing a minimum segment length below.

While we will generally be reticent to provide physical explanations for the estimated changepoints, the upwards shift in 1931 is often attributed to modern-day hurricane data collection, including aircraft reconnaissance (Landsea et al, 1999, Neumann et al, 1999). The strong increase circa 1995 will repeatedly surface below.

TABLE 2.1: MDL model fits for tropical cyclones by changepoint numbers. The best configuration has seven changepoints and is bolded

m	MDL objective	Changepoint times
0	−4093.48	—
1	−4171.04	1931
2	−4189.96	1931, 1995
3	−4193.04	1931, 1960, 1995
4	−4194.29	1886, 1888, 1931, 1995
5	−4197.55	1886, 1888, 1931, 1960, 1995
7*	**−4198.38**	**1886, 1888, 1914, 1915, 1931, 1960, 1995**

Results

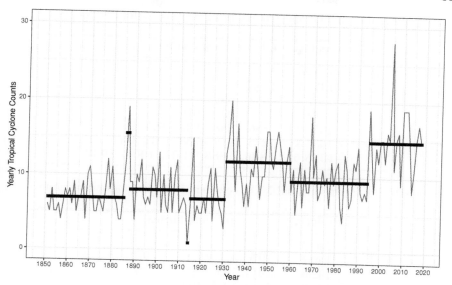

FIGURE 2.3: The optimal MDL segmentation for North Atlantic tropical cyclones.

2.4.2 Hurricanes and major storms

The yearly storm counts that achieve hurricane status (sustained winds of 64 knots or higher), and major hurricane status (categories 3, 4, and 5 on the Saffir–Simpson scale, those with sustained winds of 96 knots or higher) were also analyzed separately. A summary of the MDL fits are provided in Tables 2.3 and 2.4 with Figure 2.4 displaying the optimal segmentations.

The optimal segmentation for all hurricanes and major hurricanes (strong storms) both have seven regimes. In both fits, the optimal model has several short segments, suggestive of outliers from a Poisson model. However, in both

TABLE 2.2: Summary statistics by regime for the tropical cyclone counts

Regime	Mean	Var	Min	Median	Max
1851–1885	6.86	4.42	4.00	7.00	12.00
1886–1887	15.50	24.50	12.00	15.50	19.00
1888–1913	8.00	6.80	4.00	7.00	13.00
1914	1.00	—	1.00	1.00	1.00
1915–1930	6.88	10.25	3.00	6.00	15.00
1931–1959	11.90	11.67	6.00	12.00	20.00
1960–1994	9.37	8.65	4.00	9.00	18.00
1995–2018	14.79	18.61	8.00	15.00	28.00

TABLE 2.3: The optimal MDL segmentations for hurricanes

m	Objective	Changepoint times
0	−1336.6	—
1	−1352.1	1995
2	−1351.4	1932, 1995
3	−1353.2	1895, 1932, 1995
4	−1355.0	1886, 1888, 1932, 1995
5	−1354.5	1886, 1888, 1933, 1934, 1995
6*	**−1355.5**	**1886, 1888, 1907, 1908, 1932, 1995**

TABLE 2.4: The optimal MDL segmentations for major hurricanes

m	Objective	Changepoint times
0	230.2	—
1	198.7	1926
2	192.6	1915, 1995
3	192.9	1913, 1915, 1995
4	189.8	1861, 1866, 1926, 1995
5	189.4	1861, 1866, 1913, 1915, 1995
6*	**187.7**	**1861, 1866, 1893, 1895, 1915, 1995**

analyses, a more recent upward shift circa 1995 is evident; moreover, the last two shifts have served to increase the counts.

2.4.3 Analyses with segment-length restrictions

In the previous sections, several short segments were found, particularly during the early years of the record when the data is considered less reliable. As a follow-up, we reestimate changepoint configurations where the minimum regime length is set to be six years.

Table 2.5 provides results when regimes must be "6+" years. Consistent with previous results, shifts circa 1931, 1960, and 1995 are seen in this analysis. While the optimal segmentation has only four regimes now, increases in activity levels occurred in both 1931 and 1995 as is seen in Figure 2.5. This analysis, however, contains a regime from 1960–1994 with less activity.

Restricting to storms that attain hurricane strength only, the 6+ year restriction's optimal model puts changepoints at 1878, 1894, 1932, and 1995. The optimal segmentation for the major hurricanes has six segments in the optimal model, with changepoints occurring at 1857, 1869, 1948, 1965, and 1995.

It is worth considering the Poisson assumption for the storm counts. This can be assessed by checking whether the sample mean and variance are equal (the Poisson distribution's mean is also its variance; that is, its dispersion is

Results

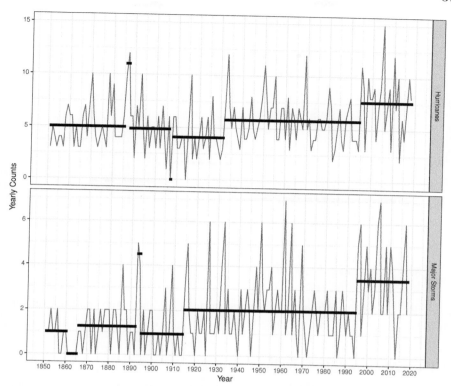

FIGURE 2.4: The optimal MDL segmentations for hurricanes and major hurricanes.

unity). As seen in Table 2.2, although means and variances may differ slightly in certain segments, there is no clear pattern to indicate that a non-unit dispersion is present across all segments. See Livsey et al (2018) for a more detailed analysis of the major hurricanes only.

TABLE 2.5: The optimal MDL segmentations for tropical cyclones with a 6+ year segment length restriction

m	MDL objective	Changepoint times
0	−4093.48	—
1	−4171.04	1931
2	−4189.96	1931, 1995
3*	**−4193.04**	**1931, 1960, 1995**
4	−4191.36	1859, 1931, 1960, 1995
5	−4193.02	1885, 1910, 1931, 1960, 1995

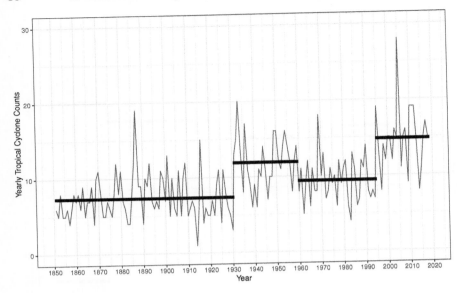

FIGURE 2.5: The optimal MDL segmentations for hurricanes and major hurricanes.

2.4.4 Accumulated cyclone energy

We now turn to the ACE series. Based on preliminary segmentations and correlation calculations with the residuals, we determined that the ACE series is close to white noise (uncorrelated) when mean shifts are taken into account in computing year-to-year correlations. As a conservative measure (it may not be needed at all), we used the simple first-order autoregressive (AR(1)) ARMA structure and optimized its associated Gaussian MDL objective function. Unfortunately, the ACE data does not appear Gaussian. Figure 2.6 shows a histogram of the ACE series and indicates a heavy right tail. How this would affect the MDL segmentation was initially unclear to us, but a large/small ACE value from the tails could induce two changepoints that demarcate an outlier (Gaussian distributions have so-called "light tails").

Indeed, attempts at segmenting the ACE series without imposing a minimum segment length were largely uninformative, with a GA preferring over 30 segments. As such, we only report results when a minimum segment length of 6+ years is imposed. When a segment length restriction is imposed in the model, the MDL procedure will discriminate more on mean shifts and less on marginal distributions. Table 2.6 displays results and shows an oscillating pattern, with 1995 again a shift to one of higher activity. This pattern involves alternating up-down shifts.

Table 2.7 provides summary statistics for the optimal six-segment fit. Figure 2.7 plots the segmentation against the series, which seems visually

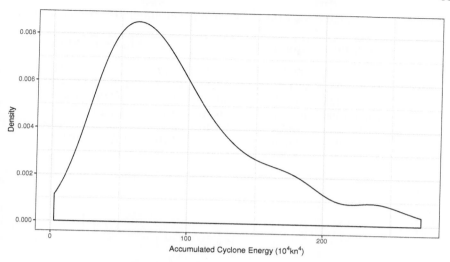

FIGURE 2.6: Histogram of annual ACE values.

TABLE 2.6: Optimal MDL segmentations as a function of the number of changepoints for the accumulated cyclone energy series with a 6+ year restriction imposed on segment lengths. The optimal model is bolded

m	MDL objective	Changepoint times
0	1821.04	—
1	1807.71	1995
2	1805.99	1878, 1995
3	1806.44	1878, 1970, 1995
4	1807.33	1878, 1950, 1970, 1995
5*	**1804.28**	**1878, 1902, 1926, 1970, 1995**

pleasing. Based on this segmentation, there is evidence of oscillating more-active/less-active periods in the ACE values.

2.5 Comments and conclusions

Several climate findings appear consistently across the different analyses presented here. First and foremost, the Atlantic Basin's hurricane record has endured many changepoints, and is far from stationary in time. Second, all analyses indicate that the Atlantic basin is currently in a record-high period of activity, and that that period began circa 1995. The "1995 changepoint" has

TABLE 2.7: Summary statistics by regime for accumulated cyclone energy

Regime	Mean	Std. dev.	Min	Median	Max
1851–1877	56.71	18.91	18.12	51.31	92.02
1878–1901	113.95	52.45	35.00	106.14	244.59
1902–1925	67.16	43.76	2.53	57.96	165.96
1926–1969	110.07	56.26	30.48	91.19	272.63
1970–1994	70.20	35.40	17.40	69.22	150.73
1995–2018	144.59	65.38	42.70	151.54	262.18

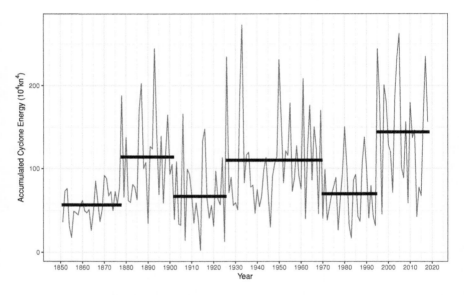

FIGURE 2.7: Optimal segmentation for North-accumulated cyclone energy.

been identified previously by several authors; Elsner et al (2000) remarkably note the shift using only 5 years of post-shift data, and Elsner et al (2004), Robbins et al (2011b) statistically verify the shift. This shift is likely climatic; specifically, it is not a consequence of changes in techniques used to monitor cyclones.

A variety of changepoints were discovered in earlier years of each series, many of which can be explained to some degree through technological advancements that led to more accurate detection and tracking of storms. For the hurricane and major hurricane counts, earlier changepoints were generally marked by an increase in storm activity. For the total cyclone series, the 1995 changepoint was preceded by a comparatively inactive period that began in 1960, and that inactive period was itself preceded by a period of higher activity, beginning in 1931. This behavior is perhaps indicative of a multi-decadal cycle, whose existence is reinforced by the ACE segmentation.

Our ACE optimal segmentation had three separate segments of "reduced activity," each of which was followed by a segment of higher activity. The segments are approximately 20–25 years on average, with the exception of a high-activity segment spanning the 1920s through the late 1960s. The ACE series does not exhibit the increasing trend that is seen in the count series; this perhaps indicates that the ACE series is less sensitive to undercounting of storms in early years of the data (or that the record has been reanalyzed and adjusted). Periodic behavior in Atlantic basin tropical cyclones was previously noted in Chylek and Lesins (2008), discovered via a metric akin to ACE using data through 2007. However, in our ACE analysis, the current segment is the most active segment on record, a phenomenon inconsistent with Chylek and Lesins (2008). Furthermore, Chylek and Lesins (2008) conclude that "we can expect… a decreasing trend taking over a few years after 2010." Our findings indicate that such a trend has not yet commenced.

Statistically, time series models for non-Gaussian data are needed. We conjecture that a gamma-type marginal distribution would describe the ACE data more appropriately than a Gaussian model. Also, in our modeling, once a new regime commences, the system is forced to enter a completely new regime, unlike any previous regime. Hidden Markov models would extend our work, allowing the processes to move back to former levels of activity. This is perhaps more commensurate with the notion of synoptic modes of the atmosphere. Such techniques are currently being developed by the authors.

For examples of analysis of economic losses associated with hurricanes, see Chapters 8, 9, and 11.

References

Brockwell PJ, Davis RA (1991) Time Series: Theory and Methods, 2nd edn. Springer, New York

Casella G, Berger RL (2002) Statistical Inference, 2nd edn. Duxbury, Pacific Grove, CA

Chylek P, Lesins G (2008) Multidecadal variability of Atlantic hurricane activity: 1851–2007. Journal of Geophysical Research: Atmospheres 113:D22106

Davis RA, Lee TCM, Rodriguez-Yam GA (2006) Structural break estimation for nonstationary time series models. Journal of the American Statistical Association 101(473):223–239

Elsner JB, Jagger TH (2006) Prediction models for annual US hurricane counts. Journal of Climate 19(12):2935–2952

Elsner JB, Jagger TH (2009) Hurricanes and Climate Change. Springer, New York

Elsner JB, Jagger T, Niu XF (2000) Changes in the rates of North Atlantic major hurricane activity during the 20th century. Geophysical Research Letters 27(12):1743–1746

Elsner JB, Niu X, Jagger TH (2004) Detecting shifts in hurricane rates using a Markov chain Monte Carlo approach. Journal of Climate 17(13):2652–2666

Elsner JB, Kossin JP, Jagger TH (2008) The increasing intensity of the strongest tropical cyclones. Nature 455:92–95

Emanuel K (2005) Divine Wind: The History and Science of Hurricanes. Oxford University Press, Auckland, New Zealand

Gallagher C, Lund R, Robbins M (2013) Changepoint detection in climate time series with long-term trends. Journal of Climate 26(14):4994–5006

Giddens A (2009) The Politics of Climate Change. Polity Press, Cambridge, UK

Hodges K, Cobb A, Vidale PL (2017) How well are tropical cyclones represented in reanalysis datasets? Journal of Climate 30(14):5243–5264

Knutson TR, Sirutis JJ, Garner ST, Vecchi GA, Held IM (2008) Simulated reduction in Atlantic hurricane frequency under twenty-first-century warming conditions. Nature Geoscience 1(6):359–364

Knutson TR, McBride JL, Chan J, Emanuel K, Holland G, Landsea C, Held I, Kossin JP, Srivastava AK, Sugi M (2010) Tropical cyclones and climate change. Nature Geoscience 3:157–163

Landsea CW (2007) Counting Atlantic tropical cyclones back to 1900. Eos 88(18):197–202

Landsea CW, Franklin JL (2013) Atlantic hurricane database uncertainty and presentation of a new database format. Monthly Weather Review 141(10):3576–3592

Landsea CW, Pielke RA, Mestas-Nunez AM, Knaff JA (1999) Atlantic basin hurricanes: Indices of climatic changes. Climatic Change 42(1):89–129

Landsea CW, Glenn DA, Bredemeyer W, Chenoweth M, Ellis R, Gamache J, Hufstetler L, Mock C, Perez R, Prieto R, Sanchez-Sesma J, Thomas D, Woolcock L (2008) A reanalysis of the 1911–20 Atlantic hurricane database. Journal of Climate 21(10):2138–2168

Li S, Lund RB (2012) Multiple changepoint detection via genetic algorithms. Journal of Climate 25(2):674–686

Livsey J, Lund RB, Kechagias S, Pipiras V (2018) Multivariate integer-valued time series with flexible autocovariances and their application to major hurricane counts. The Annals of Applied Statistics 12(1):408–431

Lu Q, Lund RB, Seymour PL (2005) An update of US temperature trends. Journal of Climate 18(22):4906–4914

Lu Q, Lund RB, Lee TCM (2010) An MDL approach to the climate segmentation problem. The Annals of Applied Statistics 4(1):299–319

Lund RB, Wang XL, Lu Q, Reeves J, Gallagher C, Feng Y (2007) Changepoint detection in periodic and autocorrelated time series. Journal of Climate 20:5178–5190

References

Mann ME, Zhang Z, Hughes MK, Bradley RS, Miller SK, Rutherford S, Ni F (2008) Proxy-based reconstructions of hemispheric and global surface temperature variations over the past two millennia. Proceedings of the National Academy of Sciences 105(36):13252–13257

McDonnell KA, Holbrook NJ (2004) A Poisson regression model of tropical cyclogenesis for the Australian–southwest Pacific Ocean region. Weather and Forecasting 19(2):440–455

Mooley DA (1981) Applicability of the Poisson probability model to the severe cyclonic storms striking the coast around the Bay of Bengal. Sankhyā: The Indian Journal of Statistics, Series B 43:187–197

Mooney CC (2007) Storm World: Hurricanes, Politics, and the Battle over Global Warming. Harcourt, New York

Neumann CJ, Jarvinen BR, McAdie CJ, Elms JD (1999) Tropical Cyclones of the North Atlantic Ocean, 1871–1998. National Climatic Data Center, Asheville, NC

Ohio Supercomputer Center (1987) Ohio Supercomputer Center. Ohio Supercomputer Center, Columbus, OH, URL http://osc.edu/ark:/19495/f5s1ph73

R Core Team (2019) R: A Language and Environment for Statistical Computing. R Foundation for Statistical Computing, Vienna, Austria, URL https://www.R-project.org/

Robbins M, Gallagher C, Lund RB, Aue A (2011a) Mean shift testing in correlated data. Journal of Time Series Analysis 32(5):498–511

Robbins MW, Lund RB, Gallagher CM, Lu Q (2011b) Changepoints in the North Atlantic tropical cyclone record. Journal of the American Statistical Association 106(493):89–99

Robbins MW, Gallagher CM, Lund RB (2016) A general regression changepoint test for time series data. Journal of the American Statistical Association 111:670–683

Scrucca L (2013) GA: a package for genetic algorithms in R. Journal of Statistical Software 53(4):1–37

Scrucca L (2017) On some extensions to GA package: hybrid optimisation, parallelisation and islands evolution. The R Journal 9(1):187–206

Trenberth KE (1990) Recent observed interdecadal climate changes in the Northern Hemisphere. Bulletin of the American Meteorological Society 71(7):988–993

Truchelut RE, Hart RE, Luthman B (2013) Global identification of previously undetected pre-satellite-era tropical cyclone candidates in NOAA/CIRES twentieth-century reanalysis data. Journal of Applied Meteorology and Climatology 52(10):2243–2259

Wanner H, Beer J, Bütikofer J, Crowley TJ, Cubasch U, Flückiger J, Goosse H, Grosjean M, Joos F, Kaplan JO, Küttel M, Müller SA, Prentice IC, Solominia O (2008) Mid-to Late Holocene climate change: an overview. Quaternary Science Reviews 27(19–20):1791–1828

3
Fire-Weather Index and Climate Change

Zuzana Hubnerova
Brno University of Technology, Brno, Czech Republic

Sylvia Esterby
University of British Columbia Okanagan, Kelowna, BC, Canada

Steve Taylor
Canadian Forest Service, Pacific Forestry Centre, Victoria, BC, Canada

CONTENTS

3.1	Introduction	45
3.2	Statistical modeling of the fire-weather index monthly maxima	48
	3.2.1 Separate modeling	49
	3.2.2 Spatial modeling	51
3.3	Summary and discussion	56
References		61

3.1 Introduction

Forest fire danger is a term which encompasses both the static and dynamic factors of the fire environment in the assessment of the ease of ignition, rate of spread, difficulty of control and impact of wildland fires (Wotton, 2009). Fire danger rating systems such as the Canadian Forest Fire Danger Rating System (CFFDRS) provide the means of transferring scientific knowledge of wildland fire to operational fire management (Taylor and Alexander, 2006). The Fire Weather Index (FWI) system, a subsystem of the CFFDRS, uses basic physical models of moisture in forest-floor fuel layers calibrated with field-based empirical observations and in situ measurements of four weather variables to calculate three moisture codes and three fire behavior indexes (Van Wagner, 1987). Temperature, relative humidity, wind speed, and 24-h accumulated precipitation are recorded at noon local standard time, and they are used to calculate conditions at the site in late afternoon, the peak fire danger period. The Fine Fuel Moisture Code (FFMC) represents the moisture content of the surface litter, where ignition and fire spread occur, the Duff Moisture Code (DMC) and the Drought Code (DC) represent the moisture content of shallow and deep organic layers, respectively, and are important to surface fire intensity and crowning potential. The Initial Spread Index (ISI) is calculated from FFMC and wind speed, the Buildup Index (BUI) representing fuel availability is calculated from DMC and DC, and FWI combines ISI and BUI to give an estimate of the fire potential.

Increasing temperatures, which are expected to result from climate change, are of concern since they could alter forest fire regime characteristics including frequency of severe fire weather, extended fire seasons, and duration of large fire activity (Weber and Stocks, 1998). Most studies that have addressed the impact of climate change on fire weather and forest fire behavior in Canada have used values of weather variables generated from global circulation models (GCMs) to calculate components of the FWI system and to further infer characteristics of the fire regime (Price et al, 2013). For example, Flannigan et al (2005) obtained relationships between historical observations of weather or fire danger and area burned to estimate area burned for projected meteorological variables from two GCMs under a $3 \times CO_2$ scenario. They projected a 74%–118% increase in area burned by 2100. However, the relationships between FWI system indexes and characteristics of fire regimes (Wotton, 2009) require many considerations to be taken into account. Examples of these are the need to consider lightning-caused and human-caused fires separately and to include in the modeling process the fact that as climate changes so does the wildland-urban interface.

Following FWI at a location over time makes it possible to follow an indicator of fire potential based on weather variables free of the complications of the many confounders that are present when we look at fire regime characteristics over time. As with the Canadian studies referred to above, two European studies generated weather variables using GCMs. The Canadian FWI was used to study changes in fire danger in Europe under extreme future climate scenarios (de Rigo et al, 2017). Fire danger was found to increase around the Mediterranean, the moderate danger region moved northward to central Europe, but there was little change across northern Europe. The Daily Severity Rating (DSR), where $DSR = 0.0272 \cdot FWI^{1.77}$, was used in the Burnt Area Model (BAM), a linear regression model of monthly area burned as a function of pre-fire season DSR and DSR for the particular month (DaCamara et al, 2014). Area burnt by vegetation fires in Portugal were projected from weather variables generated by GCMs under different future climate scenarios. Unlike the previous studies, Jolly et al (2015) use three daily global meteorological data sets spanning the period 1979 to 2013 that integrate observations of different types, but all are observed, not calculated, values. They use three danger indexes: US Burning Index, the Canadian FWI, and the Australian (or McArthur) Forest Fire Danger Index, and identify global and regional patterns of change in fire-weather season length, change in the frequency of long fire-weather seasons, and change in the area affected by long fire-weather seasons.

Introduction

Many of the largest fires in Canada have started on a few critical days with extreme fire weather (Flannigan and Wotton, 2001), which suggests that modeling extreme values of fire weather indexes and fire characteristics would be informative. Beverly and Martell (2005) used the statistics of extremes to gain insight into the potential for extreme fire weather to produce large and intense fires. They followed the methods of Moritz (1997) to fit extreme value models to dry spell extremes (1963–1998) and fire size extremes (1976–1999) using data from the Boreal Shield ecozone in Ontario. Regional differences were detected and return periods reported. Sanabria et al (2013) fitted extreme value distributions to data sets of McArthur Forest Fire Danger Index (FFDI) observed June 1972 to June 2010 at 78 recording stations around Australia. They chose the peaks-over-threshold technique and the Generalised Pareto Distribution. Spatial interpolation methods were used to obtain the spatial distribution of return periods and produce maps of Australia showing the FFDI level corresponding to 50-year and 100-year return periods. Noting that extreme value statistical models are not widely used in wildfire modeling, Holmes et al (2008) provided a literature review of the methods and an example by modeling fire size determined from the perimeter of fires in the Sequoia National Forest for the years 1910–2003.

Extreme-value methods are suitable for data with long-tail distributions such as fire-weather and fire-regime data, which exhibit spikes occurring in temporal records when fire weather becomes extreme or large fires occur. Two other methods that capture this characteristic of fire-weather and fire-regime data have been used to model Ontario data. From graphical exploratory analyses of daily FWI time series, recorded over 42 fire seasons at fire-weather stations in Ontario, Canada, Albert-Green et al (2014) found that the FWI process appears to switch between nil and non-nil phases of a stochastic process. This motivated the development of a beta-based mixture of geometric random variables as a model for consecutive runs of zero and consecutive runs of positive FWI values. In a retrospective study to address the question of trends across years in lightning caused fires, Woolford et al (2014) characterize three dominant features of these observed records as periods of regular seasonal pattern, periods with more fires reported than usual (i.e., extreme behavior) and periods with no fires (i.e., zero-heavy behavior). For data from two boreal forest regions in Northwestern Ontario between 1963 and 2009, a flexible mixture modeling framework was developed which permitted the joint assessment of temporal trends in these dominant characteristics in terms of fire risk defined as the probability of a lightning-fire day.

In this chapter, we model fire-weather patterns over time and space, with particular attention to temporal changes relevant to a changing climate. An extensive historical record of FWI-system data for the Canadian province of British Columbia has been compiled, and we use these data to study temporal change in FWI while accounting for spatial heterogeneity. Since changes in fire weather over time correspond to changes in fire potential over time, the use of FWI gives us a simpler quantity to follow, at least initially. Further, since it is large values of FWI that correspond to greater potential for fire, we restrict our analysis to these values and model temporal trends in location and scale parameters of the distribution of the monthly maximum FWI at stations using extreme-value methods.

3.2 Statistical modeling of the fire-weather index monthly maxima

We obtained weather observations with calculated values of the fire weather index (FWI) together with other components (elements) of the FWI system for 861 stations operated by the BC Wildfire Service located in British Columbia, Canada for years 1970 to 2018. Some of the stations were temporary or have been closed, but a number have 30+ years of observations.

With such a rich data set, various analyses can be conducted. In the context of climate change, we focus on monthly maxima of the FWI to be able to describe the statistical distribution of the maxima parametrically. Our aim was to identify possible trends in the parameters of the theoretical distribution of the monthly FWI maxima. As noted by Flannigan et al (2002), fire-danger indexes are not measured over the whole year. Ideally, fire-danger calculations begin three days after snow has left the ground or, in areas without snow, after three consecutive days exceeding 12 °C. In practice, the fire-season end date generally corresponds to a calendar date when fire suppression agencies gear down for the winter (such as October 31). Therefore, the analysis focuses on the months May, June, July, August, and September in sequence. The stations cover the entire province of British Columbia, which has enormous climatic and orographic variation (Meyn et al, 2010), resulting in a variety of ecosystems ranging from temperate rainforests in the southwest to boreal forests in the northeast. To account for this heterogeneity, we have divided the whole data set into four subsets that are assumed to be similar within a set with respect to climate and forest fuel types (Perrakis et al, 2018), coinciding mainly with the biogeoclimatic zones described by the Biogeoclimatic Ecosystem Classification (BEC; Mackenzie and Meidinger, 2017) available for the study area (Ministry of Forests, Lands, Natural Resource Operations and Rural Development, 2018).

Figure 3.1 displays a map of analyzed stations colored to identify the set membership. Set 1 is comprised of coastal, northern, and part of the central interior of British Columbia. BEC zones include the Coastal Western Hemlock, Coastal Douglas-fir, Coastal Mountain-heather Alpine, Interior Cedar–Hemlock, Boreal Altai Fescue Alpine, Engelmann Spruce–Subalpine Fir, Spruce–Willow–Birch, Sub-Boreal Spruce, Boreal White and Black Spruce, and Sub-Boreal Pine–Spruce zones. The stations in Set 1 are spread over a huge area, however their sparsity is especially high in the north. Set 2

Statistical modeling of the fire-weather index monthly maxima

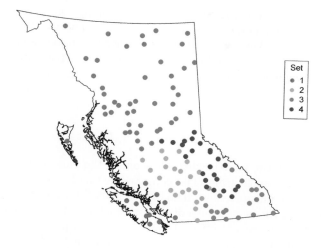

FIGURE 3.1: Map of analyzed fire-weather stations in British Columbia and their membership in the sets.

covers the interior plateau of the southwest interior where the following BEC zones appear: Sub-Boreal Pine–Spruce, Montane Spruce, Engelmann Spruce–Subalpine Fir, Interior Douglas-fir, Bunchgrass. Set 3 consists of stations covering much of the southern interior and includes Interior Cedar–Hemlock, Engelmann Spruce–Subalpine Fir, Interior Douglas-fir and Montane Spruce zones. Set 4 covers the area from Prince George to the Southeast Interior including Interior Cedar–Hemlock, Engelmann Spruce–Subalpine, Sub-Boreal Spruce zones.

3.2.1 Separate modeling

First, the stations with at least 30 years of complete measurements within a selected month were studied separately using the R package `extRemes` (Gilleland and Katz, 2016). For each station a maximum of the FWI values measured in the selected month were obtained, and these were used to estimate the parameters of the generalized extreme-value distribution (Beirlant et al, 2004, Coles, 2001) by the maximum likelihood method. There are three parameters of the generalized extreme-value distribution—location μ, scale σ, and shape ξ parameter. The distribution function of the generalized extreme-value (GEV) distribution is of the form

$$F(z) = \begin{cases} \exp\left\{-\left[1+\frac{\xi(z-\mu)}{\sigma}\right]_+^{-1/\xi}\right\} & \xi \neq 0 \\ \exp\left\{-\exp\left\{-\frac{(z-\mu)}{\sigma}\right\}\right\} & \xi = 0, \end{cases}$$

where $[u]_+$ denotes $\max(u, 0)$. See Chapter 8 for more examples of using GEV distributions. A special case, for which $\mu = 1$, $\sigma = 1$, and $\xi = 1$ is called a unit Fréchet distribution. Any variable with generalized extreme-value distribution can be transformed to a variable with unit Fréchet distribution. The model with linear dependence on time (year) in both location and scale parameters at station s

$$\mu_s(t) = \mu_{0,s} + \mu_{t,s} t$$
$$\sigma_s(t) = \sigma_{0,s} + \sigma_{t,s} t$$

was compared with the models where only one of the parameters was assumed to have a linear trend in time. The comparison was based on the likelihood ratio test at the significance level 0.05, which is used for all tests of a separate model. That way, the significance of the parameter of the linear trend in the excluded parameter was obtained. Tables 3.1 and 3.2 present the percentage of non-significant and significant temporal trends in the location and scale parameters, respectively. Moreover, if significant, positive and negative trends in the parameters are distinguished. The results are presented for the whole data set and for the considered subsets separately.

Tables 3.1 and 3.2 show that many of the trends were not significant. Significant temporal trends for the location parameter μ exceeded 50% in only 6 of the 20 month-set combinations: May Sets 3 and 4 (75% and 57%), July Set 3 (71%), and August Sets 2, 3, and 4 (83%, 71%, and 67%). However, if the temporal trends are significant, they are usually positive in location parameter μ (all parameters positive for all sets in May, July, and August and all but Set 1 in June and September). On the other hand, there were far fewer significant trends in the scale parameter in a month, ranging from 9% to 20%. Significant trends were mostly negative with the exceptions of June Set 1 (3%), July Sets 3 and 4 (6% and 5%), and September Sets 3 and 4 (13% and 13%).

For comparison and discussion of the spatial dependence of the temporal trends in the location and scale parameters, Figures 3.2 and 3.3 are presented. The symbol used to plot each station identifies the set to which it belongs and its color corresponds to the p-value of the likelihood ratio test of the temporal trend in the parameter μ and σ, respectively. To be able to distinguish between positive and negative temporal trends, the symbols are colored red or blue, respectively. Figure 3.2 displays signed p-values of the likelihood ratio test of the linear temporal trend in location parameter μ in July (a) and August (b) FWI maxima. In Figure 3.3, signed p-values of the likelihood ratio test of the temporal trend in scale parameter σ in July (a) and August (b) FWI maxima are presented. To complete the information on the shape parameter of the generalized extreme-value distribution of the monthly maxima, histograms of the estimate for July and August FWI maxima are given in Figure 3.4. We can conclude that the shape parameter ranges from about -0.8 to 0.6 covering all classes of the generalized extreme value distributions (Coles, 2001):

TABLE 3.1: Total number of stations analyzed in separate models of trends in monthly FWI maxima together with percentage of non-significant and significant temporal trends in *location parameter* μ of the generalized extreme-value distribution identified by the maximum likelihood test at the significance level 0.05

Month	Set	Total	Temporal trend in location (%)		
			Non-significant	Significant Positive	Negative
May	All	31	52	48	0
	1	12	58	42	0
	2	8	63	37	0
	3	4	25	75	0
	4	7	43	57	0
June	All	71	93	6	1
	1	34	91	6	3
	2	15	100	0	0
	3	12	83	17	0
	4	10	100	0	0
July	All	113	63	37	0
	1	52	81	19	0
	2	23	52	48	0
	3	17	29	71	0
	4	21	57	43	0
August	All	117	38	62	0
	1	53	53	47	0
	2	23	17	83	0
	3	17	29	71	0
	4	24	33	67	0
September	All	79	85	14	1
	1	29	93	3	3
	2	20	80	20	0
	3	15	87	13	0
	4	15	73	27	0

heavy-tailed Frechét ($\xi > 0$), light-tailed Gumbel ($\xi = 0$), and short-tailed Weibull family ($\xi < 0$).

3.2.2 Spatial modeling

Including the dependence between the monthly FWI maxima at different stations might be of advantage. Therefore, max-stable spatial processes models (Davison et al, 2012) were applied in our analysis. As explained in Ribatet (2017), every random variable with generalized extreme-value distribution with known parameters can be transformed to a random variable with unit

TABLE 3.2: Total number of stations analyzed in separate models of trends in monthly FWI maxima together with percentage of non-significant and significant temporal trends in *scale parameter* σ of the generalized extreme-value distribution identified by the maximum likelihood test at the significance level 0.05

Month	Set	Total	Temporal trend in scale (%) Non-significant	Significant Positive	Significant Negative
May	All	31	90	0	10
	1	12	100	0	0
	2	8	88	0	13
	3	4	100	0	0
	4	7	71	0	29
June	All	72	86	1	13
	1	34	88	3	9
	2	15	80	0	20
	3	12	92	0	8
	4	10	90	0	10
July	All	114	91	3	6
	1	52	100	0	0
	2	23	78	0	22
	3	17	82	6	12
	4	21	95	5	0
August	All	117	80	2	18
	1	53	89	4	8
	2	23	83	0	17
	3	17	59	0	41
	4	24	75	0	25
September	All	79	90	6	4
	1	29	93	0	7
	2	20	95	5	0
	3	15	80	13	7
	4	15	87	13	0

Fréchet distribution. Then, a max-stable process with unit Fréchet margins can be characterized by its spectral representation (Schlather, 2002). Various types of max-stable models can be obtained using different distributional assumptions on the components of the spectral representation. Description of the models available in the R package `SpatialExtremes` (Ribatet, 2018) can be found in Ribatet (2017) and Davison et al (2012). Parameters of a max-stable spatial model of interest are usually estimated by the maximum composite likelihood method (Ribatet, 2017). Following Ribatet (2013), one can perform the model selection by minimizing the composite information criterion, known as Takeuchi's information criterion (TIC). The goodness-of-fit

Statistical modeling of the fire-weather index monthly maxima 53

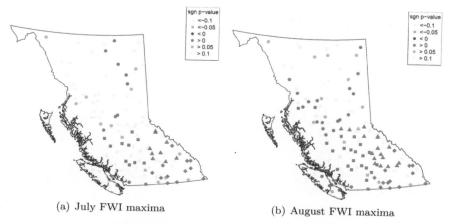

(a) July FWI maxima (b) August FWI maxima

FIGURE 3.2: Signed p-values of the temporal slope in *location parameter*. Dark blue color identifies a station with estimated significant negative temporal trend. Dark red color identifies a station with estimated significant positive temporal trend. Stations are represented by different symbols: circle for Set 1, square for Set 2, diamond for Set 3, and triangle for Set 4.

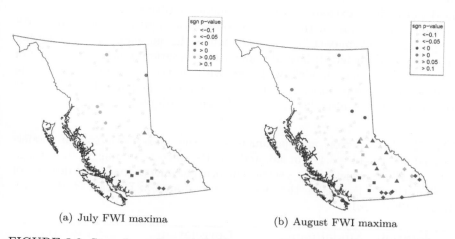

(a) July FWI maxima (b) August FWI maxima

FIGURE 3.3: Signed p-values of the temporal slope in *scale parameter*. Dark blue color identifies a station with estimated significant negative temporal trend. Dark red color identifies a station with estimated significant positive temporal trend. Stations are represented by different symbols: circle for Set 1, square for Set 2, diamond for Set 3, and triangle for Set 4.

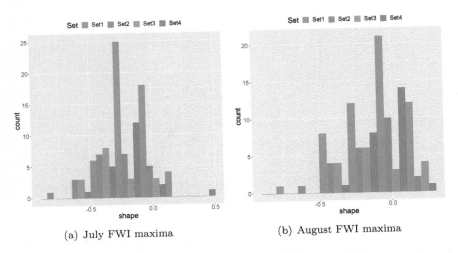

(a) July FWI maxima (b) August FWI maxima

FIGURE 3.4: Histogram of shape parameter estimates in the separate models of FWI monthly maxima in four sets of the stations.

can be also assessed by a visual comparison of the empirical F-madogram cloud to the fitted extremal coefficient function (Ribatet, 2013).

Again, the stations with at least 30 observations in the period 1970–2018 were analyzed by max-stable process models. In our models, the following covariates were included: latitude, longitude, elevation, and weather zone of the stations. Various models with and without the temporal trend in the location and scale parameters were considered and compared by TIC. Their goodness-of-fit was also checked in the F-madogram plot.

TABLE 3.3: Notation and parameters of the max-stable spatial models referred to in Tables 3.4, 3.5, 3.6, and 3.7. Parameters are nugget (γ_0), range (λ), smooth parameter (α), second smooth parameter (α_2), and degrees of freedom (DoF). Details on the models can be found in Davison et al (2012), Ribatet (2013, 2017)

Notation	Model name	Correlation	Parameters
brown	Brown–Resnick		λ, α
twhitmat	Extremal t-model	Whittle–Matérn	$\lambda, \alpha, \alpha_2$, DoF
gwhitmat	Geometric Gaussian	Whittle–Matérn	$\lambda, \alpha, \sigma^2$
powexp	Schlather model	stable	$\gamma_0, \lambda, \alpha$
whitmat	Schlather model	Whittle–Matérn	$\gamma_0, \lambda, \alpha$
cauchy	Schlather model	Cauchy	$\gamma_0, \lambda, \alpha$
caugen	Schlather model	generalized Cauchy	$\gamma_0, \lambda, \alpha, \alpha_2$
bessel	Schlather model	Bessel	$\gamma_0, \lambda, \alpha$

TABLE 3.4: Estimates (standard errors are in parentheses) of the temporal slopes in location (μ_t) and scale (σ_t) parameters in **Set 1** with N stations for the models selected by TIC

Month	Model	N	μ_t	σ_t	γ_0	λ	α
May	cauchy	12	0.199 (0.031)	0.013 (0.020)	0.313 (0.531)	73.252 (187.001)	1.345 (3.728)
June	powexp	35	0.040 (0.046)	−0.053 (0.015)	0.038 (0.053)	77.220 (6.352)	1.992 (0.514)
July	brown	52				93.205 (24.023)	0.571 (0.031)
August	brown	53	0.278 (0.056)	0.003 (0.022)		81.717 (18.793)	0.510 (0.021)
September	twhitmat[a]	29			0.094 (0.057)	947.190 (500.680)	0.415 (0.136)

TABLE 3.5: Estimates (standard errors are in parentheses) of the temporal slopes in location (μ_t) and scale (σ_t) parameters in **Set 2** with N stations for the models selected by TIC

Month	Model	N	μ_t	σ_t	γ_0	λ	α
May	brown	8	0.197 (0.059)	−0.038 (0.045)		21.819 (6.770)	0.757 (0.133)
June	cauchy	15			0.392 (0.074)	118.848 (75.825)	0.711 (0.662)
July	caugen[b]	23	0.469 (0.090)	−0.030 (0.043)	0.142 (0.268)	54.610 (27.377)	0.743 (0.444)
August	brown	23	0.511 (0.083)	−0.130 (0.037)		5.681 (6.158)	0.203 (0.062)
September	bessel	20			0.522 (0.065)	41.560 (175.234)	9.548 (88.134)

Tables 3.4, 3.5, 3.6, and 3.7 display estimates and standard errors of the slope of the assumed linear temporal trends in the location and scale parameter of the generalized extreme-value distribution in the spatial max-stable model for all four sets in sequence. Models of the spectral representation selected by the TIC and referred to in the Tables 3.4, 3.5, 3.6, and 3.7 are summarized in Table 3.3. The significance of the temporal trend in location and scale parameter was also tested by the likelihood ratio test as in Ribatet (2013) at the significance level 0.05.

From Tables 3.4, 3.5, 3.6, and 3.7, we can conclude that a positive trend in location parameter (μ_t) of the generalized extreme-value distribution is significant in Set 1—May, June and August, Sets 2 and 4—May, July, and August, and Set 3—May, August and September.

---
[a] Estimate of degrees of freedom in twhitmat model was 3.569 (0.790).
[b] Estimate of α_2 of caugen model was 1.975 (2.532).

TABLE 3.6: Estimates (standard errors are in parentheses) of the temporal slopes in location (μ_t) and scale (σ_t) parameters in **Set 3** with N stations for the models selected by TIC

Month	Model	N	μ_t	σ_t	γ_0	λ	α
May	brown	4	0.145 (0.082)	−0.122 (0.045)		38.327 (38.383)	0.241 (0.304)
June	caugen[c]	12			0.214 (15.997)	18.203 (199.717)	0.905 (4.372)
July	whitmat	17			0.012 (0.629)	129.422 (149.461)	0.334 (0.571)
August	powexp	18	0.493 (0.077)	−0.151 (0.031)	0.120 (4.676)	21.329 (62.930)	1.888 (7.660)
September	powexp	15	0.221 (0.089)	0.105 (0.041)	0.026 (4.281)	26.693 (266.254)	0.406 (1.168)

TABLE 3.7: Estimates (standard errors are in parentheses) of the temporal slopes in location (μ_t) and scale (σ_t) parameters in **Set 4** with N stations for the models selected by TIC

Month	Model	N	μ_t	σ_t	γ_0	λ	α
May	twhitmat[d]	7	−0.0004 (0.043)	−0.101 (0.006)	0.000 (0.334)	120.199 (150.259)	0.749 (1.327)
June	brown	10				0.390 (1.796)	0.101 (0.074)
July	gwhitmat[e]	21	0.140 (0.093)	−0.100 (0.050)	0.252 (0.085)	130.432 (192.425)	3.856 (7.461)
August	powexp	24	0.395 (0.059)	−0.127 (0.037)	0.183 (0.263)	88.956 (30.770)	0.746 (0.433)
September	brown	15				126.885 (37.347)	0.582 (0.079)

3.3 Summary and discussion

The data used here were drawn from records of FWI spanning up to 49 years (1970 to 2018) and 861 stations covering the Canadian province of British Columbia. FWI is an indicator of the fire potential which is calculated from weather measurements and thus provides an indicator that should

---

[c] Estimate of α_2 of caugen model was 1.281 (33.010).
[d] Estimate of degrees of freedom in twhitmat model was 3.483 (1.182).
[e] Estimate of σ^2 of gwhitmat model was 2.164 (0.721).

Summary and discussion

be responsive to changes in climate. Since it is high fire potential that provides hospitable conditions for fire, models of maximum FWI have been fitted. To account for the enormous climatic and orographic variation in British Columbia, a mountainous province with the Pacific Ocean coastline as its western boundary, the stations have been divided into four geographic sets. The fire potential is also expected to differ over the fire season. To increase the sensitivity of the analysis to temporal changes over years the monthly maximum FWI have been modeled for each of the months May to September. First, temporal models for each station in each month have been developed. Then, spatial models have been fitted to each set of stations to capture any advantage to the analysis gained by including spatial dependence.

The results of separate modeling show that for all stations in a particular month, the percentage of stations with a significant linear time trend in the location parameter differs considerably among months (7% to 62%) but is low for the scale parameter (9% to 20%). Temporal trends with p-value not greater than 0.05 are referred to as being significant in this discussion. Significant trends for the location parameter are almost entirely positive and those for the scale parameter predominantly negative. A positive value of the temporal trend in the location parameter corresponds to the annual rate of change in monthly maximum FWI, where maximum FWI is increasing over time. A negative value of the temporal trend in the scale parameter means a decrease in the variance of the monthly FWI maxima over time.

Note that opposite trends in the location and scale parameter might result in non-significant trend or opposite trend in quantiles of the distribution. However, in our case, the estimated trends in median agreed in sign with the estimated trend in the location parameter of the generalized extreme value distribution. Moreover, the sign of the trend in upper quartile agreed with the sign of the trend in location parameter in most of the cases except for 2 stations in May, 3 stations in July, and 12 stations in August. Allowing for trends in both location and scale parameter enabled us to capture more complex changes in the distribution of monthly FWI maxima.

Considering location parameter by month, the highest percentage of stations with significant positive trends are May, July, and August (48%, 37%, and 62%). When region is taken into account (Figure 3.5), the percentage of positive significant trends for Set 3, in order by month, is 75%, 17%, 71%, 71%, and 13%. June has low percentages for all sets (6%, 0%, 17%, and 0%), while in July Set 3 is highest (71%) and in August Sets 2 and 3 are high (83% and 71%) but drop in September (20% and 13%). These positive temporal trends in the location parameter are consistent with the findings of Wan et al (2019) who used homogenized Canadian temperature data from 1900 to present and reported that warm seasons and hot extremes are getting warmer in British Columbia.

Set 3 is in the southeastern part of the province, and Set 2 sits above and to the west but excludes the coastal area (Figure 3.1). Set 1 is comprised of stations north of Sets 2, 3, and 4 plus coastal stations. The location of a set

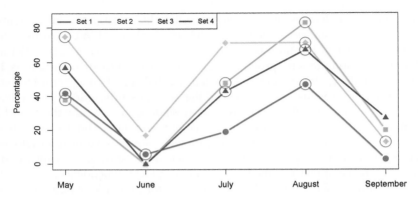

FIGURE 3.5: Percentages of significant positive temporal trends in location parameter μ of the generalized extreme-value distribution in separate models as given in Table 3.1. Circles identify the combination of months and sets where the temporal trend was identified as significant by the spatial modeling as listed in Tables 3.4, 3.5, 3.6, and 3.7. Color of the circle reflects the sign of the estimated temporal slope in the location parameter μ_t in the spatial model—red (positive) and blue (negative).

partially determines the values of the weather variables used in calculation of FWI. To compare the results for temporal trends in the parameters of maximum FWI with maximum FWI, plots of the set average FWI maximum vs year for each month were created (not shown here). The plots show that average maximum FWI for Sets 2 and 3 are generally higher than average maximum FWI for Sets 1 and 4. Since Sets 2 and 3 had more positive trends in the location parameter, this suggests that the hotter, drier regions show more positive trends in location parameter. To examine this more closely, the signed p-value for a station was plotted versus both the average maximum FWI and the overall maximum for the particular month and set. This confirmed the above statement and provided more insight into the relationship between trends in the location parameter and FWI. For all sets there was a FWI value below which the scatter of signed p-values covered the range from -1 to $+1$. In May, June, and September, the scatter between -1 and $+1$ covered the entire range up to the highest value of average maximum FWI, which was about 45, 55, and 50, respectively. In July and August, there is a very different picture. The scatter of signed p-values for FWI below about 30 covers the range -1 to $+1$, and above this, between 30 and the largest average maximum FWI of about 62, the signed p-values are much closer to 0 and are all positive, and the stations were in Sets 2 and 3 except for 3 or 4 stations in Set 1. The plots using overall maximum FWI showed similar patterns except for higher values of FWI.

Summary and discussion

May shows an atypical pattern in the percentage of significant positive trends in location parameter with Set 1 relative to the other sets being higher than in the other months, and Set 3 showing a high proportion of significant positive trends similar to July and August as opposed to the low proportion in September. The number of stations in May is lower than in the other months since a weather station opens in the spring once the snow is gone or a criterion on consecutive-day temperature is met. In May, Set 1 has few of the northern-most stations open, and in all sets stations at higher elevation will also have later snow melt and thus not be open. Thus May has relatively more southerly or lower stations than in other months, which may explain the deviation in pattern. June, which had the lowest percentages of significant positive trends, is usually a wet month in British Columbia.

The interesting observation from Table 3.2 and Figure 3.3 is that, where there is an indication of significant trend in the scale parameter, the direction is predominantly negative, i.e., variability in maximum FWI is decreasing. Considering the scale parameter by month, the highest percentage of stations with significant negative trends are May, June, and August (10%, 13%, and 16%). When region is taken into account, the consistent patterns seen for location parameter trends are not present. The higher percentages of negative trends occur as follows: May Set 4 (29%), July Set 2 (22%), and August Sets 2, 3, and 4 (17%, 41%, and 25%). Small percentages of significant positive trends occur in Set 1 in June and August (3% and 4%) and in Sets 3 and 4 in July (6% and 5%) and September (13% and 13%), but these positive trends in Sets 3 and 4 are not present in August. For August, the month with the highest number of significant negative trends, increasing temporal trends in location parameter for Sets 2, 3, and 4 (83%, 71%, and 67%) are accompanied by decreasing temporal trends in scale parameter for these sets (17%, 41%, and 25%).

The plots of station p-value for slope on the BC map for both location and scale parameters (shown only for July and August) provide a more descriptive view of where changes over time are occurring, in which direction, and, by viewing the maps for all 5 months (May, June, and September not shown), how this is changing over the fire season. The p-values from the separate models have been used rather than parameter estimates to account for differing numbers of observations among stations and should be considered a tool for looking at patterns.

The simulation study by Westra and Sisson (2011) clearly demonstrates the advantages of explicitly considering spatial information in the detection and attribution of trends in extremes. Therefore, we applied the max-stable process models to the monthly FWI maxima for stations from this same British Columbia data set. Nevertheless, as found by Ribatet (2013), fitting spatial temporal models of extremes requires considerable care and trade-offs. As more elements or layer variability are added, computations become more challenging (Davison et al, 2012). For these data, the best form of the max-stable model varied with month-set combination (Tables 3.4–3.7). Some of the models allow for additional parameters of the spatial dependence and therefore are more flexible. Note also, that unlike the other models, Schlather models do not accommodate independence with increasing distance of the stations (Davison et al, 2012).

Fitting a model to an individual station captures local behavior, whereas fitting a spatial model to a group of contiguous stations should tell us about the regional behavior, assuming that the group of stations does possess some regional characteristics. A method of comparison that could be applied to the results on trends in the location parameter is to compare the percentage of positive trends in location parameter from the separate modeling for a particular month-set combination with the estimate of location parameter in the corresponding spatial model. A high percentage of positive trends could be considered consistent with a significant positive location trend parameter in the spatial model. The percentage of positive trends in separate models for each month-set combination are shown in Figure 3.5 and the existence of a positive trend (red circle) or negative trend (blue circle) in the location parameter of the spatial model is indicated by the circle around the symbol, if the term is significant in the model. A red circle and high percentage of positive trends would indicate consistency and a blue circle with high percentage indicates disagreement. The absence of a circle where the percentage of positive trends is low also indicates consistency. The major inconsistencies are May Set 4, June Set 1, July Set 3, and September Set 3.

There are several possible explanations for these inconsistencies. An important consideration is the local effect at some stations which may truly differ from a more general regional characteristic of a set of stations, leading to different conclusions about changes in FWI over the years from the two approaches. An alternative way of choosing sets may improve the results of the spatial modeling. It is encouraging that the results of the two approaches agree with respect to positive trends in the location parameter for May (Sets 1, 2, and 4) and August. May is an important month because one of the concerns with changing climate is the lengthening fire season which would be expected to then show increasing FWI in May as temperatures increase. The results of separate modeling were very striking for August with a high proportion of significant positive trends in the location parameter and negative trends in the scale parameter for Sets 2, 3, and 4, which comprise the more southerly locations. The results from the plots of the signed p-values for the location parameter versus average maximum FWI show that, for August, above an average maximum FWI of about 30, trends in the location parameter are positive with p-values typically much smaller than obtained for stations with lower FWI, and this is occurring for stations in Sets 2 and 3. The behavior in July is very similar to August, but p-values are somewhat higher for average maximum FWI above about 30.

The results presented here can be considered preliminary with regard to conclusions about extreme FWI values for British Columbia. The analyses conducted demonstrate that the described extreme value methods have potential for providing more definitive conclusions about the changes over time in historical FWI. To do this, we have work underway to use the features of the data which have been uncovered in the present study to focus our efforts, for example, to refining the regions used and further considering the form of change over time. Longer records and local-effect covariates will also be sought. With respect to methodology, inclusion of goodness-of-fit tests in the separate models is of interest. Regarding future research on spatial models, a true distribution of the monthly maximal FWI can be approximated with the simulations from the fitted max-stable process models Ribatet (2017, 2018). Continuing with this approach is important, since modeling the extremes in a spatial context allows one to assess risks that involve simultaneous rare events (Shang et al, 2011).

References

Albert-Green A, Braun JW, Martell DL, Woolford DG (2014) Visualization tools for assessing the Markov property: sojourn times in the forest Fire Weather Index in Ontario. Environmetrics 25(6):417–430

Beirlant J, Goegebeur Y, Segers J, Teugels J, De Waal D, Ferro C (2004) Statistics of Extremes: Theory and Applications. Wiley Series in Probability and Statistics, John Wiley & Sons, Chichester, GB

Beverly JL, Martell DL (2005) Characterizing extreme fire and weather events in the Boreal Shield ecozone of Ontario. Agricultural and Forest Meteorology 133(1):5–16

Coles S (2001) An Introduction to Statistical Modeling of Extreme Values. Springer, New York

DaCamara CC, Pereira MG, Calado TJ, Calheiros T (2014) Impacts of climate change on the fire regime in Portugal. In: Impacts of Climate Change on the Fire Regime in Portugal, Imprensa da Universidade de Coimbra, Coimbra, 1193–1206

Davison AC, Padoan SA, Ribatet M (2012) Statistical modeling of spatial extremes. Statistical Science 27(2):161–186

Flannigan MD, Wotton BM (2001) Climate, weather, and area burned. In: Forest Fires—Behavior and Ecological Effects, Academic Press, New York, pp 351–373

Flannigan MD, Wotton BM, Todd B, Cameron H, Logan K (2002) Climate change implications in British Columbia: assessing past, current and future fire occurrence and fire severity in BC. Tech. rep., Canadian Forest Service and British Columbia Ministry of Forests, Victoria, BC

Flannigan MD, Logan KA, Amiro BD, Skinner WR, Stocks BJ (2005) Future area burned in Canada. Climatic Change 72(1):1–16

Gilleland E, Katz RW (2016) extRemes 2.0: An extreme value analysis package in R. Journal of Statistical Software 72(8):1–39

Holmes TP, Huggett RJ, Westerling AL (2008) Statistical analysis of large wildfires. In: Holmes TP, Prestemon JP, Abt KL (eds) The Economics of Forest Disturbances: Wildfires, Storms, and Invasive Species, Springer Netherlands, Dordrecht, 59–77

Jolly WM, Cochrane MA, Freeborn PH, Holden ZA, Brown TJ, Williamson GJ, Bowman DM (2015) Climate-induced variations in global wildfire danger from 1979 to 2013. Nature Communications 6(7537):545–550

Mackenzie W, Meidinger D (2017) The Biogeoclimatic Ecosystem Classification Approach: an ecological framework for vegetation classification. Phytocoenologia 48

Meyn A, Schmidtlein S, Taylor SW, Girardin MP, Thonicke K, Cramer W (2010) Spatial variation of trends in wildfire and summer drought in British Columbia, Canada, 1920–2000. International Journal of Wildland Fire 19(3):272–283

Ministry of Forests, Lands, Natural Resource Operations and Rural Development (2018) Biogeoclimatic zones of British Columbia. map. 1:7,500,000. URL `https://www.for.gov.bc.ca/ftp/hre/external/!publish/becmaps/PaperMaps/BGCzones.8x11.pdf`

Moritz MA (1997) Analyzing extreme disturbance events: Fire in Los Padres National Forest. Ecological Applications 7(4):1252–1262

Perrakis D, Eade G, Hicks D (2018) British Columbia wildfire fuel typing and fuel type layer description. Tech. Rep. Information report BC-X-444, Natural Resources Canada, Canadian Forest Service, Pacific Forestry Centre, Victoria, British Columbia

Price D, Alfaro R, Brown K, Flannigan M, Fleming R, Hogg E, Girardin M, Lakusta T, Johnston M, McKenney D, Pedlar J, Stratton T, Sturrock R, Thompson I, Trofymow J, Venier L (2013) Anticipating the consequences of climate change for Canada's boreal forest ecosystems. Environmental Reviews 21:322–365

Ribatet M (2013) Spatial extremes: Max-stable processes at work. Journal de la Société Française de Statistique 154(2):156–177

Ribatet M (2017) Modelling spatial extremes using max-stable processes. In: Franzke CLE, O'Kane TJ (eds) Nonlinear and Stochastic Climate Dynamics, Cambridge University Press, pp 369–391

Ribatet M (2018) SpatialExtremes: Modelling Spatial Extremes. URL `https://CRAN.R-project.org/package=SpatialExtremes`, R package version 2.0-7

de Rigo D, Libertà G, Houston Durrant T, Artés Vivancos T, San-Miguel-Ayanz J (2017) Forest fire danger extremes in Europe under climate change: variability and uncertainty. Publication Office of the European Union, Luxembourg

References

Sanabria L, Qin X, Li J, Cechet R, Lucas C (2013) Spatial interpolation of McArthur's Forest Fire Danger Index across Australia: Observational study. Environmental Modelling and Software 50:37–60

Schlather M (2002) Models for stationary max-stable random fields. Extremes 5(1):33–44

Shang H, Yan J, Zhang X (2011) El Niño—Southern Oscillation influence on winter maximum daily precipitation in California in a spatial model. Water Resources Research 47: W11507

Taylor SW, Alexander ME (2006) Science, technology, and human factors in fire danger rating: the Canadian experience. International Journal of Wildland Fire 15(1):121–135

Van Wagner CE (1987) Development and structure of the Canadian Forest Fire Weather Index System. In: Forest Technology Report 35, Canadian Forestry Service, Ottawa

Wan H, Zhang X, Zwiers F (2019) Human influence on Canadian temperatures. Climate Dynamics 52: 479–494

Weber MG, Stocks BJ (1998) Forest fires and sustainability in the boreal forests of Canada. Ambio 27(7):545–550

Westra S, Sisson S (2011) Detection of non-stationarity in precipitation extremes using max-stable process model. Journal of Hydrology 406:119–128

Woolford DG, Dean C, Martell DL, Cao J, Wotton B (2014) Lightning-caused forest fire risk in Northwestern Ontario, Canada, is increasing and associated with anomalies in fire weather. Environmetrics 25(6):406–416

Wotton BM (2009) Interpreting and using outputs from the Canadian Forest Fire Danger Rating System in research applications. Environmental and Ecological Statistics 16(2):107–131

4

Probabilistic Projections of High-Tide Flooding for the State of Maryland in the Twenty-First Century

Ming Li, Fan Zhang, Yijun Guo
University of Maryland Center for Environmental Science, Cambridge, MD, USA

Xiaohong Wang
Salisbury University, Salisbury, MD, USA

CONTENTS

4.1	Introduction	65
4.2	Methods	69
	4.2.1 Regional ocean model	69
	4.2.2 Design of numerical experiments	70
	4.2.3 Inundation impact analysis	71
4.3	Results	72
	4.3.1 Bay-wide response	73
	4.3.2 Dorchester County	75
	4.3.3 Annapolis and Baltimore	78
4.4	Conclusions	80
References		83

4.1 Introduction

The small area occupied by the coastal zone belies its importance to human affairs and the potential risks posed by climate change. Humans are concentrated in the coastal zone; three-quarters of the global population lives within 50 km of the sea and 50% of the US population lives within 50 miles (∼80 km) of the sea. Climate change is expected to increase the rate of sea-level rise and coastal inundation (Church and Clark, 2013), putting coastal communities in jeopardy of significant property damage, sociocultural and economic disruption, and loss of life. The number of medium-to-large coastal municipalities in the United States affected by flooding is estimated to exceed 33 in 2050 and 90 in 2100 (Kulp and Strauss, 2017). Globally, 0.2%–4.6% of the population is expected to be flooded annually in 2100 under 0.25–1.23 m of global mean sea level rise, with expected annual losses of 0.3%–9.3% of global gross domestic product (Hinkel et al, 2014). New elevation data triple estimates of global vulnerability to sea level rise and coastal flooding: about 340/630 million people will live in land below annual flood level by 2050/2100 (Kulp and Strauss, 2019). Therefore, there is an urgency to quantify the flooding risks faced by coastal communities, their resilience to rising sea levels, and what should be done to reduce the coastal risks.

Maryland, with over 3000 miles (4828 km) of tidal shoreline along both the Chesapeake Bay and the state's Atlantic Ocean shoreline, is highly vulnerable to sea level rise. Recurrent flooding is already a major problem in Chesapeake Bay (Mitchell et al, 2013) and will likely become more frequent in the future as sea level rises (Spanger-Siegfried et al, 2014). For example, "nuisance" tidal flooding that occurred just a very few days per year in Annapolis in the 1950s now occurs 40 or more days per year (Boesch et al, 2018).

Tide gauge records and satellite altimetry reveal that global-mean sea level (GSML) rose at a rate of 1.2 ± 0.2 mm yr^{-1} between 1900 and 1990 and at a much faster rate of 3.0 ± 0.7 mm yr^{-1} between 1993 and 2012 (Church and White, 2011, Dangendorf et al, 2017, Hay et al, 2015). The rate of sea level rise is accelerating in the twenty-first century. According to IPCC AR5 (Fifth Assessment Report of the Intergovernmental Panel on Climate Change), GMSL will rise 0.52–0.98 m by 2100 for the highest emission scenario considered—Representative Concentration Pathway RCP 8.5 (Church and Clark, 2013). Probabilistic sea level projections suggest a very likely (90% probability) GMSL rise of 0.5–1.2 m under RCP 8.5 (Kopp et al, 2014). If the rapid collapse of Antarctic ice sheet as projected in some climate models is taken into consideration, the median projected GMSL for 2100 will increase from 0.79 to 1.46 m under RCP 8.5 (Kopp et al, 2017). (For an overview of climate models, see Chapter 1.)

Tide-gauge records in Chesapeake Bay show that sea levels rose by 3–4 mm per year over the twentieth century (Zervas, 2001, 2009), twice that of the global average. Land subsidence associated with glacial isostatic adjustment is a major contributor to the high relative sea level rise in the Bay (Miller et al, 2013). Ocean dynamics, arising from changing ocean circulation, may also contribute to higher sea levels at the coast. The weakening of the Gulf Stream over the past decade may have contributed to the higher rates of sea level rise along the Mid-Atlantic coast (Ezer et al, 2013, Kopp, 2013, Sallenger et al, 2012). However, recent analysis showed that sea level declined north of Cape Hatteras between 2010 and 2015, and this decline was caused by an increase in atmospheric pressure combined with shifting wind patterns (Domingues et al, 2018).

With respect to coastal inundation, the height of the highest waters, the sum of local mean sea level and tidal amplitude, is more relevant than the mean

Introduction

sea level alone. Müller et al (2011) showed that the response of the oceans to tidal forces changed significantly during the last century. Flick et al (2003) examined long-term records at US tide gauges and found significant changes in the tidal range. Semi-enclosed bays such as the Bay of Fundy have natural resonance periods that are close to those for semidiurnal or diurnal tides. In these bays, tide at the head of the bay is greatly amplified as compared to that at the mouth (Garrett, 1972). The resonant period in Chesapeake Bay is about 48 hours. Raising sea level by 1 m shortens it to 36 hours, moves diurnal tides inside the resonance band, and increases tidal ranges in the upper Bay (Zhong et al, 2008). Similar results are found for Delaware Bay: tidal ranges in the upper part increased 100% over the past 4000 years (Hall et al, 2013). However, such calculations ignore the fact that flooding of adjacent low-lying areas introduces frictional, intertidal regions that may serve as energy sinks for incoming tidal waves (Holleman and Stacey, 2014). While sea level rise is accompanied by larger tidal ranges in the Bay of Fundy due to steep rocky coastlines (Greenberg et al, 2012), net tidal amplification in most areas of San Francisco is predicted to be lower in most sea level rise scenarios because many low-lying areas around the northern branch of San Francisco Bay are tidal marshlands (Holleman and Stacey, 2014). Similarly, Lee et al (2017) found that tidal ranges in the upper reaches of Chesapeake and Delaware Bays decrease with sea level rise if the low-lying land, consisting mostly of salt marshes and agricultural fields, is allowed to flood. Therefore, it is important to consider tidal response to sea level rise when projecting flooding in the future climate. The peak tidal sea level is not simply a linear sum of sea level rise and historical tidal height.

There are two approaches to generating sea level rise projections. One develops scenarios spanning a range of possible future scenarios (Sweet and Park, 2014). The other estimates the probability of future sea level changes, either through a central projection with an associated range or through a probability distribution. Kopp et al (2014) synthesized several lines of evidence to produce probability distributions for global and local sea level changes. The probability distribution of relative sea level rise over 2000 is provided over time and for three greenhouse gas emissions pathways or Representative Concentration Pathways (RCP): Growing Emissions (RCP 8.5), Stabilized Emissions (RCP 4.5), and meeting the Paris Agreement (RCP 2.6). This framework has been adopted by California (Griggs et al, 2017), Oregon (Dalton et al, 2017), Washington, and most recently Maryland (Boesch et al, 2018). The likely range (66% chance) of sea level rise in Maryland between 2000 and 2050 is 0.24 to 0.48 m, with 5% chance exceeding 0.61 m and 1% chance exceeding 0.70 m (Boesch et al, 2018, Figure 4.1). Later this century, sea level rise rates are highly sensitive to the emission pathway. Between 2000 and 2100, the likely range for the relative sea level rise in Maryland is 0.36 to 0.91 m under RCP 2.6, 0.49 to 1.04 m under RCP 4.5, and is 0.61 to 1.28 m under RCP 8.5 (Figures 4.1a and 4.1b).

The probabilistic sea level projection is the most appropriate approach for use in planning and regulation, infrastructure siting, design, etc. However,

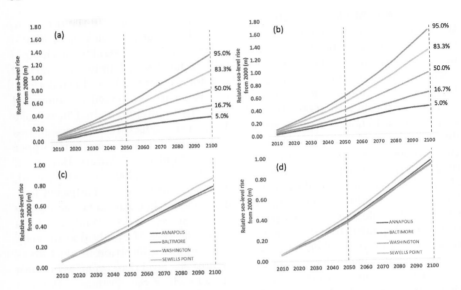

FIGURE 4.1: Probabilistic projections of the relative sea level rise in Annapolis under climate change scenario RCP 4.5 (a) and RCP 8.5 (b). Median projections of the relative sea level rise in Chesapeake Bay under RCP 4.5 (c) and 8.5 (d).

these sea level rise predictions must be projected onto low-lying land areas in order to assess the flooding risks faced by coastal communities. Projections of sea level rise onto land areas were mostly based on static images (e.g., bathtub approach) and did not consider dynamical processes of tides in rising seas. These graphic products may have underestimated the inundation risks faced by coastal community and infrastructure. Statistical approaches were developed to characterize coastal flood risk by using long-term sea level observations at tidal gauges and superimposing the time series with the sea level rise projected for the future climate (Ghanbari et al, 2019, Moftakhari et al, 2015). These analyses led to useful estimates of flood frequency at certain coastal locations but did not provide a direct estimate of the flooded land areas. To account for the full dynamic effect of sea level rise on coastal inundation, an ocean model capable of simulating tides and currents in rising seas is required.

In this study we used a regional ocean model to examine flooding at high tides around Chesapeake Bay, especially over low-lying land areas in the State of Maryland. Three sites were selected as focus studies areas: the City of Baltimore and City of Annapolis are the two largest cities in Maryland; the Dorchester County on the Eastern Shore of Maryland is among the most vulnerable rural areas to sea level rise. Our goal is to produce a probabilistic projection of high tide flooding in 2050 and 2100, and develop dynamics-based inundation

Methods

graphics that can prepare coastal communities for the rising inundation risks in the twenty-first century.

4.2 Methods

To assess the impacts of sea level rise on tidal water levels and coastal inundation in the twenty-first century, we used the Finite Volume Coastal Ocean Model (FVCOM) and forced it with the probabilistic projections for the relative sea level rise in Chesapeake Bay.

4.2.1 Regional ocean model

The unstructured-grid FVCOM was used to simulate tidal flows and intertidal flooding over low-lying land (Chen et al, 2003, 2006). The model domain covers Chesapeake Bay and the eastern US continental shelf (Figure 4.2a). The horizontal resolution ranges from ~1 km in the inner shelf to ~10 km near the open boundaries. The model resolves Chesapeake Bay and its surrounding lands (up to 5 m height above the current mean sea level) at a resolution of 0.2–1.0 km. Finer resolutions are placed over the City of Baltimore, City of Annapolis (5–10 m) and the Dorchester County on the rural eastern shore of Maryland (100–200 m), three focus areas in this study. The model is run in three-dimensional barotropic mode in which temperature and salinity are kept constant. In the vertical direction, five sigma layers are used. At the offshore open boundary, the tidal sea level is prescribed using ten tidal constituents according to the Oregon State University global tidal model TOPEX/POSEIDON 7.1 (Egbert and Erofeeva, 2002). A quadratic stress is exerted at the bed, with the bottom roughness height set to be 2 mm in Chesapeake Bay and 2 cm on the adjacent shelf (Lee et al, 2017). As a simplification the roughness heights are assumed to be the same between the sea beds and the surrounding lands.

To simulate overland inundation, coastal lands up to 5 m above the mean sea level are included in the model domain. High-resolution (10 m horizontal resolution) digital elevation data in land areas surrounding Chesapeake Bay are obtained from US Geological Survey National Elevation Data Set (Gesch, 2009). Fine-resolution LIDAR data,[1] with a horizontal resolution of 1 foot (~0.3 m) and a vertical resolution of 1 cm, are used for the digital elevation over Maryland. Bathymetry data are acquired from the NOAA 1 arc-second resolution Bathymetric Digital Elevation Model in the estuary, the 3 arc-second Coastal Relief Model on the continental shelf, and the 1 arc-minute ETOPO1 Global Relief Model in the deep ocean (Amante and Eakins,

---

[1] https://imap.maryland.gov/Pages/lidar-dem-download-files.aspx

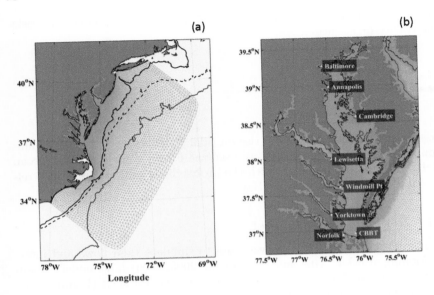

FIGURE 4.2: (a) FVCOM model grids (red). (b) Zoomed-in view of FVCOM grids over Chesapeake Bay and the surrounding coastal plains.

2009). Raw elevation and bathymetry data referenced to different vertical datum are converted to the same vertical coordinate system (NAVD88) using the V-Datum program (Lee et al, 2017, Yang et al, 2008). Wetting and drying of grid cells is implemented to simulate overland inundation. FVCOM uses a point treatment technique in which numerical grids consist of wet and dry points with a boundary defined as an interface line between the water and land, respectively (Chen et al, 2011). A grid is treated as a wet point when the water depth exceeds the threshold h_c (set to be 5 cm in our model).

4.2.2 Design of numerical experiments

To project the impact of sea level rise on high tide flooding in 2050 and 2100, we make use of the IPCC AR5. The IPCC AR5 projections are based on a set of greenhouse gas concentration scenarios called Representative Concentration Pathways that reflect the updated greenhouse gas emission reduction possibilities and climate change stabilization goals (Moss et al, 2010, Van Vuuren et al, 2011). Under RCP 2.6 (Paris Agreement), emissions begin to decline now and become net zero later in the century, thus offering a reasonably good probability of keeping the increase in global mean temperature to less than 2 °C above pre-industrial levels in line with the Paris Climate Agreement. Under RCP 4.5 (Stabilized Emissions), emissions stabilize around their current levels slowly and then begin to decline after 2050. Under RCP 8.5 (Growing Emissions),

Methods

emissions continue to grow until the end of the century. We selected RCP 4.5 and 8.5, representative of medium (delayed action) and high (growing) emission scenarios, respectively.

At the offshore boundary, the FVCOM model was forced with the projected increase in the mean sea level superimposed onto the astronomical tides. This is a simplified representation of the sea level rise, which changes coastlines gradually, but previous studies by Bilskie et al (2016) and Ross et al (2017) suggested that forcing these sea level rise projections at the offshore boundary of a regional ocean model produces essentially the same results as more elaborate modeling approaches in which land subsidence and sea level rise are accounted for through bathymetry changes. The sea level projections used at the offshore boundary are based on the averages over the entire Chesapeake Bay, as regional differences in the future sea level rise projections are much smaller than the projected changes themselves (Kopp et al, 2014, Figures 4.1c and 4.1d). About 25% of the Chesapeake Bay shoreline is hardened, but these structures mostly use shoreline stabilization techniques such as riprap and bulkheading and do not provide much protection against flooding (Palinkas et al, 2018, Patrick et al, 2014). These small engineered structures are not resolved in the FVCOM model.

For each RCP scenario (RCP 4.5 or RCP 8.5) and for both 2050 and 2100, we considered the median (50%), the likely range (17%–83%) and very likely range (5%–95%) of the relative sea level rise projections (Kopp et al, 2014). A total of 20 numerical experiments were conducted.

4.2.3 Inundation impact analysis

Google Map and Google Earth are used to visualize inundations over the land areas surrounding Chesapeake Bay, including Annapolis, Baltimore, and Dorchester County in Maryland. Water level data from FVCOM were imported and overlaid on Google Map and Google Earth. Google Earth allows users to add and view 3D buildings, thus enabling 3D views of inundations over buildings and structures. Inundation depths are obtained by subtracting the LIDAR digital elevation data from the water level in each grid cell. The result is a wet/dry profile of inundation. To improve the accuracy of the profile, a layer representing buildings is used as a mask if one is available for the local jurisdiction. The resulting grid is then converted into vector polygons and stored in the geodatabase. The polygons in the geodatabase can be converted into KML files.

The inundation analysis focused on three local regions. Dorchester County was chosen as a representative rural site (Figure 4.3a). It is the largest county in Maryland and has a total area of 983 square miles (2550 km^2), including land areas of 1400 km^2 and water areas of 1140 km^2. According to the census in 2010, the county had a population of 32,618 and a population density of 55 people per square mile. There were 14,681 housing units at an average density of 26 per square mile, with the average home value of $188,000. The City of

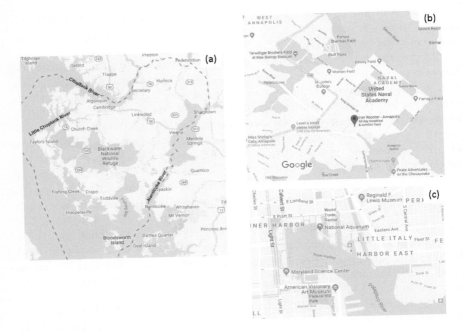

FIGURE 4.3: Maps of Dorchester County (a), downtown Annapolis (b), and Baltimore (c), Maryland.

Annapolis is the capital of the state of Maryland (Figure 4.3b). Its population was estimated to be 38,394 by the 2010 census. The population density was 5350 inhabitants per square mile. There were 17,850 housing units at an average density of 2485 per square mile. Annapolis is home to the US Naval Academy and many historical buildings such as the Maryland State House. The City of Baltimore was chosen as a representative urban site (Figure 4.3c). It is the largest city in Maryland, with a population of 2.81 million in the Baltimore metropolitan area. Baltimore is densely populated, with approximately 7671 people per square mile. Baltimore has about 50,800 firms where many of these firms and businesses are located on or near the waterfront. A majority of the properties in downtown Baltimore are commercial buildings.

4.3 Results

The probabilistic projections for high tidal flooding in 2050 and 2100 are presented for RCP 4.5 and 8.5. The Bay-wide response is presented first, followed by detailed analyses on Dorchester County, Annapolis, and Baltimore.

Results

4.3.1 Bay-wide response

Figure 4.4 shows the projected inundated areas at high tide over the entire region of Chesapeake Bay in 2050. The Eastern Shore of Maryland and Virginia as well as the Atlantic coast of Delmarva Peninsula are the two regions most vulnerable to inundation. However, the extent of the flooding depends on the climate change scenario and projected relative sea level rise within each scenario. The median projection corresponds to the 50% probability that high tide will flood the areas (the middle column). The projected flooded areas for the 17% and 83% probability represent the likely range where the actual water boundary will lie between the contours of the two projections. The flooded areas for the 5% and 95% probability represent the very likely range for the high tide flooding. For example, land areas outside the flooded areas marked in the rightmost column will have less than a 5% chance of getting flooded in 2050. On the other hand, there is less than a 5% chance that the flooded areas will be smaller than those marked in the leftmost column in 2050. When the flooded areas are summed up over the entire Chesapeake Bay region, there is a 50% probability that the total inundated areas exceed 1285 km^2 under RCP 4.5 and 1303 km^2 under RCP 8.5 (Figures 4.6a and 4.6b). The difference between the two climate change scenarios is modest at the mid-twenty-first century, as reflected in the small differences in the projected relative sea level rise between RCP 4.5 and 8.5 (Figures 4.1a and 4.1b). The likely range for the flooded areas, as defined by the 17% and 83% probability, lies between and 1,168/1,190 and 1,397/1,463 km^2 under RCP 4.5/8.5. The difference in the total inundated area between the upper and lower limit of the likely range

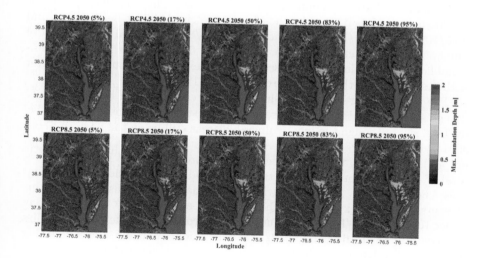

FIGURE 4.4: Probabilistic projections of inundated areas over Chesapeake Bay at 2050 under climate change scenarios RCP 4.5 and RCP 8.5.

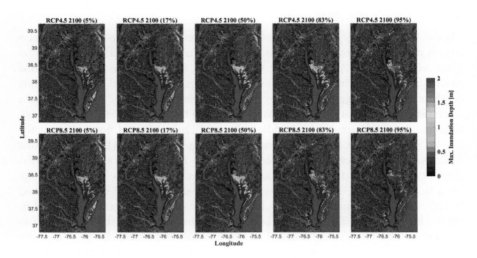

FIGURE 4.5: Probabilistic projections of inundated areas over Chesapeake Bay at 2100 under climate change scenarios RCP 4.5 and RCP 8.5.

is about 20%, even though the difference in the relative sea level rise reaches 100% (0.32 m versus 0.68 m). The inundation depends not only on the sea level rise but also on how land topography varies in low-lying areas, such that 100% increase in the relative sea level rise only translates to a 20% increase in the inundated areas around the Chesapeake Bay. The very likely range for the flooded areas, as defined by the 5% and 95% probability, lies between and 1085/1099 and 1540/1594 km^2 under RCP 4.5/8.5. The total surface area of Chesapeake Bay is currently estimated to be 11,600 km^2. Therefore, the additional flooded areas in 2050 represent 9%–14% expansion in the surface water of the estuary, with the median projection at 11%.

The inundated areas in 2100 show large spreads between the two climate change scenarios and among different probabilistic projections of the relative sea level rise, although the most vulnerable areas still lie on the Eastern Shore of Maryland and Virginia and the Atlantic Coast of Delmarva Peninsula (Figure 4.5). Under the median projection (50% probability) of RCP 4.5/8.5, a total of 1757/1912 km^2 are projected to be flooded by high tide in 2100 (Figures 4.6c and 4.6d). Compared with the median projections for 2050, this presents 37%/46% expansion of the inundated area around Chesapeake Bay under RCP 4.5/8.5. There is a much larger spread in the likely range: it lies between and 1489/1642 and 2012/2241 km^2 under RCP 4.5/8.5, amounting to 35%–36% difference in the total inundated area under each climate change scenario. Moreover, the total inundated area is 153–229 km^2 larger under RCP 8.5 than under RCP 4.5. The very likely range (5% to 95%) covers an

Results

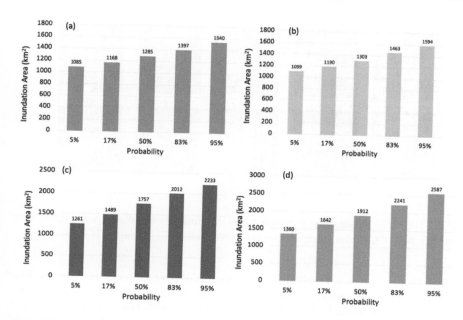

FIGURE 4.6: Total projected inundated areas over Chesapeake Bay at 2050 (a)/(b) and 2100 (c)/(d) under climate change scenarios RCP 4.5 and RCP 8.5.

even larger spread: ranging from 1261 to 2233 km² under RCP 4.5 and 1360 to 2587 km² under RCP 8.5.

4.3.2 Dorchester County

Figure 4.7 shows the inundated areas in Dorchester County at high tide in 2050. A large swath of land areas in southern Dorchester County will be flooded under most projections of the relative sea level rise. The inundated areas expand eastward and northward at higher water level projections. The median (50% probability) projection for the total inundated area in Dorchester County is nearly identical between RCP 4.5 and 8.5, at 581/589 km² (Figures 4.9a and 4.9b). This is equivalent to about 42% of the total land areas. In other words, over 40% of Dorchester County will be subjected to high tide flooding in 2050. The likely range of the flooded areas, as defined by the 17% and 83% probability, is between 540/547 and 619/632 km² under RCP 4.5/8.5. The very likely range of the flooded areas, as defined by the 5% and 95% probability, is between 508/513 to 654/671 km² under RCP 4.5/8.5. It is interesting to note the minor differences between RCP 4.5 and 8.5 and the narrow range of the projected areas as bracketed by different probabilistic

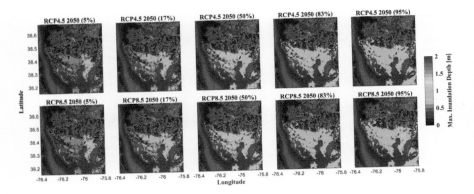

FIGURE 4.7: Probabilistic projections of inundated areas over Dorchester county at 2050 under climate change scenarios RCP 4.5 and RCP 8.5.

projections. This is a result of land topography over Dorchester County. The southern part of the county has low elevations but land elevation rises steeply further north and east. In contrast to the relative sensitivity of the inundated areas to climate change scenarios, the average inundation depth displays a wide range, reaching 0.45 m for the median projection and spanning 0.37 to 0.53 m for the likely range and 0.32 to 0.60 m for the very likely range (Figures 4.10a and 4.10b). Once again, the differences between RCP 4.5 and 8.5 are small at 2050.

By 2100, the flooded areas expand towards higher grounds in the northward direction (Figure 4.8). In particular, the northwest corner of Dorchester County, including the town of Cambridge, will be exposed to extensive tidal flooding. More flooding is projected under the higher end projections of the relative sea level rise, especially the 83% and 95% probabilistic projections. Moreover, there are significantly more flooded areas under RCP 8.5 than RCP 4.5. The median (50% probability) projection for the total inundated area in Dorchester County is 711/746 km^2 under RCP 4.5/8.5 (Figures 4.9c and 4.9d). This is 23%–27% larger than the corresponding projections in 2050. The likely range of the flooded areas is between 637/682 and 761/806 km^2 under RCP 4.5/8.5. The very likely range of the flooded areas is between 573/607 to 804/843 km^2 under RCP 4.5/8.5. Unlike 2050, there are significant differences in the total inundated areas between RCP 4.5 and 8.5. This reflects a wider range in the projected relative sea level rise rates in 2100 (Figures 4.1a and 4.1b), as well as the fact that higher water levels are now reaching new areas in the northwest corner of Dorchester County. There is 5% probability that over 60% of Dorchester County will be lost to tidal flooding and sea level rise in 2100 under the RCP 8.5 (business as usual) climate change scenario, with huge implications for the coastal communities.

Results

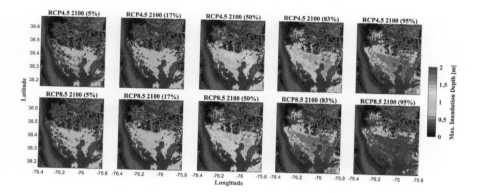

FIGURE 4.8: Probabilistic projections of inundated areas over Dorchester county at 2100 under climate change scenarios RCP 4.5 and RCP 8.5.

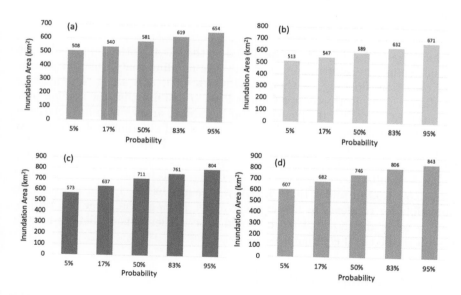

FIGURE 4.9: Total projected inundated areas over Dorchester County at 2050 (a)/(b) and 2100 (c)/(d) under climate change scenarios RCP 4.5 and RCP 8.5.

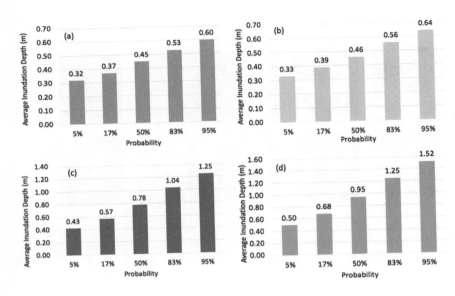

FIGURE 4.10: Probabilistic projections for average inundation depth over Dorchester County at 2050 (a)/(b) and 2100 (c)/(d) under climate change scenarios RCP 4.5 and RCP 8.5.

Such dire projections are compounded by the fact that the inundated areas will not simply be subject to minor nuisance flooding that is usually associated with tidal flooding, as shown in Figures 4.10c and 4.10d. The average inundation depth in Dorchester County is 0.78/0.95 m under the median projection of RCP 4.5/8.5. Unlike the total inundated areas which are relatively insensitive to different climate change scenarios and different probabilistic sea level rise projections, the average inundation depth spans a wide range. Its likely range spans 0.57–1.04 m and very likely range spans 0.43–1.25 m under RCP 4.5. Similarly, its likely ranges span 0.68–1.25 m and very likely range spans 0.50–1.52 m under RCP 8.5. At water depths 0.8–1.5 m, it would be impossible for residents to live in those areas. Even at the lower end projections, a water depth of 0.4–0.5 m would pose tremendous challenges for the livelihood of coastal communities.

4.3.3 Annapolis and Baltimore

Unlike the flat coastal plains on the eastern shore, the City of Annapolis has relatively steep topographic changes. Most of the tidal flooding areas are limited to the downtown waterfront areas and US Naval Academy (Figures 4.11 and 4.3b). At the upper end (83% and 95% probability) projections for 2100 under either RCP 4.5 or RCP 8.5, a large part of those areas

Results

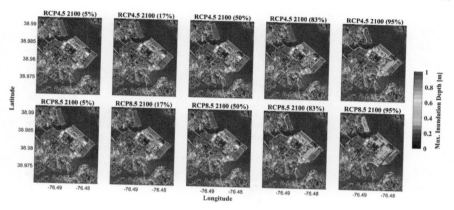

FIGURE 4.11: Probabilistic projections of inundated areas over City of Annapolis at 2100 under climate change scenarios RCP 4.5 and RCP 8.5.

will be under water. Many low-lying coastlines along the two creeks off the Sevens River will also subject to tidal flooding. In comparison, little areas will be flooded at high tide at the lower-end projections of the relative sea level rise. Only the downtown dock and a small part of the Naval Academy will be flooded in 2100 under the median projection of RCP 4.5 and 8.5. In terms of the total inundated areas for Annapolis, it only adds up to about 9000 m^2 in the median RCP 4.5 projection for 2050 and ranges from 5500 to 15,300 m^2 for the likely range (Figure 4.12a). The total flooded areas are only marginally higher under RCP 8.5 (Figure 4.12b). However, the average water depth in the flooded areas is about 0.45 m in all scenarios (Figures 4.13a and 4.13b), thus posing serious challenges for access and usage. Overall, these are relatively small flooding damages. In 2100, the total inundated area expands by 10–30 times (Figures 4.12c and 4.12d). The median projection reaches 90,000/16,500 m^2 under RCP4.5/8.5. There are wide spreads in the probabilistic projections for the inundated areas: the likely range spans from 19,600/42,500 to 256,000/506,500 m^2 under RCP 4.5/8.5. On the other hand, the average inundated depth for all scenarios falls into a narrow range of 0.44 to 0.51 m, with the exception of 0.70 m under the high-end projection (95%) of RCP 8.5 (Figures 4.13c and 4.13d). This offers an interesting contrast with the rural eastern shore where the inundated areas do not change much among the climate change scenarios, but the inundation depths are highly sensitive.

Tidal flooding in downtown Baltimore in 2100 is limited to the Inner Harbor, which is connected to Patapsco River, a tributary of Chesapeake Bay (Figure 4.3c). Hundreds of businesses are found in the downtown financial district, including skyscrapers like the Bank of America building and the Baltimore World Trade Center. Both Charles Street and Pratt Street are signifi-

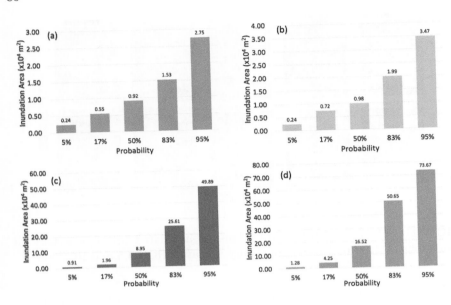

FIGURE 4.12: Total projected inundated areas over City of Annapolis at 2050 (a)/(b) and 2100 (c)/(d) under climate change scenarios RCP 4.5 and RCP 8.5.

cant avenues of commercial and cultural activity. To the northeast of the Inner Harbor lies in Fells Point and Little Italy featuring residential buildings and restaurants, with many low-lying areas. Figure 4.14 shows that a significant part of the downtown Inner Harbor and Little Italy districts will be flooded at high tide in 2100 under the higher end (the 83% and 95%) projections of RCP 4.5 and 8.5. No significant flooding is projected beyond the immediate boundary of the Inner Harbor under other scenarios.

4.4 Conclusions

Using the climate model projections to drive a regional ocean model, we have investigated how sea level rise affects high-tide flooding and coastal inundation in Chesapeake Bay. In 2050, there is a 50% probability that the total inundated areas will exceed ~1300 km², equivalent to 11% of the current surface area of Chesapeake Bay. The likely range for the flooded areas, as defined by the 17% and 83% probability, lies between ~1180 and 1420 km². In 2100, the projected inundated areas depend critically on the climate change scenario. Under the

Conclusions

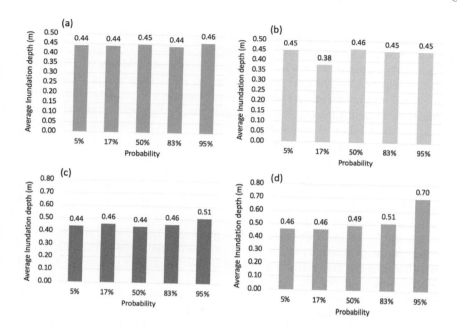

FIGURE 4.13: Probabilistic projections for average inundation depth over City of Annapolis at 2050 (a)/(b) and 2100 (c)/(d) under climate change scenarios RCP 4.5 and RCP 8.5.

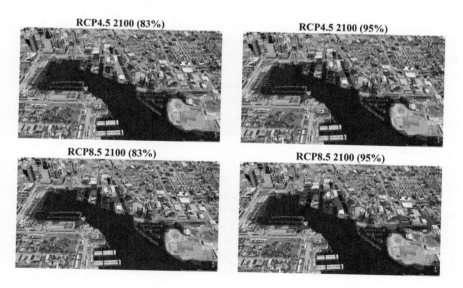

FIGURE 4.14: Projections of inundated areas over City of Baltimore at 2100 due to sea level rise under climate change scenarios RCP 4.5 and RCP 8.5.

median projection (50% probability) of RCP 4.5/8.5, a total of 1757/1912 km^2 are projected to be flooded. The likely range lies between and 1489/1642 and 2012/2241 km^2 under RCP 4.5/8.5, amounting to 35%–36% difference in the total inundated area under each climate change scenario. Moreover, the total inundated area is 153–229 km^2 larger under RCP 8.5 than under RCP 4.5.

The rural and urban areas show different responses to climate change, due to differences in land topography. Over the rural Dorchester County, the inundated areas show minor differences between different climate change scenarios and only moderate gains in 2100 than in 2050. However, the average inundation depth is ~70%–100% higher in 2100 than in 2050. In comparison, the inundated areas in the City of Annapolis is projected to expand 10–30 times from 2050 to 2100: the median projection increases from 9800 m^2 in 2050 to 165,000 m^2 under RCP 8.5. On the other hand, the average inundated depth for all scenarios falls into a narrow range of 0.44 to 0.51 m, with the exception of 0.70 m under the high-end projection (95%) of RCP 8.5. In downtown Baltimore, no extensive tidal flooding is projected beyond the immediate neighborhood of the Inner Harbor except under the higher end projections of the relative sea level rise for 2100.

Although a number of inundation maps are available, none of them have adequately addressed the effects of climate change on coastal flooding. Projections of sea level rise onto low-lying land areas are mostly based on static images (e.g., bathtub approach) and do not consider dynamical processes of tides in rising seas. This study applies the latest research findings on sea level rise and develops dynamics-based inundation graphics that may better prepare coastal communities for the rising inundation risks in the twenty-first century. The State of Maryland has taken the threats of sea level rise seriously. In 2018, the Maryland General Assembly passed HB 1350/ SB 1006—Sea Level Rise Inundation and Coastal Flooding—Construction, Adaptation, and Mitigation, which was signed into law by the governor. Maryland expanded its "Coast Smart" siting and design criteria in order to better manage sea level rise and improve coastal adaptation efforts. The legislation also requires the state to establish a plan to adapt to saltwater intrusion, and to build criteria for hazard mitigation funding for sea level rise and coastal flooding. Coastal inundation projections described in this chapter may be useful to the state and local agencies tasked to execute the latest legislation on coastal flooding in Maryland.

Although this study focused on Chesapeake Bay and the State of Maryland, the same approach could be used to make probabilistic projections of overland inundation in other coastal regions. Kopp et al (2014) provided probabilistic sea level rise projections at locations around the world, and their projections could be used to drive models of other estuaries and coastal regions. Future model working could also consider a scenario of accelerating sea level rise in the late twenty-first century that might be caused by rapid melt of the Antarctic ice (DeConto and Pollard, 2016, Kopp et al, 2017).

Future inundation studies will also need to consider the impact of climate change on storm surge flooding. Knutson et al (2013) conducted dynamic downscaling projections of the twenty-first-century Atlantic hurricane activity and found a significant increase in the frequency of intense storms. The combination of stronger storms and sea level rise will likely result in higher water levels and more extensive inundation in the future climate. Lin et al (2016) found that Hurricane-Sandy levels of flooding are becoming significantly more frequent in New York City compared to the scenario with sea level rise alone. Similarly, Zhang and Li (2019) found that a Category 2 storm like Hurricane Isabel (2013) will generate much higher sea levels in 2050 and 2100 due to the combined effect of sea level rise and warming ocean. To make a probabilistic prediction of storm-induced flooding, one would need to combine probabilistic sea level rise projections with model simulations of storms of different intensity, track, and size.

References

Amante C, Eakins BW (2009) ETOPO1 Global Relief Model converted to PanMap layer format. Boulder, CO

Bilskie MV, Hagen SC, Alizad K, Medeiros SC, Passeri DL, Needham HF, Cox A (2016) Dynamic simulation and numerical analysis of hurricane storm surge under sea level rise with geomorphologic changes along the northern Gulf of Mexico. Earth's Future 4(5):177–193

Boesch DF, Boicourt WC, Cullather RI, Ezer T, Galloway Jr GE, Johnson ZP, Kilbourne KH, Kirwan ML, Kopp RE, Land S, Li M, Nardin W, Sommerfield CK, Sweet WV (2018) Sea-level rise: projections for Maryland 2018. University of Maryland Center for Environmental Science, Cambridge, MD

Chen C, Liu H, Beardsley RC (2003) An unstructured grid, finite-volume, three-dimensional, primitive equations ocean model: application to coastal ocean and estuaries. Journal of Atmospheric and Oceanic Technology 20(1):159–186

Chen C, Beardsley RC, Cowles G (2006) An unstructured-grid, finite-volume coastal ocean model (FVCOM) system. Oceanography 19:78–89

Chen C, Beardsley RC, Cowles G, Qi J, Lai Z, Gao G, Stuebe D, Xu Q, Xue P, Ge J, Ji R, Hu S, Tian R, Huang H, Wu L, Lin H (2011) An unstructured-grid, finite-volume community ocean model FVCOM user manual, 3rd edn. SMAST/UMASSD, New Bedford, MA, USA

Church JA, Clark PU (2013) Climate change 2013: The physical science basis. In: Stocker TF, Qin D, Plattner GK, Tignor M, Allen SK, Boschung J, Nauels A, Xia Y, Bex V, Midgley PM (eds) Contribution of Working Group I to the Fifth Assessment Report of the Intergovernmental Panel on Climate Change, Cambridge University Press, Cambridge, UK, 1137–1216

Church JA, White NJ (2011) Sea-level rise from the late 19th to the early 21st century. Surveys in Geophysics 32(4–5):585–602

Dalton MM, Dello KD, Hawkins L, Mote PW, Rupp DE (2017) The third Oregon climate assessment report. Oregon Climate Change Research Institute, College of Earth, Ocean and Atmospheric Sciences, Oregon State University, Corvallis, OR

Dangendorf S, Marcos M, Wöppelmann G, Conrad CP, Frederikse T, Riva R (2017) Reassessment of 20th century global mean sea level rise. Proceedings of the National Academy of Sciences 114(23):5946–5951

DeConto RM, Pollard D (2016) Contribution of Antarctica to past and future sea-level rise. Nature 531(7596):591–597

Domingues R, Goni G, Baringer M, Volkov D (2018) What caused the accelerated sea level changes along the US East Coast during 2010–2015? Geophysical Research Letters 45(24):13–367

Egbert GD, Erofeeva SY (2002) Efficient inverse modeling of barotropic ocean tides. Journal of Atmospheric and Oceanic Technology 19(2):183–204

Ezer T, Atkinson LP, Corlett WB, Blanco JL (2013) Gulf Stream's induced sea level rise and variability along the US mid-Atlantic coast. Journal of Geophysical Research: Oceans 118(2):685–697

Flick RE, Murray JF, Ewing LC (2003) Trends in United States tidal datum statistics and tide range. Journal of Waterway, Port, Coastal, and Ocean Engineering 129(4):155–164

Garrett C (1972) Tidal resonance in the Bay of Fundy and Gulf of Maine. Nature 238(5365):441–443

Gesch DB (2009) Analysis of Lidar elevation data for improved identification and delineation of lands vulnerable to sea-level rise. Journal of Coastal Research 2009(10053):49–58

Ghanbari M, Arabi M, Obeysekera J, Sweet W (2019) A coherent statistical model for coastal flood frequency analysis under nonstationary sea level conditions. Earth's Future 7(2):162–177

Greenberg DA, Blanchard W, Smith B, Barrow E (2012) Climate change, mean sea level and high tides in the Bay of Fundy. Atmosphere–Ocean 50(3):261–276

Griggs G, Árvai J, Cayan D, DeConto R, Fox J, Fricker HA, Kopp RE, Tebaldi C, Whiteman EA (2017) Rising seas in California: an update on sea-level rise science. California Ocean Science Trust, Oakland, CA, USA

Hall GF, Hill DF, Horton BP, Engelhart SE, Peltier WR (2013) A high-resolution study of tides in the Delaware Bay: past conditions and future scenarios. Geophysical Research Letters 40(2):338–342

Hay CC, Morrow E, Kopp RE, Mitrovica JX (2015) Probabilistic reanalysis of twentieth-century sea-level rise. Nature 517(7535):481–484

Hinkel J, Lincke D, Vafeidis AT, Perrette M, Nicholls RJ, Tol RS, Marzeion B, Fettweis X, Ionescu C, Levermann A (2014) Coastal flood damage and adaptation costs under 21st century sea-level rise. Proceedings of the National Academy of Sciences 111(9):3292–3297

References

Holleman RC, Stacey MT (2014) Coupling of sea level rise, tidal amplification, and inundation. Journal of Physical Oceanography 44(5):1439–1455

Knutson TR, Sirutis JJ, Vecchi GA, Garner S, Zhao M, Kim HS, Bender M, Tuleya RE, Held IM, Villarini G (2013) Dynamical downscaling projections of twenty-first-century Atlantic hurricane activity: CMIP3 and CMIP5 model-based scenarios. Journal of Climate 26(17):6591–6617

Kopp RE (2013) Does the mid-Atlantic United States sea level acceleration hot spot reflect ocean dynamic variability? Geophysical Research Letters 40(15):3981–3985

Kopp RE, Horton RM, Little CM, Mitrovica JX, Oppenheimer M, Rasmussen D, Strauss BH, Tebaldi C (2014) Probabilistic 21st and 22nd century sea-level projections at a global network of tide-gauge sites. Earth's future 2(8):383–406

Kopp RE, DeConto RM, Bader DA, Horton RM, Hay CC, Kulp S, Oppenheimer M, Pllard D, Strauss BH (2017) Implications of Antarctic ice-cliff collapse and ice-shelf hydrofracturing mechanisms for sea-level projections. Earth's Future 5(12):1217–1233

Kulp S, Strauss BH (2017) Rapid escalation of coastal flood exposure in US municipalities from sea level rise. Climatic Change 142(3-4):477–489

Kulp SA, Strauss BH (2019) New elevation data triple estimates of global vulnerability to sea-level rise and coastal flooding. Nature Communications 10(1):1–12

Lee SB, Li M, Zhang F (2017) Impact of sea level rise on tidal range in Chesapeake and Delaware Bays. Journal of Geophysical Research: Oceans 122(5):3917–3938

Lin N, Kopp RE, Horton BP, Donnelly JP (2016) Hurricane Sandy's flood frequency increasing from year 1800 to 2100. Proceedings of the National Academy of Sciences 113(43):12071–12075

Miller KG, Kopp RE, Horton BP, Browning JV, Kemp AC (2013) A geological perspective on sea-level rise and its impacts along the US mid-Atlantic coast. Earth's Future 1(1):3–18

Mitchell M, Herschner CH, Herman JD, Schatt DE, Eggington E, Stiles S (2013) Recurrent flooding study for Tidewater Virginia. The Virginia Institute of Marine Science, Center for Coastal Resources Management, Old Dominion University, the Hampton Roads Planning District Commission, the City of Norfolk, the Accomack-Northampton Planning District Commission and Wetlands Watch, Richmond, VA

Moftakhari HR, AghaKouchak A, Sanders BF, Feldman DL, Sweet W, Matthew RA, Luke A (2015) Increased nuisance flooding along the coasts of the united states due to sea level rise: past and future. Geophysical Research Letters 42(22):9846–9852

Moss RH, Edmonds JA, Hibbard KA, Manning MR, Rose SK, Van Vuuren DP, Carter TR, Emori S, Kainuma M, Kram T, Meehl GA, Mitchell JFB, Nakicenovic N, Riahi K, Smith SJ, Stouffer RJ, Thomson AM, Weyant JP,

Wilbanks TJ (2010) The next generation of scenarios for climate change research and assessment. Nature 463(7282):747–756

Müller M, Arbic BK, Mitrovica JX (2011) Secular trends in ocean tides: observations and model results. Journal of Geophysical Research: Oceans 116:C05013

Palinkas CM, Sanford LP, Koch EW (2018) Influence of shoreline stabilization structures on the nearshore sedimentary environment in mesohaline Chesapeake Bay. Estuaries and Coasts 41(4):952–965

Patrick CJ, Weller DE, Li X, Ryder M (2014) Effects of shoreline alteration and other stressors on submerged aquatic vegetation in subestuaries of Chesapeake Bay and the mid-Atlantic coastal bays. Estuaries and Coasts 37(6):1516–1531

Ross AC, Najjar RG, Li M, Lee SB, Zhang F, Liu W (2017) Fingerprints of sea level rise on changing tides in the Chesapeake and Delaware Bays. Journal of Geophysical Research: Oceans 122(10):8102–8125

Sallenger AH, Doran KS, Howd PA (2012) Hotspot of accelerated sea-level rise on the Atlantic coast of North America. Nature Climate Change 2(12):884–888

Spanger-Siegfried E, Fitzpatrick M, Dahl K (2014) Encroaching tides: How sea level rise and tidal flooding threaten US East and Gulf Coast communities over the next 30 years. Union of Concerned Scientists, Cambridge, MA

Sweet WV, Park J (2014) From the extreme to the mean: Acceleration and tipping points of coastal inundation from sea level rise. Earth's Future 2(12):579–600

Van Vuuren DP, Edmonds J, Kainuma M, Riahi K, Thomson A, Hibbard K, Hurtt GC, Kram T, Krey V, Lamarque JF, Masui T, Meinshausen M, Nakicenovic N, Smith SJ, Rose SK (2011) The representative concentration pathways: an overview. Climatic Change 109(1–2):5

Yang Z, Myers EP, Wong AM, White SA (2008) VDatum for Chesapeake Bay, Delaware Bay, and adjacent coastal water areas tidal datums, and sea surface topography. Tech. Rep. NOS CS 15, NOAA, Silver Spring, MD

Zervas CE (2001) Sea level variations of the United States 1854–1999. Tech. Rep. NOS CO-OPS 36, NOAA, Silver Spring, MD, USA

Zervas CE (2009) Sea level variations of the United States, 1854-2006. Tech. Rep. NOS CO-OPS 53, NOAA, Silver Spring, MD, USA

Zhang F, Li M (2019) Impacts of ocean warming, sea level rise, and coastline management on storm surge in a semienclosed bay. Journal of Geophysical Research: Oceans 124(9):6498–6514

Zhong L, Li M, Foreman M (2008) Resonance and sea level variability in Chesapeake Bay. Continental Shelf Research 28(18):2565–2573

5

Response of Benthic Biodiversity to Climate-Sensitive Regional and Local Conditions in a Complex Estuarine System

Ryan J. Woodland and Jeremy M. Testa
Chesapeake Biological Laboratory, University of Maryland Center for Environmental Science, Solomons, MD, USA

CONTENTS

5.1	Introduction	87
5.2	Methods	89
	5.2.1 Data sources	89
	5.2.2 Biodiversity-climate modeling	92
5.3	Results	96
	5.3.1 Benthic biodiversity patterns	96
	5.3.2 Biodiversity-climate modeling results	98
	5.3.3 Multivariate assemblage analysis	103
5.4	Discussion	104
	5.4.1 Long-term trends in Chesapeake Bay benthic biodiversity	106
	5.4.2 Climate drivers of benthic biodiversity	108
	5.4.3 Regional climate outlook for Chesapeake Bay	111
	5.4.4 Global outlook for estuarine communities in the face of climate forcing	113
5.5	Conclusions	115
References		115

5.1 Introduction

Coastal ecosystems are particularly vulnerable to climate change due to their exposure and sensitivity to multiple external stressors including sea level rise, altered seasonal temperature and precipitation patterns, and increased storm frequency and severity (Najjar et al, 2000, Scavia et al, 2002). Future projections of climate include monotonic increases in the magnitude of many of these external stressors (e.g., temperature, sea level), and elevated variability for others. The effects of these stressors are exacerbated by anthropogenic activities in coastal areas and upstream watersheds, often interacting to degrade the physical, environmental, and biological conditions available to aquatic flora and fauna through eutrophication, elevated "flashiness" in freshwater discharge, and land-use changes. For example, coastal areas are particularly vulnerable to hypoxia due to their proximity to major urban centers, receipt of high nutrient loads from rivers, limited water exchange, and propensity toward water column stratification. Coastal hypoxia is a particularly compelling problem because its influence permeates biogeochemical nutrient cycling, habitat availability, consumer community dynamics, food-web interactions, and the growth, reproduction, and survival of metazoan life. The vulnerability of bottom waters to degradation caused by oxygen depletion is important because bottom-associated (benthic) habitats and the communities of organisms that live in benthic habitats are directly involved in facilitating many of those key ecological roles in coastal ecosystems (Ihde et al, 2015, Levin et al, 2009, Rosenberg, 2001).

Biodiversity is often considered an important metric of the health of biotic communities because the diversity of naturally occurring species in a given habitat typically declines as the habitat becomes degraded. As species are lost, the species-specific suite of traits (e.g., foraging mode, burrowing activity, productivity) that facilitate those species' ecological functions are lost from the community. Eventually, these losses in species diversity can compromise the total range of traits available to the community to fulfill ecological functions (i.e., functional diversity, Tilman, 2001). In addition to species losses, increased abundance or biomass of ruderal (tolerant) species or invasion by non-native species can influence biodiversity values and alter community dynamics and ecological functions (Airoldi et al, 2008). Communities with high species-level biodiversity typically have higher functional diversity, although some communities can maintain relatively high functional diversity in the face of species losses (e.g., Gallagher et al, 2013, Törnroos et al, 2015), and some studies have highlighted the dominant role of individual species on certain ecological functions (e.g., Norling et al, 2007).

Multidecade time series for ecological conditions in coastal waters have been emerging recently and provide the opportunity to understand long-term changes in biological communities in relation to chemical and physical alterations. For example, declines in wastewater inputs of nutrients to Boston Harbor and Tampa Bay over the past three decades have clearly shown reductions in sediment oxygen uptake and nutrient release, the recovery of autotrophic benthic communities, or a response of benthic communities (Greening and Janicki, 2006, Taylor et al, 2011, Tucker et al, 2014). In areas less impacted by large external changes, variability in long-term benthic communities may not follow a discernible temporal trajectory (Tsikopoulou et al, 2019). In estuarine environments where multiple biophysical factors are influential at any given

Methods

time or location, benthic community change is often responsive to multiple, often dynamical factors (Zettler et al, 2017). In Chesapeake Bay, multi-decade, spatially resolved time series of benthic invertebrate abundance, biomass, and diversity have revealed key insights into changes in benthic communities in response to ambient conditions, but the interactions between climatic variability and water-column conditions in driving long-term change in benthic diversity have yet to be achieved.

In this study, we analyzed the response of the Chesapeake Bay benthic community to a suite of climate-relevant factors. The robust, long-term physical, environmental, and biological monitoring programs established in Chesapeake Bay make this ecosystem uniquely suitable for analysis of climate effects. We have purposefully selected a flexible, nonlinear modeling framework to best capture the complex relationships that exist between benthic communities, climate variables, and site-level covariates that are known to structure spatial and temporal patterns in those communities. While our analysis focuses on Chesapeake Bay, the processes and relationships present within this estuary are likely to be similar to other coastal ecosystems.

5.2 Methods

5.2.1 Data sources

The Chesapeake Bay Program's long-term Benthic Monitoring Program conducts an annual survey at fixed and random locations throughout Chesapeake Bay. The random component of the survey was implemented in 1994, but the current random sampling scheme was implemented in 1995 in Maryland waters and in 1996 in Virginia waters of Chesapeake Bay. Each year, 25 station locations are randomly selected within each of 10 spatial strata throughout the Bay. Areas deeper than 12 m in the mesohaline middle reach of the mainstem are often azoic due to the persistence of hypoxia or anoxia and are not sampled (Figure 5.1). Stations are visited once during the mid-summer months of July–September, although sampling logistics occasionally result in sampling occurring during late June or early October. For this analysis, we analyzed survey data from $n = 9$ of those strata (Figure 5.1). We excluded one surveyed stratum because the highly urbanized watersheds of several estuaries within that stratum could potentially confound our analysis of climate variables on benthic conditions.

At each station, a single bottom sample of the benthic community is collected using a Young benthic grab (440 cm^2 sampling area). The sediment from the benthic grab is sieved through a 500-μm mesh, and the retained organisms and material are stored in a preservative (formalin) with a vial stain (Rose Bengal) to aid in laboratory identification. A second deployment

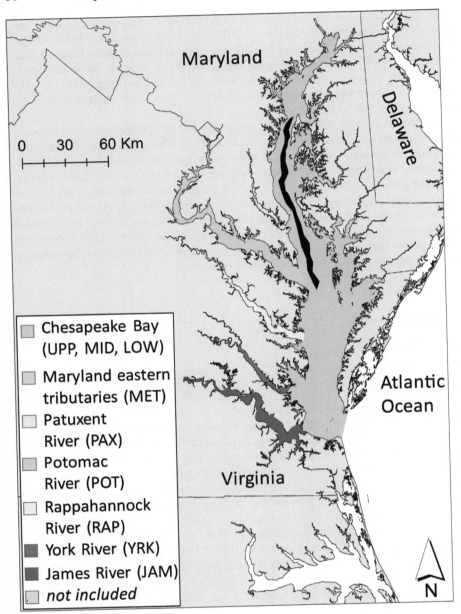

FIGURE 5.1: Map of Chesapeake Bay showing the three mainstem regions and six tributary regions included in this study (black region in the MID Chesapeake Bay mainstem region is not sampled by the Chesapeake Bay Program's Benthic Monitoring Survey due to azoic conditions arising from prevalent deep water hypoxia and anoxia).

Methods

of the grab is used to collect a sample of surficial bottom sediment for analysis of sediment grain size, total carbon (TC), and total nitrogen (TN) content. Additional data collected at each station include geolocation (latitude and longitude, decimal degrees), total water depth (m), and water-column biological, environmental, and biogeochemical variables. These additional data sampling programs include measurements collected just below the water surface and just above the sediment surface in bottom waters (and also at several intermediate depths depending on the variable). We extracted a subset of these variables from the available data set that have been shown in previous studies to be relevant to benthic community dynamics, including those measured with a multiparameter sonde (e.g., YSI 6600 or EXO) including dissolved oxygen concentration (DO, mg/l), salinity (ppt), and temperature (°C), as well as filtered water samples later measured for chlorophyll-a concentration (chl-a, μg/l) in the laboratory using standard methods. Dissolved oxygen saturation was not used because this measurement was not available for many stations.

In the laboratory, benthic community samples are sorted to the lowest possible taxon (typically species-level for most taxa) and enumerated. The sorted taxa are then dried and combusted to obtain ash-free dry-weight biomass (AFDW, g). Sediment nutrient content is analyzed with an elemental analyzer and presented as the percent TC or TN of sediment dry weight. Sediment grain size is determined by wet sieving, drying, and weighing samples. We use percentage of sandy sediment, the fraction of the dry weight of the sediment retained by a 63-μm sieve, as an indicator of bottom sediment conditions.

Regional climate-associated data were obtained from online data repositories. Mean monthly discharge data (ft^3 s^{-1}) for the major tributary in each stratum were downloaded from the United States Geological Survey monitoring station data hub (https://waterdata.usgs.gov/nwis). Discharge for two rivers, the Mattaponi and Pamunkey, were downloaded to represent the combined freshwater input to the York River stratum. These discharge data were used to calculate two stratum-specific flow indices (see below). Water column DO and chl-a concentration data are collected monthly at fixed monitoring stations and were obtained from the Chesapeake Bay Program's mainstem and tidal tributary Water Quality Monitoring survey (1995–2017; https://chesapeakebay.net/data). Surface and bottom measurements of DO and chl-a were averaged for each station to yield an integrated water column mean, then station means were averaged to yield stratum-level estimates of monthly conditions. These monthly values were used to calculate seasonal DO and chl-a indices for each stratum. In the case of the Maryland eastern tributaries (MET) stratum, discharge, DO, and chl-a indices were all derived from Choptank River data, given its central location, relatively large size, and robust monitoring history.

Two degree day (DD) indices were calculated from daily water temperature data to serve as thermal climate indicators on a Chesapeake Bay–wide scale. Daily water temperature data were obtained from four centralized monitoring stations, including three stations near the mouth of the York River (i.e.,

YKTV2 [National Oceanographic and Atmospheric Administration/National Ocean Service, NOAA/NOS], Virginia Institute of Marine Science Ferry Pier, CBVGI [Goodwin Islands National Estuarine Research Reserve System]), and one station near the mouth of the Patuxent River (SLIM2 [NOAA/NOS]). The York River water temperature data sets were integrated into a single water temperature record by using linear regressions derived from paired monthly mean water temperatures to adjust between-station differences in daily temperatures:

$$WTemp_{\text{CBVGI}} = 1.0212 \times WTemp_{\text{VIMS-Ferry}} + 0.6173, \ n = 72, \ R^2 = 0.98;$$

$$WTemp_{\text{CBVGI}} = 0.9745 \times WTemp_{\text{YKTV2}} + 0.9758, \ n = 36, \ R^2 = 0.99.$$

Water and air temperatures are highly correlated in Chesapeake Bay (Ding and Elmore 2015), and an analysis of paired monthly mean water and air temperatures at the SLIM2 station supported this relationship in a third-order polynomial regression

$$WTemp_{\text{SLIM2}} = -0.0008 \times AirTemp_{\text{SLIM2}}^3 + 0.037 \times AirTemp_{\text{SLIM2}}^2$$
$$+ 0.5105 \times AirTemp_{\text{SLIM2}} + 2.0561; \ n = 529, \ R^2 = 0.96.$$

Therefore, gaps in daily water temperatures at SLIM2 were reconstructed using air temperature records from SLIM2 or from a proximal weather station at Royal Oak, MD

$$WTemp_{\text{SLIM2}} = -0.0008 \times AirTemp_{\text{RoyalOak}}^3 + 0.0401 \times AirTemp_{\text{RoyalOak}}^2$$
$$+ 0.4846 \times AirTemp_{\text{RoyalOak}} + 2.681; \ n = 748, \ R^2 = 0.95.$$

Gaps in the integrated York River daily water temperature data set were reconstructed using water temperature records from SLIM2

$$WTemp_{\text{YRK}} = 1.0314 \times WTemp_{\text{SLIM2}} - 1.1047; \ n = 126, \ R^2 = 0.98.$$

Finally, these two reconstructed daily water temperature time series were averaged to yield a single time series of mean daily water temperature from 1950–2017 that is assumed to be broadly representative of the Chesapeake Bay region.

5.2.2 Biodiversity-climate modeling

Semi-parametric generalized additive models (GAMs) were used to model the response of three different metrics of benthic biodiversity to a suite of predictor variables. Generalized additive models fit flexible, non-parametric smoothing functions (splines) to model the relationship between the predictor variables and the response variable (Hastie and Tibshirani, 1990). Semi-parametric GAMs include parametric model terms for class or continuous (linear) predictor variables in addition to spline terms. These models can accommodate error

Methods

distributions from the exponential family and a range of link functions (Quinn and Keough, 2003).

The three biodiversity response metrics we considered were total species richness, and two biodiversity indices (Shannon–Wiener index, Simpson's Index of Diversity). Species richness (S) is the total number of unique species encountered per site. The Shannon–Wiener index (H') is calculated as:

$$H' = \sum_{i=1}^{S} p_i \ln p_i,$$

where p_i is the proportional abundance of species i in a given sample (Pielou, 1974). Simpson's Index of Diversity (D) is calculated as $D = 1 - \sum_i p_i^2$, where p and i are defined as for H' (Pielou, 1974). As formulated, each of these indices will increase as the number of species encountered increases and, in the case of H' and D, as the relative abundances of species in a sample become more even. Readers are referred to any basic ecology text for additional information on these and other biodiversity indices (e.g., Begon et al, 2006, Pielou, 1974).

Site-specific predictor variables were included as covariates in the models to account for known or suspected local-scale factors that could influence observed biodiversity values. These included depth, percentage of sandy sediment (*sand*), water column averages of DO, and salinity at the time of sampling. The latitude and longitude of each site were included in the model to account for spatial patterns in benthic biodiversity not captured by the other site-specific predictors. These site-level predictors were included in a "null" model formulation, to compare the performance of these site-focused models with the alternative model formulations that included a range of indicators representative of climate phenomena acting at broader spatiotemporal scales. We also tested several potential error distributions (Gaussian, Poisson, negative binomial, and gamma) and link functions (identity, log, and reciprocal) for each null model. Initial testing of the optimal parameterization of the null models was conducted using Akaike's Information Criterion corrected for small sample size (AIC_C). Values of AIC_C decline as model prediction error declines but increase as the number of model parameters increase. Therefore, AIC_C provides a relative indicator of the most parsimonious model formulation given the available data and a defined suite of potential models (Burnham and Anderson, 2002). We used AIC_C rather than AIC because AIC_C is more conservative and converges with AIC at large sample sizes (Burnham et al, 2011). Based on our initial model selection testing, null model formulations for S, H', and D were as follows (Table 5.1):

$$\begin{aligned} g(S) = {} & \beta_0 + \beta_1 sand + s_1(DO) + s_2(latitude \times longitude) \\ & + s_3(depth \times salinity) + \epsilon, \end{aligned}$$

TABLE 5.1: Slopes and standard errors (in parentheses) from linear regression of annual biodiversity index estimates against year for deep (> 4 m depth) and shallow (< 4 m depth) zones in each spatial region. Italicized slope and errors correspond to *p*-values of 0.05–0.10; bold slopes and errors correspond to *p*-values < 0.05

Region		S	H'	D
		> 4 m depth		
Mainstem	UPP	−0.10 (0.06)	−0.008 (0.006)	−0.001 (0.002)
	MID	−0.01 (0.08)	−0.002 (0.009)	0.001 (0.002)
	LOW	*0.24 (0.13)*	**0.014 (0.007)**	*0.003 (0.001)*
Tributaries	MWT	−0.11 (0.06)	−0.011 (0.01)	−0.001 (0.003)
	PAX	−0.14 (0.07)	**−0.022 (0.01)**	−0.004 (0.002)
	POT	**−0.13 (0.05)**	**−0.019 (0.008)**	0 (0.004)
	RAP	−0.15 (0.09)	−0.013 (0.011)	−0.005 (0.004)
	YRK	**−0.12 (0.05)**	*−0.01 (0.006)*	−0.003 (0.002)
	JAM	**−0.28 (0.13)**	**−0.016 (0.007)**	**−0.005 (0.002)**
		< 4 m depth		
Mainstem	UPP	−0.03 (0.06)	0.006 (0.006)	0.003 (0.002)
	MID	*0.19 (0.10)*	**0.024 (0.009)**	0.003 (0.003)
	LOW	0.15 (0.16)	0.013 (0.013)	**0.007 (0.002)**
Tributaries	MWT	−0.05 (0.05)	−0.003 (0.005)	−0.001 (0.002)
	PAX	**−0.13 (0.05)**	−0.006 (0.007)	0 (0.002)
	POT	0.01 (0.05)	0.01 (0.006)	0.003 (0.002)
	RAP	0.04 (0.06)	−0.002 (0.005)	−0.002 (0.002)
	YRK	0.03 (0.07)	**−0.007 (0.003)**	**−0.003 (0.001)**
	JAM	−0.03 (0.07)	**−0.017 (0.006)**	**−0.006 (0.002)**

where $g(S)$ has a negative binomial error distribution with a log link, and

$$g(H') = \beta_0 + \beta_1 sand + s_1(DO) + s_2(latitude \times longitude) + s_3(depth \times salinity) + \epsilon;$$

$$g(D) = \beta_0 + \beta_1 sand + s_1(DO) + s_2(latitude \times longitude) + s_3(depth \times salinity) + \epsilon,$$

where both $g(H')$ and $g(D)$ have Gaussian error distributions and identity link functions g. For all models, β_i denotes a parametric (linear) term, s_i denotes a nonparametric spline function for individual variables or a bivariate thin-plate spline for interactions, and ϵ is the error term. (A model of similar structure was implemented in Chapter 14 for predicting weather-related traffic accidents.)

Climate factors included six indicators: two river discharge indices, an early summer DO (DO_{ES}, mg/l) index, a spring chlorophyll-a (chl-a_{Spring}, μg/l) bloom intensity index, and two DD temperature indices. The discharge indices include a late winter-to-spring metric ($Flow_{Spring}$, ft^3 s^{-1}) calculated as the grand mean of the January–April monthly average discharge each year, and a previous fall metric ($Flow_{Fall}$, ft^3 s^{-1}) calculated as the grand mean of the September–December monthly average discharge from the previous year. Discharge is an important environmental variable in estuarine ecosystems, influencing biological and chemical conditions during the subsequent summer period (e.g., Wingate and Secor, 2008, Woodland et al, 2019). The DO_{ES} index is the grand mean of the monthly May–July average DO concentrations calculated from the CBP Water Quality Monitoring survey. The $chl\text{-}a_{Spring}$ index is calculated as the grand mean of the monthly January–April station chl-a concentrations collected during the CBP Water Quality Monitoring survey. The degree day (DD) indices were based on a 5°C DD minimum temperature threshold and are calculated as the sum of the average daily water temperature anomalies above 5°C (daily temperatures $\leqslant$ 5°C have $DD = 0$). One DD index is representative of cumulative annual warming before the onset of mid-summer (5°C DD_{Cum}), and is the sum of daily 5°C DD from Jan 1 to July 1 each year (units are DD). The second DD index is a phenology index (5°C DD_{Time}) representative of the relative rate of warming each year and is calculated as the number of days from January 1 required in a given year to accumulate 500 5°C DD (units are days [d]).

A backward model selection approach was applied to identify the most parsimonious models for each biodiversity metric. The AIC$_C$ were calculated for null model formulations and each tested model variant for each biodiversity metric (Wagenmakers and Farrell, 2004). The difference between each model variant's AIC$_C$ (including the null model) and the lowest (best) observed model AIC$_C$ (ΔAIC$_C$) was calculated and the associated relative model weights (Wt_{AICc}) computed (higher Wt_{AICc} means higher model relative probability). These AIC$_C$-based criteria were used as baseline performance metrics to select the most parsimonious model from among those tested. During iterative model selection, model terms were either removed if not significant ($p > 0.05$) or spline terms were replaced with linear terms if fitted splines displayed a linear pattern. Interactions between flow indices and DD indices were also explored and compared to model formulations with separate terms for each variable. Nelder–Mead Simplex optimization was used to avoid convergence failures during smoother fitting. All GAM fitting and modeling were conducted in SAS (v 9.4).

Multivariate analysis of assemblage composition was used to determine how, or if, community composition was changing along with species biodiversity under changing 5°C DD annual thermal regimes identified during GAM analysis. Constrained canonical correspondence analysis (CCA; Leguendre and Leguendre, 2012, ter Braak, 1986) was used to test for assemblage composition differences at the whole-of-ecosystem scale between years associated with rapid (< 130 d) or slow (> 130 d) vernal warming (5°C DD_{Time}) and between years associated with high ($> 1400\ DD$), medium ($1300–1400\ DD$), or low ($< 1300\ DD$) total accumulated warming (5°C DD_{Cum}). Permutation-based analysis of variance under the constrained CCA model was used to test for the significance of group effects in the presence of conditional variables (salinity, depth, region). Indicator species associated with group-differences of interest were identified by calculating the Indicator Value index ($IndVal$) for species, a measure of the relationship between each species and each group. High $IndVal$ indicates a strong association with sites within a grouping, and significance is determined using a permutation test (Dufrene and Legendre 1997). Multivariate species assemblage analysis was conducted in R (v 3.6.1), using the packages `vegan` (Oksanen et al, 2019) and `indicspecies` (De Cáceres and Jansen, 2019).

5.3 Results

5.3.1 Benthic biodiversity patterns

Benthic biodiversity indices showed evidence of spatial and temporal patterns within and across regions. Regional estimates of annual S values ranged from 9.4 ± 1.5 (UPP [mean $\pm$ standard deviation]) to 22.5 ± 3.8 (LOW) in the mainstem regions of Chesapeake Bay, and from 6.4 ± 1.4 (POT) to 12.8 ± 1.8 (JAM) in the tributaries (Figure 5.2). Species richness was typically higher in shallow waters (< 4 m depth), but this relationship varied from year to year in some systems and was reversed in the lower Chesapeake Bay and James River (Figure 5.2). A declining temporal trend in shallow water S was present in the Patuxent River (linear regression, $n = 23$, $R^2_{adj} = 0.17$); whereas, declining deep water trends (> 4 m depth) in S were present in the Potomac ($n = 23$, $R^2_{adj} = 0.19$), York ($n = 22$, $R^2_{adj} = 0.17$), and James ($n = 22$, $R^2_{adj} = 0.15$) rivers (Table 5.1). No temporal trends in S in the mainstem regions were identified, and no positive trends in S were identified.

Annual estimates of H' also differed among regions, ranging from 1.54 ± 0.15 (UPP) to 2.21 ± 0.21 (LOW) in the mainstem and from 1.01 ± 0.20 (POT) to 1.59 ± 0.12 (YRK) in the tributaries (Figure 5.3). Depth-related patterns in H' were similar to S, with higher values typically occurring in shallow waters. The lower Chesapeake Bay and James River were the exceptions to this pattern and showed higher mean H' in deep waters (again similar to S). Declining temporal trends in H' were present in shallow waters of the York ($n = 22$, $R^2_{adj} = 0.14$) and James ($n = 22$, $R^2_{adj} = 0.25$) rivers (Table 5.1). Deepwater declines in H' over the time series were present in the Patuxent ($n = 23$, $R^2_{adj} = 0.15$), Potomac ($n = 22$, $R^2_{adj} = 0.18$), and James ($n = 22$, $R^2_{adj} = 0.14$) rivers. In the mainstem regions, H' increased in shallow waters of the mid-Chesapeake Bay ($n = 22$, $R^2_{adj} = 0.22$) and deep waters of the lower Chesapeake Bay ($n = 22$, $R^2_{adj} = 0.16$).

Spatial and temporal patterns for D differed somewhat from patterns in S and H' (Figure 5.4). Annual estimates of average D ranged from 0.70 ± 0.05

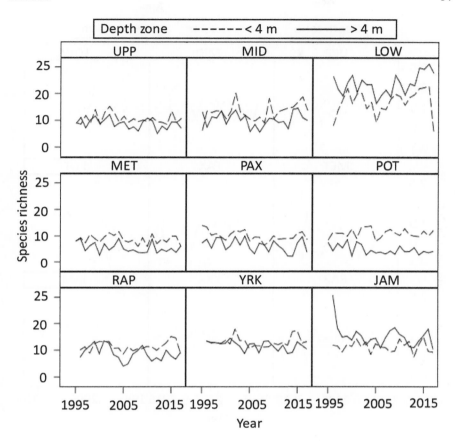

FIGURE 5.2: Time series of annual estimates of species richness from each study region of Chesapeake Bay. Time series are shown separately for shallow (< 4 m) and deep (> 4 m) zones. Please refer to Figure 5.1 for full region names and locations.

(MID) to 0.80 ± 0.05 (LOW) in the mainstem regions, and from 0.64 ± 0.06 (JAM) to 0.70 ± 0.03 (MET) in the tributaries. Depth-related patterns were less pronounced, due to stronger variability and higher overlap of shallow and deepwater estimates (Figure 5.3). Temporal trends, where present, were similar to those of S and H', in that significant tributary trends were negative but mainstem trends were positive (Table 5.1). Declines in D were identified in the shallow waters of the York ($n = 22$, $R^2_{adj} = 0.21$) and James ($n = 22$, $R^2_{adj} = 0.20$) rivers, and in deep waters of the James River ($n = 22$, $R^2_{adj} = 0.15$). An increase in D was present in shallow waters of the lower Chesapeake Bay mainstem ($n = 22$, $R^2_{adj} = 0.26$).

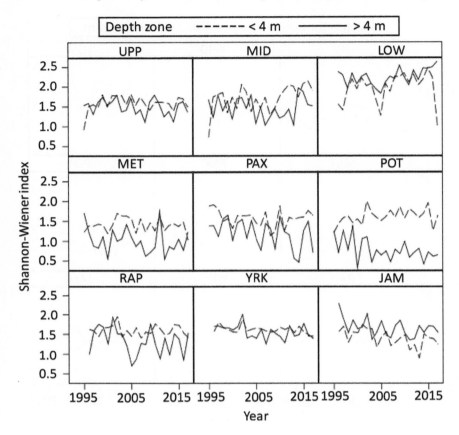

FIGURE 5.3: Time series of annual estimates of Shannon–Wiener diversity index from each study region of Chesapeake Bay. Time series are shown separately for shallow (< 4 m) and deep (> 4 m) zones. Please refer to Figure 5.1 for full region names and locations.

5.3.2 Biodiversity-climate modeling results

Generalized additive model results showed similarities and differences in how benthic biodiversity indices changed in response to climate-associated variables (Table 5.2). Among the candidate models tested for S, the most parsimonious model included a linear term for *sand* ($\hat{\beta}_1 = 0.007 \pm 0.0002$ [standard error], $\chi^2 = 1132.3$, $p < 0.0001$), spline terms for average springtime DO concentration (DO_{ES}) and DO concentration at the time of sampling (DO_{Site}), and four thin-plate spline interaction terms between: previous fall discharge and springtime discharge ($\ln Flow_{Fall} \times \ln Flow_{Spring}$), 5°C degree day cumulative and phenology (5°C $DD_{Cum} \times$ 5 °C DD_{Time}), *latitude* $\times$ *longitude*,

Results

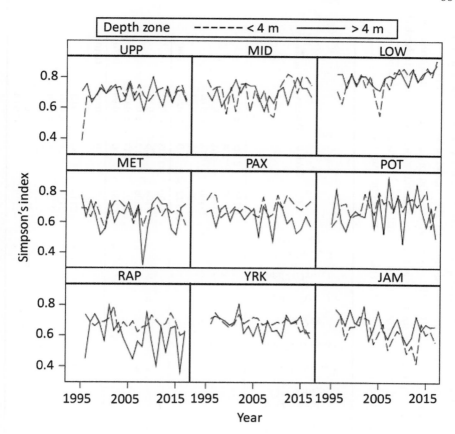

FIGURE 5.4: Time series of annual estimates of Simpson's index of diversity from each study region of Chesapeake Bay. Time series are shown separately for shallow (< 4 m) and deep (> 4 m) zones. Please refer to Figure 5.1 for full region names and locations.

and *depth* × *salinity*. Estimates from this model provided good agreement with observed S values (Pearson product-moment correlation $r_{\text{Pearson}} = 0.80$, $n = 5060$; Figure 5.5). At the site-level, S increased linearly with increasing percentage of sand and water column DO concentration (Figure 5.6D). Site-level S generally increased with salinity, particularly at locations $> 10\,m$ deep (Figure 5.6F). Spatial patterns in S indicated regional hotspots, corresponding roughly with sites located in the northwest and southeast reaches of the study area (Figure 5.6E). Species richness showed a curvilinear response to DO_{ES}, decreasing as DO_{ES} increased beyond an intermediate maximum occurring at ~ 5.0–6.5 mg/l (Figure 5.6A). Low $Flow_{\text{Fall}}$ values were associated with higher S, particularly when co-occurring with relatively low $Flow_{\text{Spring}}$ conditions

TABLE 5.2: Generalized additive modeling results for each biodiversity index. Variables and their parameterization (Linear [Lin], Spline [Spl]) present in each model variant (Model) are indicated, along with the model selection criterion (AIC$_c$ [Akaike's information criterion corrected for small sample size], ΔAIC$_c$, Wt_{AICc}) and Pearson product-moment correlation ($r_{Pearson}$) between final model predicted values and observed values for the selected model. Final model selection is indicated by bolded text. Possible linear terms that were not considered due to obvious non-linearity of relationships (e.g., Lin(DD_{Cum}) are not shown, *sand* was included as a linear term in two null models and a spline term in one null model

Index	Model	Lin or Spl(*sand*)	Spl(DO_{Site})	Spl($Sal \times depth_{Site}$)	Spl($Lat \times Long$)	Spl(ln $Flow_{Fall}$)	Spl(ln $Flow_{Spring}$)	Spl($Flow_{Fall} \times Flow_{Spring}$)	Spl($chl\text{-}a_{Spring}$)	Lin($chl\text{-}a_{Spring}$)	Spl(DO_{ES})	Spl(DD_{Cum})	Spl(DD_{Time})	Spl($DD_{Time} \times DD_{Cum}$)	AIC$_c$	ΔAIC$_c$	Wt_{AICc}	$r_{Pearson}$
Species richness	Null	×	×	×	×	×	×								32714	3592	< 0.01	
	1	×	×	×	×				×		×	×	×		29386	264	< 0.01	
	2	×	×	×	×				×		×	×			29383	261	< 0.01	
	3	×	×	×	×				×		×		×		29400	278	< 0.01	
	4	×	×	×	×	×	×			×	×		×		29133	11	< 0.01	
	5	×	×	×	×	×	×			×	×			×	**29122**	**0**	**> 0.99**	**0.80**
Shannon–Wiener index	Null	×	×	×	×	×	×		×		×				8499	1203	< 0.01	
	1	×	×	×	×			×			×	×	×		7434	138	< 0.01	
	2	×	×	×	×			×			×	×			7308	12	< 0.01	
	3	×	×	×	×			×			×		×		7429	133	< 0.01	
	4	×	×	×	×			×			×			×	**7296**	**0**	**> 0.99**	**0.70**
Simpson's index of diversity	Null	×	×	×	×	×	×		×		×				−2140	0	> 0.99	
	1	×	×	×	×				×		×	×	×		−2095	51	< 0.01	
	2	×	×	×	×				×		×	×			−2114	32	< 0.01	
	3	×	×	×	×				×		×		×		−2118	28	< 0.01	
	4	×	×	×	×				×		×			×	−2120	26	< 0.01	
	5	×	×	×	×					×	×	×	×		−2119	27	< 0.01	
	6	×	×	×	×					×	×	×			−2111	35	< 0.01	
	7	×	×	×	×					×	×			×	−2119	27	< 0.01	0.40

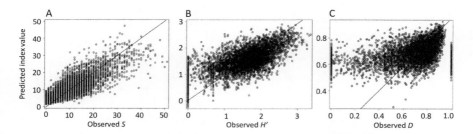

FIGURE 5.5: Observed vs predicted model results from generalized additive model fitting for A) species richness, B) Shannon–Wiener diversity, and C) Simpson's index of diversity. Dashed 1:1 line provided for reference in each panel.

(Figure 5.6B). The biggest S were associated with high 5°C DD_{Time} and intermediate 5°C DD_{Cum}; however, relatively high S values also occurred under both high and low 5°C DD_{Cum} conditions when 5°C DD_{Time} were corresponding low (Figure 5.6C).

Optimal model formulation for H' included linear parameter estimates for percentage of sand ($\hat{\beta}_1 = 0.006 \pm 0.0002$, $\chi^2 = 617.3$, $p < 0.0001$) and mean springtime chlorophyll-a concentration ($chl\text{-}a_{\text{Spring}}$; $\hat{\beta}_2 = -0.003 \pm 0.0001$, $\chi^2 = 6.25$, $p = 0.01$). Nonlinear terms in the H' model included spline terms for DO_{ES} and DO_{Site}, and the thin-plate spline interaction terms $\ln Flow_{\text{Fall}} \times \ln Flow_{\text{Spring}}$, 5°C $DD_{\text{Cum}} \times$ 5°C DD_{Time}, $latitude \times longitude$, and $depth \times salinity$ (Table 5.2). The performance of the final H' model was lower than the S model ($r_{\text{Pearson}} = 0.70$, $n = 5060$; Figure 5.5), primarily due to overestimation of H' by the model at low observed values (< 1.0). Site-level parameter estimates indicated an increase in H' with greater percentage of sand in the sediment. Salinity generally covaried positively with H' except at shallow depths below 4–5 m, where H' was reduced relative to deeper areas (Figure 5.7F). Within the study region, the greatest H' values tended to occur in the northwest and declined toward the mid-Chesapeake Bay (Figure 5.7E). A local hotspot in H' also occurred in the lower mainstem region of Chesapeake Bay, just down-estuary from the mid-Chesapeake Bay minimum. Shannon diversity index values showed a modal relationship to DO_{Site}, increasing from low to intermediate water column DO concentrations ($\sim$5–8 mg/l) before declining again at the highest observed DO_{Site} values (Figure 5.7D). An intermediate peak in H' relative to DO_{ES} conditions was also observed although the initial decline in H' at $DO_{\text{ES}} < 5$–6 was less apparent (Figure 5.7A). The combination of high $\ln Flow_{\text{Fall}}$ and $\ln Flow_{\text{Spring}}$ conditions resulted in decreased H'; however, relatively high discharge during one or the other season was associated with greater estimated H' (Figure 5.7B). The pattern in H' relative to 5°C DD_{Time} and intermediate 5°C DD_{Cum} index values matched that of S, with the highest values observed at high 5°C DD_{Time}

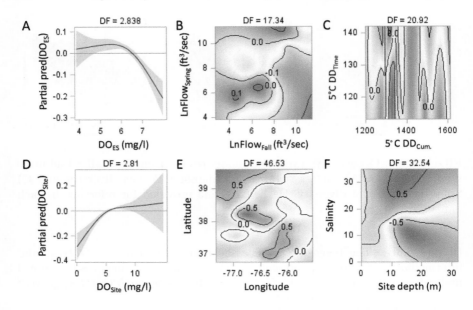

FIGURE 5.6: Species richness (S) generalized additive model results showing partial prediction splines with 95% Bayesian posterior confidence bands for individual variables in panels A and D, and contoured heat maps of S in parameter space for thin-plate spline interaction terms in panels B, C, E, and F (degrees of freedom [DF] for each variable or variable interaction provided). Panels shown are A) average spring dissolved oxygen concentration (DO_{ES}), B) ln-transformed average spring river flow ($\ln Flow_{Spring}$) × ln-transformed average fall river flow from the preceding year ($\ln Flow_{Fall}$), C) day of year at which 500 5°C degree days have accumulated (5°C DD_{Time}) × accumulated 5°C DD from January 1 to June 30 (5°C DD_{Cum}), D) site dissolved oxygen concentration (DO_{Site}), E) site latitude × site longitude, and F) site salinity × site total depth.

and intermediate 5°C DD_{Cum} conditions. Local hotspots in H' under low 5°C DD_{Time} and high 5°C DD_{Cum}, or low 5°C DD_{Time} and low 5°C DD_{Cum} were present (Figure 5.7C).

Model selection for D yielded the greatest support for the null model, inclusive of site-level predictors only. Model performance for the null model was the lowest among the three biodiversity indices and substantially overestimated D for the lower observed D values (Figure 5.5C). This overestimation led to a relatively poor correlation between model predictions and observations ($r_{Pearson} = 0.40$, $n = 5060$; Table 5.2). As with S and H', D showed a positive linear relationship with percentage of sand ($\hat{\beta}_1 = 0.001 \pm 0.0001$, $\chi^2 = 1588.4$, $p < 0.0001$). A curvilinear increase in D with increasing DO_{Site} occurred between the lowest DO_{Site} concentrations (< 1 mg/l) and intermedi-

Results

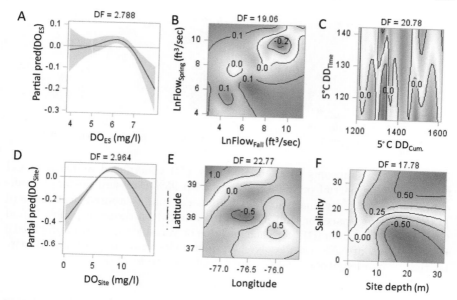

FIGURE 5.7: Shannon–Wiener diversity index (H') generalized additive model results showing partial prediction splines with 95% Bayesian posterior confidence bands for individual variables in panels A and D, and contoured heat maps of H' in parameter space for thin-plate spline interaction terms in panels B, C, E, and F (degrees of freedom [DF] for each variable or variable interaction provided). Panels shown are A) average spring dissolved oxygen concentration (DO_{ES}), B) ln-transformed average spring river flow ($\ln Flow_{Spring}$) × ln-transformed average fall river flow from the preceding year ($\ln Flow_{Fall}$), C) day of year at which 500 5°C degree days have accumulated (5°C DD_{Time}) × accumulated 5°C DD from January 1 to June 30 (5°C DD_{Cum}), D) site dissolved oxygen concentration (DO_{Site}), E) site latitude × site longitude, and F) site salinity × site total depth.

ate concentrations of ∼6-7 mg/l (Figure 5.8A). Relatively low D values were associated with the lowest latitude despite local minima located near annually hypoxic areas in the upper-to-middle Chesapeake Bay mainstem regions (Figure 5.8B). Similar to H', the modeled effect of the interaction between site depth and salinity on D indicated increasing D with increasing salinity except in shallow waters < 4-5 m depth (Figure 5.8C).

5.3.3 Multivariate assemblage analysis

The differences in S and H' associated with changing 5°C DD_{Time} and 5°C DD_{Cum} thermal regimes were indicative of structural changes in the assemblage composition. Permutation-based analysis of variance (ANOVA) of the

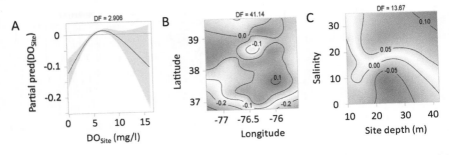

FIGURE 5.8: Simpson's index of diversity (D) generalized additive model results showing partial prediction splines with 95% Bayesian posterior confidence bands for individual variables in panel A and contoured heat maps of D in parameter space for thin-plate spline interaction terms in panels B and C (degrees of freedom [DF] for each variable or variable interaction provided). Panels shown are A) site dissolved oxygen concentration (DO_{Site}), B) site latitude × site longitude, and C) site salinity × site total depth.

constrained CCA model that included 5°C DD_{Time} and 5°C DD_{Cum} factor groupings as well as salinity, depth, and region effects showed the global model to be significant ($n = 1016$, $d.f. = 3$, $\chi^2 = 0.58$, $F = 7.24$, $p = 0.001$). Further testing of the marginal effects verified the significance of both 5°C DD_{Time} ($d.f. = 1$, $\chi^2 = 0.23$, $F = 8.67$, $p = 0.001$) and 5°C DD_{Cum} ($d.f. = 2$, $\chi^2 = 0.10$, $F = 1.86$, $p = 0.04$) as predictors of assemblage composition. Based on these results and the finding from the GAM analysis of an interaction between 5°C DD_{Time} and 5°C DD_{Cum} (specifically, evidence of high biodiversity at high and low total accumulated warming under rapid warming conditions) we analyzed the assemblage composition to identify key indicator species associated with each thermal regime. Calculation of $IndVal$ index for each species between those two thermal regimes indicates the presence of $n = 32$ unique indicator species in the high 5°C DD_{Cum} regime (all $IndVal$ values significant at the significance level $\alpha = 0.05$), and $n = 24$ unique indicator taxa in the low 5°C DD_{Cum} regime (Table 5.3 shows a subset of indicator taxa with $IndVal \geqslant 0.3$).

5.4 Discussion

Like other coastal ecosystems, Chesapeake Bay is exposed to a broad spectrum of anthropogenic stressors that arise from hydrological, physical, chemical, and climatological processes. These processes interact to generate environmental conditions that determine benthic habitat quality, and historical analyses

Discussion

TABLE 5.3: Indicator species of benthic communities (and broad taxonomic groupings to which they belong) under years with an accumulation of 5°C degree days > 1400 (↑5°C DD_{Cum}) and < 1400 by July 1 (↓5°C DD_{Cum}) in Chesapeake Bay during only those years with rapid vernal warming (5°C $DD_{\text{Time}} > 130$). For each species, the Indicator Value ($IndVal$, Dufrêne and Legendre, 1997) is given under the column associated with their thermal grouping (all values shown are significant at the level $\alpha = 0.05$)

Taxonomic group	Species	↑5°C DD_{Cum}	↓5°C DD_{Cum}
Amphipoda	*Gammarus daiberi*	0.60	
	Gammarus spp.	0.32	
	Lepidactylus dytiscus		0.49
Cirripedia	*Balanus improvisus*	0.31	
Mysidacea	*Americamysis bigelowi*		0.42
Tanaidae	*Hargeria rapax*		0.35
Bivalvia	*Gemma gemma*		0.54
	Macoma mitchelli		0.79
	Mytilopsis leucophaeata	0.41	
Gastropoda	*Haminoea solitaria*		0.46
	Littoridinops tenuipes	0.37	
Insecta	*Chaoborus punctipennis*	0.48	
	Cryptochironomus fulvus	0.38	
	Hexagenia spp.	0.30	
Chironomidae	*Chironomidae*	0.47	
	Procladius spp.	0.33	
Oligocheata	*Aulodrilus pigueti*	0.32	
	Branchiura sowerbyi	0.49	
	Ilyodrilus templetoni	0.39	
	Limnodrilus hoffmeister	0.33	
Polychaeta	*Eteone heteropoda*		0.70
	Heteromastus filiformis		0.75
	Laeonereis culveri		0.63
	Polydora cornuta		0.59

have documented negative effects on the benthos in coastal areas subject to degraded habitat (Holland et al, 1987, Karlson et al, 2002, Seitz et al, 2009, Stora and Arnoux, 1983). Despite centuries of human development and continued eutrophication of Chesapeake Bay's ecosystem (Kemp et al, 2005), recent evidence of improving DO and other water quality conditions suggests that benthic habitat conditions might be improving in some areas and times over the past 35 years (Lefcheck et al, 2018, Testa et al, 2018, Zhang et al, 2018). By coupling flexible, nonlinear modeling approaches with long-term monitoring data, we have identified temporal, spatial, and environmental trends in benthic biodiversity that covary with climate change indicators as well as local habitat characteristics. These findings have relevance to Chesapeake Bay's ecosystem dynamics as well as broader implications for the potential response of other systems to similar climate drivers.

5.4.1 Long-term trends in Chesapeake Bay benthic biodiversity

The multidecadal trends in benthic biodiversity that we identify here suggest long-term, spatially-explicit changes in benthic communities are occurring in Chesapeake Bay. Trends in biodiversity in the mainstem regions of the estuary and the tributaries showed opposing patterns, whereby significant mainstem biodiversity trends were positive and significant tributary trends were negative. Further, weaker trends (p of 0.10–0.05) in each region followed these same patterns, with only one exception (S in the upper mainstem region; Table 5.1). Rates of change are most easily interpreted for S (species/year) and in the deep waters (> 4 m depth) of several Chesapeake Bay tributaries, where fitted rates equate to total declines of 2.5–5.9 species per observation, or 0.11–0.26 species/m^2, over the duration of the survey. In the Patuxent River, a decline of 2.9 species per observation (0.13 species/m^2) occurred in shallow waters < 4 m. To place these trends in perspective, the deepwater reduction of S per sample in the James River represents a 33% decline from the 5-year average S estimated at the start of the time series (1996–2001, where mean $\pm$ a standard error is 17.8 $\pm$ 1.2) to the end in 2017. Similar calculations show that negative trends in S in other tributaries over the times-series equate to declines of 52% and 19% in the deep waters of the Potomac and York Rivers, and 29% in the shallow waters of the Patuxent River. Rates of change for H' and D are less amenable to easy interpretation at a per-unit scale due to the integration of both species richness and abundance information into each metric. Notably, the directional trends in both H' and D mirror trends in S, indicating that changes in the benthic community structure are not solely a function of changing species richness. Previously, increasing trends in S (and other benthic community condition metrics) from the 1980s to the 1990s were identified in areas of the James, York, and Rappahannock rivers, and lower Chesapeake Bay (Dauer, 1997, Dauer and Alden III, 1995). While we observed the opposite pattern in the southern tributaries, we also documented positive trends in H' and D in the middle and lower mainstem regions. The partial disagreement between our findings and those of previous studies may be attributable to differences in the period of study, study design, and analytical methods, however, it may also reflect the increasing pressures of environmental and climate-related stressors in recent decades.

It is outside the scope of this analysis to fully discern why trends differed between the tributaries and the mainstem given the same regional climate, but the discrepancy raises questions for future investigations. For example, elevated diversity in the middle and lower Bay in the most recent decade

Discussion

is consistent with improved oxygen conditions, better habitat for submerged aquatic vegetation (SAV), and relatively low flow conditions that could have led to less eutrophication and higher salinity (Orth et al, 2017, Testa et al, 2018, Zhang et al, 2018). The mainstem regions are also responsive to Susquehanna River inputs and exchange with the Atlantic Ocean, which translate larger-scale climate forcing to estuarine waters. The tributaries, in contrast, may be responding to local factors, including long-term changes in nutrient loading that are tributary-specific (Zhang et al, 2015), more rapid oxygen declines in some tributaries,[1] and spatially variable increases in water temperature (Ding and Elmore, 2015).

These negative trends in biodiversity in the tributaries are significant because species losses can alter ecological function and ecosystem properties such as secondary productivity (Duffy et al, 2007, Lotze et al, 2006). While functional redundancy is common among benthic fauna with multiple taxa engaging in functionally similar activities, some studies have demonstrated the importance of species-specific traits in regulating ecosystem processes (e.g., Heemsbergen et al, 2004, Hooper et al, 2005, Norling et al, 2007). Solan et al (2004) showed that if a species' functional traits or its rarity are correlated with their vulnerability to a stressor, the community may not be able to compensate for their loss despite the presence of functionally similar species. The pervasive reduction in ecosystem services associated with the collapse of Eastern oysters (*Crassostrea virginica*) in Chesapeake Bay is a well-documented example of functional loss arising from a single-species decline (Wilberg et al, 2011, and references therein). A corollary is that the ecological consequences of the species losses will also depend on the specific identity of the stressor (Solan et al, 2004). Thus hypoxia-induced mortality events might have different ecological consequences than thermal-stress related mortality events due to differences in the identity or functional traits possessed by species differentially vulnerable to each stressor. Conversely, the effects of functionally similar species (and their loss) on benthic ecological processes are not necessarily additive (e.g., Waldbusser et al, 2004), underscoring the potential importance of species interactions in ultimately determining net process rates and properties. Changes in biodiversity are critical given the central role of benthic communities in facilitating oxygenation of the sediments, consumption and decomposition of organic matter (especially detritus), processing of anthropogenic waste and contaminants, water-column filtration, and energy transfer to higher trophic levels (Covich et al, 2004a,b, Schratzberger and Ingels, 2018, Weslawski et al, 2004). It is unknown if the trends in biodiversity over the past 20+ years documented in this study have altered local or regional system properties in Chesapeake Bay, but this is an area of inquiry that requires additional research.

---

[1] https://www.chesapeakebay.net/channel_files/26080/do_b_summer_85o18-flow.pdf

5.4.2 Climate drivers of benthic biodiversity

Long-term patterns in benthic biodiversity in Chesapeake Bay reflect an integration of local and regional factors acting at different spatial and temporal scales. The annual timing and volume of river discharge are major drivers of inter-annual variability in community composition for many estuarine organisms, including benthos, fish, zooplankton and primary producer assemblages (Cloern et al, 1983, Holland et al, 1987, Rabalais et al, 2002, Woodland et al, 2017). In coastal ecosystems, seasonal freshwater discharge cycles influence salinity structure, water temperature, gas exchange, nutrient and sediment loading, primary production, and particle advection, all key factors influencing faunal diversity and community composition. Biodiversity minima (artenminima, sensu Remane, 1934) associated with oligohaline-to-mesohaline salinity transitions (~1-15) occur among both vertebrate and invertebrate taxa in brackish ecosystems (Deaton and Greenberg, 1986, Schaffner et al, 2001, Wagner, 1999). This pattern arises in part from the need for different, specifically adapted physiological mechanisms to maintain osmotic homeostasis at different ion concentrations in the ambient water, but can also reflect biotic responses to changes in other system properties that covary with salinity (e.g., turbidity, DO, sedimentation; Schaffner et al, 2001). In addition to direct physiological effects, discharge can modulate the survival and recruitment dynamics of benthic taxa at different life stages. For benthic taxa with pelagic egg and larval phases, flow-dependent advection and mixing can directly influence the availability of suitable water column habitat and bottom habitat at the time of settlement (Palardy and Witman, 2011, 2014, Palmer et al, 1996). During benthic life-stages, discharge effects on bottom water quality and the delivery of suspended particulate organic matter influence bottom-up (habitat quality) and top-down (predation vulnerability) processes, both of which are important controls on benthic community dynamics (Holland et al, 1987, Levin et al, 2009, Long and Seitz, 2008, Rosenberg, 2001).

The significance of climate-associated temperature, springtime oxygen concentration, and springtime chlorophyll-a (a proxy for primary production) demonstrate the important role of early season regional climate conditions on benthic community dynamics in Chesapeake Bay. Each of these variables also tend to correlate significantly with winter-spring river flow (Miller and Harding Jr, 2007, Testa and Kemp, 2014), where high winter-spring flow leads to elevated primary productivity, stratification, and earlier hypoxia onset. The potential for temperature changes to influence benthic biodiversity and community composition are likely given that time series of both DD indices indicate long-term increases in the rate and accumulation of warming before the onset of summer from 1950–2017 (Figure 5.9). These trends show that Chesapeake Bay waters accumulated an average of 235 more 5°C degree days in 2017 than they did in 1950. Similarly, waters are warming more rapidly during the late winter and early spring, accumulating 500 5°C degree days about 2 weeks earlier in 2017 than 1950. Results from the $IndVal$ analysis showed clear

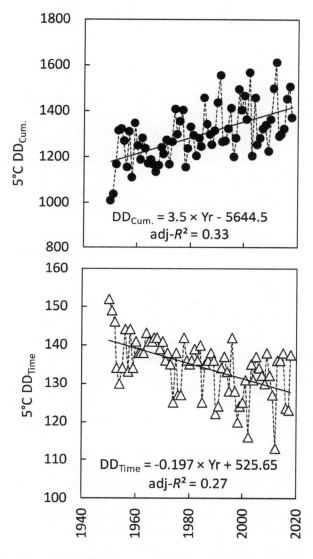

FIGURE 5.9: Time series of water temperature climate variables showing A) sum of the annual accumulated 5°C degree days from January 1 to June 30 (5°C DD_{Cum}), and B) day of year at which 500 5°C DD have accumulated (5°C DD_{Time}) from 1950–2017 in Chesapeake Bay. Least-squares linear regression fitted line given for each variable (DD_{Cum} $F = 34.7$, $p < 0.0001$; DD_{Time} $F = 26.5$, $p < 0.0001$.

differences between summer benthic communities under different spring thermal regimes (Table 5.3). Polychaete taxa were indicative of cooler years while oligochaete taxa were indicative of warmer years. Estimates of environmental tolerances of these taxa are relatively rare, but oligochaetes are generally considered tolerant of hypoxic conditions although individual species show a range of tolerances (Chapman, 2001, Giere, 2006, Reynoldson, 1987). Critical oxygen partial pressure (P_{crit}) reported for one of the oligochaete indicator taxa identified here (*Limnodrilus hoffmeister*) and several other oligochaete species at 15°C ranged 1–12.6 kPa and averaged ~4.5 kPa (< 5% O_2 saturation; Giere, 2006), values that are suggestive of hypoxia-tolerant metabolism (although see Wood, 2018 for a critique of the P_{crit} approach). Giere (2006) also provides P_{crit} values for three polychaete taxa that ranged 2.1–17 kPa with an average of 11.7 kPa, more than a twice as high as the average oligochaete P_{crit} value. Other taxonomic groups such as bivalves, gastropods, and amphipods showed species-level differences in their association with cooler and warmer conditions.

Temperature effects can interact with low DO conditions, which exert strong controls on benthic community survival and composition, particularly severe hypoxia < 0.5 mg/l and anoxia (Levin et al, 2009, Riedel et al, 2012, Seitz et al, 2009). Modal relationships between benthic biodiversity and vernal phytoplankton bloom intensity and dissolved oxygen concentrations reflect the coupling of primary production with oxygen production via photosynthesis and consumption via respiration. Increased primary production can stimulate secondary production up to threshold (i.e., a "fertilization" effect; Nixon and Buckley 2002), after which primary production outpaces the consumptive capacity of grazers. This pattern has been observed in Chesapeake Bay and in coastal systems around the world (Kemp et al, 2005, Nixon and Buckley, 2002, Rosenberg, 2001). The very high concentrations of chlorophyll that often precede or coincide with eutrophic conditions can cause very high or even supersaturated DO conditions throughout much of the water column during daylight hours (Rabalais et al, 2009) or in surface waters. For example, Dauer et al (2000) found a negative correlation between chlorophyll-a concentrations and benthic condition after accounting for the effect of low dissolved oxygen in Chesapeake Bay. Given the links between early DO and chlorophyll conditions, and summertime benthic biodiversity, further study of these relationships might yield informative metrics for resource managers interested in predicting benthic community status or productivity (e.g., fisheries managers). The benthos of Chesapeake Bay are not unique in their response to temperature and DO: a meta-analysis of temperature and hypoxia effects on survival of benthic organisms showed that survival times declined by 74% while minimum O_2-thresholds increased by 16% under warmer water temperatures (Vaquer-Sunyer and Duarte, 2011). In addition to the direct physiological stress engendered by hypoxia, redox-mediated release of ecotoxic compounds (e.g., hydrogen sulfide, Vaquer-Sunyer and Duarte, 2010) and remineralization of organic matter can feedback to further compromise benthic health and exacerbate

Discussion

hypoxia (Paerl, 2006). Under current and future warming, benthic communities are likely to become more vulnerable to environmental disturbances such as hypoxic events when and where they occur.

In coastal waters, the deposition of suspended organic matter sediment typically occurs in areas sheltered from strong current, wind or tidal forces, or in flow convergence zones (Friedrichs et al, 2000, Schaffner et al, 2001). Settling or near-bed suspended organic matter provides a basal trophic resource for benthic communities, but excessive inputs can stimulate microbial respiration and lead to local hypoxia, reductions in species richness, but potentially increases in the biomass of opportunistic or tolerant taxa (McArthur et al, 2010). In the York River, Schaffner et al (2001) found that the upper estuary was characterized by strong mixing and physical disturbance of bottom sediments and low benthic diversity. Moving down-estuary, physical disturbance declined but sedimentation increased, and communities were more representative of hypoxia-stressed environments (i.e., few large, "deep-dwelling" species; Schaffner et al, 2001). Outside the York River, physical disturbance and sedimentation decreased, and the moderate current conditions were associated with maximum benthic biodiversity and functional diversity (Schaffner et al, 2001). These observations suggest sediment organic matter concentrations during summer months should negatively covary with benthic biodiversity. A negative site-level relationship exists between sediment nutrient concentrations and predicted values of benthic biodiversity in this study (Figure 5.10). While we show the results for TN, the same relationship (albeit more variable) existed for TC (not shown). This nutrient-biodiversity relationship is present across mainstem and tributary systems, and across salinity zones within and between systems (i.e., 13 salinity-zone dependent linear regression models from 5 regions, $R^2_{adj} \geq 0.21$, $p < 0.03$). This evidence of a negative association between benthic biodiversity and accumulated organic matter aligns with the significant, positive association of biodiversity with sandy sediments (rather than fine, silty sediment) in all null model formulations. Both sediment organic matter content and grain size can influence benthic community structure, but other factors that often covary with these sediment characteristics, such as salinity, near-bed hydrodynamics, and disturbance, are also important. Untangling the relative contributions of these covarying factors to benthic communities remains a challenge, however, processes that result in large-scale sedimentation of organic-rich material such as large phytoplankton blooms or influxes of terrestrial organic matter from intense weather events are likely to adversely affect benthic biodiversity unless sufficient water movement is present to alleviate the formation or intensity of subsequent hypoxia.

5.4.3 Regional climate outlook for Chesapeake Bay

Although considerable uncertainty remains in projections of climate for the mid-Atlantic region of the United States, a growing number of reviews and

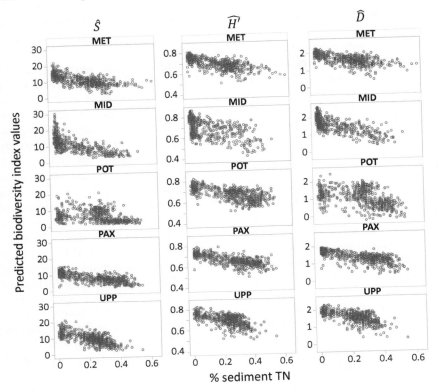

FIGURE 5.10: Model predicted values of benthic community biodiversity metrics (Species richness $[\hat{S}]$, Shannon–Wiener diversity index $[\hat{H}']$, Simpson's index of diversity $[\hat{D}]$) plotted against total nitrogen (sediment %TN) for a subset of regions in Chesapeake Bay. Please refer to Figure 5.1 for full region names and locations.

modeling analyses have suggested that precipitation and temperature are likely to increase in the coming century (Johnson et al, 2016, Najjar et al, 2010, Ni et al, 2019). For example, Ni et al (2019) analyzed six regionally-downscaled global climate model projections from the North American Regional Climate Change Assessment (NARCCAP) for the period 2014–2070, where five of the six models predicted an increase in Susquehanna River flow of 92 to 600 m^3 s^{-1} (mean flow is ~1100 m^3 s^{-1}). The projections typically predict river flow increases to occur between the months of December to February, the typical season of peak Susquehanna River discharges. Similarly, the models project air temperature increases of 1.35°C to 1.95°C by mid century and that air temperature will increase near uniformly across the spring, summer, and fall seasons. Significant warming trends in both DD indices developed for this study indi-

Discussion 113

cate these climate changes have already had an effect on thermal conditions early in the year and on benthic biodiversity during the subsequent summer. Similar studies that focused on the 1985–2017 period have also indicated warming of Chesapeake Bay surface waters (Ding and Elmore, 2015, Testa et al, 2018), but this timeframe is still longer than the benthic diversity data set used in this analysis (since 1995). The combination of such changes will clearly impact the physical environment during seasons when benthic invertebrates reproduce and reach peak biomass, given the strong relationships we found between river discharge, temperature, and the diversity indices we quantified.

5.4.4 Global outlook for estuarine communities in the face of climate forcing

Numerical model projections of elevated water temperature and river discharge suggest that the volume of oxygen-depleted water will increase over the coming century in Chesapeake Bay (Irby et al, 2018, Ni et al, 2019). These projections are supported by recent global-scale analyses that suggest an expansion of oxygen-depleted waters in estuarine regions and both the coastal and open ocean (Breitburg et al, 2018). Future projections of elevated temperature are associated with an earlier onset of hypoxia and earlier warming, both of which should be expected to lower benthic biodiversity given the results of our analyses (e.g., Figures 5.6 and 5.7). Another common feature of climate change, sea level rise (SLR), appears to have less of an impact on future hypoxia in Chesapeake Bay (e.g., Irby et al, 2018) because SLR may have compensating effects on oxygen depletion. For example, SLR may increase salinity and encourage the stratification that limits oxygen penetration to deep waters, but SLR may also increase tidal mixing rates and lead to elevated delivery of relatively cool and oxygen-rich water from more oceanic boundary waters. Thus, while SLR may have a limited impact on hypoxia, if it increases salinity in Bay waters, it will potentially favor more diverse assemblages of species (Schaffner et al, 2001, Sturdivant et al, 2014), as well as compensating for salinity-reducing impacts of elevated riverine discharges.

Given that hypoxic conditions have been generally associated with reductions in benthic biomass and productivity (Diaz and Rosenberg, 1995, Sturdivant et al, 2013), there is an expectation that these expanded future hypoxic conditions will have negative consequences for benthic invertebrate biomass, and by extension, diversity. Both our statistical model findings and past studies of oxygen impacts on benthic invertebrates indicate that as hypoxic conditions become more severe, benthic biomass is reduced. Given the diverse range of tolerances of different benthic invertebrates to oxygen conditions (Levin et al, 2009), it is possible that increases in the severity or duration of low oxygen conditions may simply alter species dominance. Short-term hypoxic stress can favor survival by infaunal or hypoxia-tolerant taxa, such as bivalves and anthozoans, over epifauna taxa, such as crustaceans and polychaetes (Riedel et al, 2012). Complete defaunation events would favor initial recovery by small, soft-bodied invertebrates with short generation times over longer-lived taxa. Recent analyses of oxygen records in Chesapeake Bay have suggested that although annually-integrated volumes of hypoxia have remained unchanged, the volume of more severely-depleted oxygen conditions has declined, and attainment of water quality standards for oxygen has improved (Testa et al, 2018, Zhang et al, 2018). It is possible, although not definitive, that recent increases in all three diversity indices in the shallow waters of the mid-bay and deeper waters of the lower bay (Figures 5.2–5.4) may be linked to recent oxygen improvements (since 2011) in these regions. This is supported by the fact that dissolved oxygen concentrations were positively associated with biodiversity metrics across all models in our analysis.

Benthic biomass, productivity, and diversity all vary in response to a multitude of factors that influence physiology, food availability, and habitat structure. The statistical models presented in this chapter reinforce the idea that external inputs (freshwater, nutrients), internal chemical conditions (dissolved oxygen, salinity), and physical structure (sediment composition) all interact to control benthic diversity. The complexity of these relationships is clear given that linear trends in the climate indices were few ($n = 3$) despite the presence of robust linear trends in biodiversity in several areas of Chesapeake Bay during the study period. Linear regression analysis of climate indices in each spatial region found significant increasing trends in $chl\text{-}a_{\text{Spring}}$ ($F_{1,21} = 4.48$, $p = 0.045$; $R^2_{adj} = 0.14$) in the upper Bay, increasing DO_{ES} ($F_{1,21} = 5.08$, $p = 0.04$; $R^2_{adj} = 0.16$) in the Potomac River, and declining DO_{ES} in the York River ($F_{1,21} = 5.62$, $p = 0.03$; $R^2_{adj} = 0.17$). These patterns do not clearly align with the observed trends in biodiversity except for the York River, in which deepwater declines in S and shallow water declines in H' and D were observed. The challenge for predicting future changes in benthic invertebrate diversity stems not only from the difficulty in predicting future physical and chemical conditions, but also from the fact that there can be compensating impacts on benthic communities from any given forcing variable. For example, elevated freshwater inputs lower salinity and support oxygen depletion, both of which can have negative consequences for diversity, but these freshwater inputs may also enhance the generation of labile organic material and associated food availability to support additional benthic production (e.g., Kemp et al, 2005), if not diversity. Vulnerability to various external inputs may also vary substantially across space in Chesapeake Bay, where higher salinity waters typified by stronger currents and reduced organic matter deposition are also hotbeds of diversity and typically do not accommodate oxygen depletion, whereas tributary and middle bay waters are highly vulnerable to oxygen depletion.

5.5 Conclusions

We found evidence of long-term patterns in benthic biodiversity in Chesapeake Bay and evidence that two of three metrics of biodiversity were related to climate factors in Chesapeake Bay. These climate-relevant factors included environmental indices of river flow, water temperatures (both the timing and integrated sum of vernal water warming), dissolved oxygen concentrations, and phytoplankton biomass (a proxy for primary production). Modeled relationships between biodiversity and climate indices ranged from linear responses to complex, nonlinear responses with evidence of biodiversity changing in response to interactions among some climate indices. Despite the relatively long time series of benthic data available for this study (1995–2017) and clear evidence of temporal trends in biodiversity in different regions of the estuary, there were very few concurrent linear trends among the climate variables. Absence of highly correlated climate indices with the benthic biodiversity is indicative of a complex biotic response integrating not only the conditions represented by the modeled predictors, but also (1) the effects of hydrodynamics and recruitment processes, both in the water column and at the seabed interface, (2) interactions with environmental conditions at different spatiotemporal scales, (3) species interactions such as competition and predation, (4) event-scale disturbances (e.g., hurricanes and extreme precipitation), and (5) other environmental conditions not explicitly considered here such as quality of deposited organic matter, ecotoxicological conditions associated with land use patterns or sediment contamination, and shoreline development. Future work that builds on this analysis should consider the potential role of these and other predictors, evaluate the importance of scale-dependence on the explanatory power of climate indices, and investigate functional diversity and species-specific responses to climate forcing.

Acknowledgments

The authors would like to thank Lora Harris for providing thoughtful discussion on some of the material in this chapter. This work was partially funded by Chesapeake Bay Trust award #13663 to RJW and National Science Foundation grant CBET-1360395 to JMT. This is UMCES publication #5753.

References

Airoldi L, Balata D, Beck MW (2008) The gray zone: relationships between habitat loss and marine diversity and their applications in conservation. Journal of Experimental Marine Biology and Ecology 366(1–2):8–15

Begon M, Townsend C, Harper JL (2006) Ecology: From Individuals to Ecosystems. Blackwell Publishing, Malden, MA

Breitburg D, Levin LA, Oschlies A, Grégoire M, Chavez FP, Conley DJ, Garçon V, Gilbert D, Gutiérrez D, Isensee K, Jacinto GS, Limburg KE, Montes I, Naqvi SWA, Pitcher GC, Rabalais NN, Roman MR, Rose KA, Seibel BA, Telszewski M, Yasuhara M, Zhang J (2018) Declining oxygen in the global ocean and coastal waters. Science 359(6371):eaam7240

Burnham KP, Anderson DR (2002) Model Selection and Multimodel Inference: A Practical Information-Theoretic Approach, 2nd edn. Springer, New York

Burnham KP, Anderson DR, Huyvaert KP (2011) AIC model selection and multimodel inference in behavioral ecology: some background, observations, and comparisons. Behavioral Ecology and Sociobiology 65(1):23–35

Chapman PM (2001) Utility and relevance of aquatic oligochaetes in ecological risk assessment. In: Aquatic Oligochaete Biology VIII, Springer, Netherlands, 149–169

Cloern JE, Alpine AE, Cole BE, Wong RL, Arthur JF, Ball MD (1983) River discharge controls phytoplankton dynamics in the northern San Francisco Bay estuary. Estuarine, Coastal and Shelf Science 16(4):415–429

Covich AP, Austen MC, Bärlocher F, Chauvet E, Cardinale BJ, Biles CL, Inchausti P, Dangles O, Solan M, Gessner MO, Statzner B, Moss B (2004a) The role of biodiversity in the functioning of freshwater and marine benthic ecosystems. BioScience 54(8):767–775

Covich AP, Ewel KC, Hall RO, Giller PE, Goedkoop W, Merritt DM (2004b) Ecosystem services provided by freshwater benthos. In: Wall DH (ed) Sustaining Biodiversity and Ecosystem Services in Soils and Sediments, vol 64, Island Press, Washington, DC

Dauer DM (1997) Dynamics of an estuarine ecosystem: long-term trends in the macrobenthic communities of Chesapeake Bay. Oceanologica Acta 20:291–298

Dauer DM, Alden III RW (1995) Long-term trends in the macrobenthos and water quality of the lower Chesapeake Bay (1985–1991). Marine Pollution Bulletin 30(12):840–850

Dauer DM, Ranasinghe JA, Weisberg SB (2000) Relationships between benthic community condition, water quality, sediment quality, nutrient loads, and land use patterns in Chesapeake Bay. Estuaries 23(1):80–96

De Cáceres M, Jansen F (2019) indicspecies: Relationship Between Species and Groups of Sites. URL https://CRAN.R-project.org/package=indicspecies, R package version 1.7.8

Deaton LE, Greenberg MJ (1986) There is no horohalinicum. Estuaries 9(1):20

Diaz RJ, Rosenberg R (1995) Marine benthic hypoxia: a review of its ecological effects and the behavioural responses of benthic macrofauna. Oceanography and Marine Biology An annual review 33:245–303

Ding H, Elmore AJ (2015) Spatio-temporal patterns in water surface temperature from Landsat time series data in the Chesapeake Bay, USA. Remote Sensing of Environment 168:335–348

Duffy JE, Cardinale BJ, France KE, McIntyre PB, Thébault E, Loreau M (2007) The functional role of biodiversity in ecosystems: incorporating trophic complexity. Ecology Letters 10(6):522–538

Dufrêne M, Legendre P (1997) Species assemblages and indicator species: the need for a flexible asymmetrical approach. Ecological Monographs 67(3):345–366

Friedrichs CT, Wright LD, Hepworth DA, Kim SC (2000) Bottom-boundary-layer processes associated with fine sediment accumulation in coastal seas and bays. Continental Shelf Research 20(7):807–841

Gallagher RV, Hughes L, Leishman MR (2013) Species loss and gain in communities under future climate change: consequences for functional diversity. Ecography 36(5):531–540

Giere O (2006) Ecology and biology of marine oligochaeta—an inventory rather than another review. Hydrobiologia 564(1):103–116

Greening H, Janicki A (2006) Toward reversal of eutrophic conditions in a subtropical estuary: water quality and seagrass response to nitrogen loading reductions in Tampa Bay, Florida, USA. Environmental Management 38(2):163–178

Hastie TJ, Tibshirani RJ (1990) Generalized Additive Models, 1st edn. Chapman & Hall/CRC, New York

Heemsbergen DA, Berg MP, Loreau M, Van Hal JR, Faber JH, Verhoef HA (2004) Biodiversity effects on soil processes explained by interspecific functional dissimilarity. Science 306(5698):1019–1020

Holland AF, Shaughnessy AT, Hiegel MH (1987) Long-term variation in mesohaline Chesapeake Bay macrobenthos: spatial and temporal patterns. Estuaries 10(3):227–245

Hooper DU, Chapin FS, Ewel JJ, Hector A, Inchausti P, Lavorel S, Lawton JH, Lodge DM, Loreau M, Naeem S, Schmid B, Setälä H, Symstad AJ, Vandermeer J, Wardle DA (2005) Effects of biodiversity on ecosystem functioning: a consensus of current knowledge. Ecological Monographs 75(1):3–35

Ihde TF, Houde ED, Bonzek CF, Franke E (2015) Assessing the Chesapeake Bay forage base: existing data and research priorities. Tech. Rep. 15-005, Chesapeake Bay Program Scientific and Technical Advisory Committee, Edgewater, MD

Irby ID, Friedrichs MAM, Da F, Hinson KE (2018) The competing impacts of climate change and nutrient reductions on dissolved oxygen in Chesapeake Bay. Biogeosciences 15(9):2649–2668

Johnson Z, Bennett M, Linker L, Julius S, Najjar R, Mitchell M, Montali D, Dixon R (2016) The development of climate projections for use in Chesapeake Bay Program assessments (16-006)

Karlson K, Rosenberg R, Bonsdorff E (2002) Temporal and spatial large-scale effects of eutrophication and oxygen deficiency on benthic fauna in Scandinavian and Baltic waters: a review. In: Gibson RN, Barnes M, Atkinson R (eds) Oceanography and Marine Biology: an Annual Review, vol 40, Taylor & Francis, New York

Kemp WM, Boynton WR, Adolf JE, Boesch DF, Boicourt WC, Brush G, Cornwell JC, Fisher TR, Glibert PM, Hagy JD, Harding LW, Houde ED, Kimmel DG, Miller WD, Newell RIE, Roman MR, Smith EM, Stevenson JC (2005) Eutrophication of Chesapeake Bay: historical trends and ecological interactions. Marine Ecology Progress Series 303:1–29

Lefcheck JS, Orth RJ, Dennison WC, Wilcox DJ, Murphy RR, Keisman J, Gurbisz C, Hannam M, Landry JB, Moore KA, Patrick CJ, Testa JM, Weller DE, Batiuk RA (2018) Long-term nutrient reductions lead to the unprecedented recovery of a temperate coastal region. Proceedings of the National Academy of Sciences 115(14):3658–3662

Leguendre P, Leguendre L (2012) Numerical Ecology, vol 24. Elsevier, Amsterdam, Netherlands

Levin LA, Ekau W, Gooday AJ, Jorissen F, Middelburg JJ, Naqvi SWA, Neira C, Rabalais NN, Zhang J (2009) Effects of natural and human-induced hypoxia on coastal benthos. Biogeosciences 6:2063–2098

Long WC, Seitz RD (2008) Trophic interactions under stress: hypoxia enhances foraging in an estuarine food web. Marine Ecology Progress Series 362:59–68

Lotze HK, Lenihan HS, Bourque BJ, Bradbury RH, Cooke RG, Kay MC, Kidwell SM, Kirby MX, Peterson CH, Jackson JBC (2006) Depletion, degradation, and recovery potential of estuaries and coastal seas. Science 312(5781):1806–1809

McArthur MA, Brooke BP, Przeslawski R, Ryan DA, Lucieer VL, Nichol S, McCallum AW, Mellin C, Cresswell ID, Radke LC (2010) On the use of abiotic surrogates to describe marine benthic biodiversity. Estuarine, Coastal and Shelf Science 88(1):21–32

Miller WD, Harding Jr LW (2007) Climate forcing of the spring bloom in Chesapeake Bay. Marine Ecology Progress Series 331:11–22

Najjar RG, Walker HA, Anderson PJ, Barron EJ, Bord RJ, Gibson JR, Kennedy VS, Knight CG, Megonigal JP, O'Connor RE, Polsky CD, Psuty NP, Richards BA, Sorenson LG, Steele EM, Swanson RS (2000) The potential impacts of climate change on the mid-Atlantic coastal region. Climate Research 14(3):219–233

Najjar RG, Pyke CR, Adams MB, Breitburg D, Hershner C, Kemp M, Howarth R, Mulholland MR, Paolisso M, Secor D, Sellner K, Wardrop D, Wood R (2010) Potential climate-change impacts on the Chesapeake Bay. Estuarine, Coastal and Shelf Science 86(1):1–20

Ni W, Li M, Ross AC, Najjar RG (2019) Large projected decline in dissolved oxygen in a eutrophic estuary due to climate change. Journal of Geophysical Research: Oceans 124(11):8271–8289

Nixon SW, Buckley BA (2002) "A strikingly rich zone"–nutrient enrichment and secondary production in coastal marine ecosystems. Estuaries 25(4):782–796

Norling K, Rosenberg R, Hulth S, Grémare A, Bonsdorff E (2007) Importance of functional biodiversity and species-specific traits of benthic fauna for ecosystem functions in marine sediment. Marine Ecology Progress Series 332:11–23

Oksanen J, Blanchet FG, Friendly M, Kindt R, Legendre P, McGlinn D, Minchin PR, O'Hara RB, Simpson GL, Solymos P, Stevens MHH, Szoecs E, Wagner H (2019) vegan: Community Ecology Package. URL https://CRAN.R-project.org/package=vegan, R package version 2.5-6

Orth RJ, Dennison WC, Lefcheck JS, Gurbisz C, Hannam M, Keisman J, Landry JB, Moore KA, Murphy RR, Patrick CJ, Testa J, Weller DE, Wilcox DJ (2017) Submersed aquatic vegetation in Chesapeake Bay: sentinel species in a changing world. Bioscience 67(8):698–712

Paerl HW (2006) Assessing and managing nutrient-enhanced eutrophication in estuarine and coastal waters: Interactive effects of human and climatic perturbations. Ecological Engineering 26(1):40–54

Palardy JE, Witman JD (2011) Water flow drives biodiversity by mediating rarity in marine benthic communities. Ecology Letters 14(1):63–68

Palardy JE, Witman JD (2014) Flow, recruitment limitation, and the maintenance of diversity in marine benthic communities. Ecology 95(2):286–297

Palmer MA, Allan JD, Butman CA (1996) Dispersal as a regional process affecting the local dynamics of marine and stream benthic invertebrates. Trends in Ecology & Evolution 11(8):322–326

Pielou EC (1974) Population and Community Ecology: Principles and Methods. CRC Press, New York

Quinn GP, Keough MJ (2003) Experimental design and data analysis for biologists. Cambridge University Press, Cambridge, UK

Rabalais NN, Turner RE, Wiseman Jr WJ (2002) Gulf of Mexico hypoxia, aka "the dead zone". Annual Review of Ecology and Systematics 33(1):235–263

Rabalais NN, Turner RE, Díaz RJ, Justić D (2009) Global change and eutrophication of coastal waters. ICES Journal of Marine Science 66(7):1528–1537

Remane A (1934) Die brackwasserfauna. Verhandlungen Der Deutschen Zoologischen Gesellschaft 36:34–74

Reynoldson TB (1987) The role of environmental factors in the ecology of tubificid oligochaetes: an experimental study. Ecography 10(4):241–248

Riedel B, Zuschin M, Stachowitsch M (2012) Tolerance of benthic macrofauna to hypoxia and anoxia in shallow coastal seas: a realistic scenario. Marine Ecology Progress Series 458:39–52

Rosenberg R (2001) Marine benthic faunal successional stages and related sedimentary activity. Scientia Marina 65(S2):107–119

Scavia D, Field JC, Boesch DF, Buddemeier RW, Burkett V, Cayan DR, Fogarty M, Harwell MA, Howarth RW, Mason C, Reed DJ, Royer TC,

Sallenger AH, Titus JG (2002) Climate change impacts on US coastal and marine ecosystems. Estuaries 25(2):149–164

Schaffner LC, Dellapenna TM, Hinchey EK, Friedrichs CT, Neubauer MT, Smith ME, Kuehl SA (2001) Physical energy regimes, seabed dynamics and organism-sediment interactions along an estuarine gradient. In: Aller JY, Woodin SA, Aller RC (eds) Organism-Sediment Interactions, University of South Carolina Press, Columbia, SC, 159–179

Schratzberger M, Ingels J (2018) Meiofauna matters: the roles of meiofauna in benthic ecosystems. Journal of Experimental Marine Biology and Ecology 502:12–25

Seitz RD, Dauer DM, Llansó RJ, Long WC (2009) Broad-scale effects of hypoxia on benthic community structure in Chesapeake Bay, USA. Journal of Experimental Marine Biology and Ecology 381:S4–S12

Solan M, Cardinale BJ, Downing AL, Engelhardt KAM, Ruesink JL, Srivastava DS (2004) Extinction and ecosystem function in the marine benthos. Science 306(5699):1177–1180

Stora G, Arnoux A (1983) Effects of large freshwater diversions on benthos of a Mediterranean lagoon. Estuaries 6(2):115–125

Sturdivant SK, Brush MJ, Diaz RJ (2013) Modeling the effect of hypoxia on macrobenthos production in the lower Rappahannock River, Chesapeake Bay, USA. PloS One 8(12):e84140

Sturdivant SK, Díaz RJ, Llansó R, Dauer DM (2014) Relationship between hypoxia and macrobenthic production in Chesapeake Bay. Estuaries and Coasts 37(5):1219–1232

Taylor DI, Oviatt CA, Borkman DG (2011) Non-linear responses of a coastal aquatic ecosystem to large decreases in nutrient and organic loadings. Estuaries and Coasts 34(4):745–757

ter Braak CJF (1986) Canonical correspondence analysis: a new eigenvector technique for multivariate direct gradient analysis. Ecology 67(5):1167–1179

Testa JM, Kemp WM (2014) Spatial and temporal patterns of winter–spring oxygen depletion in Chesapeake Bay bottom water. Estuaries and Coasts 37(6):1432–1448

Testa JM, Murphy RR, Brady DC, Kemp WM (2018) Nutrient- and climate-induced shifts in the phenology of linked biogeochemical cycles in a temperate estuary. Frontiers in Marine Science 5:114

Tilman D (2001) Functional diversity. In: Levin S (ed) Encyclopedia of Biodiversity, vol 3, Academic Press, San Diego, CA, 587–596

Törnroos A, Bonsdorff E, Bremner J, Blomqvist M, Josefson AB, Garcia C, Warzocha J (2015) Marine benthic ecological functioning over decreasing taxonomic richness. Journal of Sea Research 98:49–56

Tsikopoulou I, Moraitis ML, Geropoulos A, Papadopoulou KN, Papageorgiou N, Plaiti W, Smith CJ, Karakassis I, Eleftheriou A (2019) Long-term changes in the structure of benthic communities: revisiting a sampling transect in Crete after 24 years. Marine Environmental Research 144:9–19

Tucker J, Giblin AE, Hopkinson CS, Kelsey SW, Howes BL (2014) Response of benthic metabolism and nutrient cycling to reductions in wastewater loading to Boston Harbor, USA. Estuarine, Coastal and Shelf Science 151:54–68

Vaquer-Sunyer R, Duarte CM (2010) Sulfide exposure accelerates hypoxia-driven mortality. Limnology and Oceanography 55(3):1075–1082

Vaquer-Sunyer R, Duarte CM (2011) Temperature effects on oxygen thresholds for hypoxia in marine benthic organisms. Global Change Biology 17(5):1788–1797

Wagenmakers EJ, Farrell S (2004) AIC model selection using Akaike weights. Psychonomic Bulletin & Review 11(1):192–196

Wagner CM (1999) Expression of the estuarine species minimum in littoral fish assemblages of the lower Chesapeake Bay tributaries. Estuaries 22(2):304–312

Waldbusser GG, Marinelli RL, Whitlatch RB, Visscher PT (2004) The effects of infaunal biodiversity on biogeochemistry of coastal marine sediments. Limnology and Oceanography 49(5):1482–1492

Weslawski JM, Snelgrove PVR, Levin LA, Austen MC, Kneib RT, Iliffe TM, Carey JR, Hawkins SJ, Whitlatch RB (2004) Marine sedimentary biota as providers of ecosystem goods and services. In: Sustaining Biodiversity and Ecosystem Services in Soils and Sediment, Island Press, Washington, DC, 73–98

Wilberg MJ, Livings ME, Barkman JS, Morris BT, Robinson JM (2011) Overfishing, disease, habitat loss, and potential extirpation of oysters in upper Chesapeake Bay. Marine Ecology Progress Series 436:131–144

Wingate RL, Secor DH (2008) Effects of winter temperature and flow on a summer-fall nursery fish assemblage in the Chesapeake Bay, Maryland. Transactions of the American Fisheries Society 137(4):1147–1156

Wood CM (2018) The fallacy of the P_{crit} – are there more useful alternatives? Journal of Experimental Biology 221(22):jeb163717

Woodland RJ, Houde ED, Buchheister A, Latour RJ, Lozano C, Fabrizio MC, Tuckey T, Sweetman C (2017) Environmental, spatial and temporal patterns in Chesapeake Bay forage population distributions and predator consumption. Final Report to Chesapeake Bay Trust. University of Maryland Center for Environmental Science Chesapeake Biological Laboratory, Solomons, MD

Woodland RJ, Warry FY, Zhu Y, Mac Nally R, Reich P, Jenkins GP, Brehm D, Cook PLM (2019) Role of benthic habitat structure and riverine connectivity in controlling the spatial distribution and ecology of estuarine fish. Marine Ecology Progress Series 630:197–214

Zettler ML, Friedland R, Gogina M, Darr A (2017) Variation in benthic long-term data of transitional waters: Is interpretation more than speculation? PloS One 12(4):e0175746

Zhang Q, Brady DC, Boynton WR, Ball WP (2015) Long-term trends of nutrients and sediment from the nontidal Chesapeake Watershed: an assessment of progress by river and season. Journal of the American Water Resources Association 51(6):1534–1555

Zhang Q, Murphy RR, Tian R, Forsyth MK, Trentacoste EM, Keisman J, Tango PJ (2018) Chesapeake Bay's water quality condition has been recovering: Insights from a multimetric indicator assessment of thirty years of tidal monitoring data. Science of the Total Environment 637:1617–1625

6

Using Structural Comparisons to Measure the Behavior of Complex Systems

Ryan E. Langendorf
University of Colorado, Boulder, CO, USA

CONTENTS

6.1	Introduction	123
6.2	Data	125
6.3	Network alignment	126
6.4	Visualization	127
6.5	Example: the Chesapeake Bay	128
6.6	Critical considerations	130
6.7	Recipe	132
	6.7.1 Ingredients	132
	6.7.2 Step 1/3: Data	132
	6.7.3 Step 2/3: Network alignment	133
	6.7.4 Step 3/3: Visualization	134
6.8	Final thought	135
References		135

6.1 Introduction

Do complex systems need protection? Many of the conservation challenges we expect to face in this century will involve not only declining species, but degrading ecosystems (Montoya and Raffaelli, 2010). To protect such complex systems we need measures of their behavior that we can monitor. This includes changes in the numbers of their components but also in the structures of interactions connecting them. This chapter explores one way to track these systemic structures using a network alignment approach applied to the Chesapeake Bay ecosystem.

The intuition here is that many of the systems we care about have emergent functioning not simply ascribed to their structure. Consider an ecosystem's structure and its collective set of interactions, analogous to the rules of a game. Then, its functioning is an instance of the game being played (Odum, 1964). As with human consciousness, complex system functioning emerges from underlying structure, but is more than the sum of these structural parts. And, because of this, they cannot be entirely understood by reduction.

Emergent functioning sounds abstract and even fantastical but has been debated by ecologists going back to Clements's holism (Clements, 1905) and Gleason's individualism (Gleason, 1927). One of the more salient demonstrations of emergent ecological functioning comes from a series of colonization experiments conducted by Simberloff and Wilson in the 1960s when they defaunated six small mangrove islands in Florida Bay (Simberloff and Wilson, 1969). The trophic structures originally present on the islands were reestablished but with different species. It may be that these structures are themselves causal such that their components, say species in an ecosystem, depend on them being in a specific state (Langendorf and Doak, 2019). Recognizing this, there have been calls to protect systemic properties like species (Tylianakis et al, 2010), and some actual legislation that does so (Auditor-General, 2007). It is a recognition that tracking systems by individually watching components of them can fail to usefully capture their functioning, and as a result yields shorter and less accurate predictions. We must instead try to describe changes in the system's behavior as a whole.

Our planet's biosphere is one of these emergent systems. It is comprised of components interacting in stochastic and chaotic ways across orders of space and time. On top of this complexity, these component variables are simultaneously and differently being affected by human activity, directly and as a result of climatic changes. To write effective climate policy we need accurate and specific ecological predictions, which have been elusive because of the degree to which the planet's climate and biosphere are emergent systems.

We can do better by first improving the way we measure systemic behavior. Scientists are already tracking many of our planet's components individually, looking for harmful deteriorations. What if we also tracked systemic properties? As you will see in this chapter, this would not require additional observations, only some computation and a willingness to consider that, as Ulanowicz (2012) put it, the "development [of complex systems] was not entirely determined by events and entities at smaller scales."

Check today's weather forecast. Mine lists the temperature highs for the coming week: 92°F, 87°F, 81°F, 82°F, 84°F, 87°F, and 79°F. Google even plots these numbers for me as a line showing how it will gradually cool down in the coming days. Imagine visualizing the functioning of an entire ecosystem in the same way. We could then watch as it changed, tracking the challenges we face and the successes of our interventions. So far this has remained elusive, despite a long history of attempts to invent a thermometer for systems that can reduce systemic structures and their dynamics to a single easily tracked number (e.g., Ulanowicz, 2012).

This chapter demonstrates a way of creating a thermometer for complex systems, which is possible if we consider relative measures of system dynamics that have no scale (e.g., degrees Celsius). One way to do this is make pairwise comparisons of every pair of observations. With data stored as a table (e.g., a spreadsheet), with columns of variables and rows of observations, we can calculate the Euclidean distance between each pair of rows. The meaning of these distances is less intuitive, but we can still use them to understand the system's behavior, from identifying rare observations to destabilizing trends that can result in critical transitions. The rest of this chapter shows one way to do this.

6.2 Data

To measure changes in systems we must have systemic data. Networks are a natural choice for systemic data:

1. Networks are visually intuitive. This makes it easier to collaborate with people from different backgrounds and with different goals.
2. Speaking of collaboration, almost all other kinds of systemic data can be translated into a network. Networks are such a general framework that they tend to be not only intuitive but also applicable.
3. Network science has become a large and robust field distinct from graph theory with a whole suite of tools designed to tackle practical questions about networks.

Let's spend a moment on the building blocks of networks. Having an intuition for their design will be helpful throughout this chapter, and will help you envision how to adapt these ideas to your own needs.

At their core, networks are really a way of encoding interactions. Because of this, every network has two kinds of components: nodes (interacting variables) and edges (their interactions). Use the toy ecosystem in Figure 6.1 as an example.

Each variable in the system is assigned to a node (also called a vertex in graph theory). Here each variable is a species, but the variables can be anything, even combinations of observations or unobserved latent variables. While the example in Figure 6.1 does not show it, nodes can have quantities, such as the number of individuals of each of the four species.

The edges, the other component of a network, are the interactions between the nodes. These are represented by arrows, each connecting a pair of nodes. Notice that edges can be unidirectional or bidirectional. We could also add weight to these interactions, to distinguish stronger ones. We could even turn each edge into a function where the interaction's strength varies through time, or with changes in the rest of the network's composition. In this way networks can describe most systems.

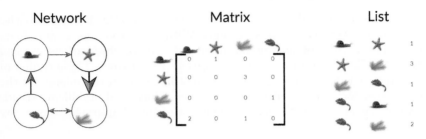

FIGURE 6.1: Example of systemic data, showing how networks are equivalent to matrices and lists of interactions. Note that arrows can represent any kind of interaction, in this case competition rather than trophic relationships.

As Figure 6.1 illustrates, networks are one of three ways to encode systemic data. The same system can also be stored as a matrix or a list of interactions. Each has advantages: Networks help us visually learn about a system. Matrices are amenable to powerful mathematics, as the rest of this chapter will show. And, lists are efficient. This may seem trivial but for large systems like social media or even the internet, storing information efficiently matters.

6.3 Network alignment

You may be hung up on the thought *Why can't we just use changes in the individual variables to track changes in the system at large?*, thinking *How wrong will we really be if we stick to measuring changes in individual variables?*. Unfortunately, we cannot know in general because the answer is context-dependent. This is an area of research in need of attention, in large part because macrobiologists are still debating the merits of reductionism. Component variables, especially those correlated with many of the system's other variables, will surely change as the whole system changes. They just may not give much insight into the functioning of the system, or offer early warning signs of critical transitions (Scheffer et al, 2012).

So then, how can we measure a system's behavior? Rather than try to distill its important structures and functions down to a single number, what if we merely compare it to itself through time? This relative way of measuring system behavior works by building an image of the system's behavior one comparison at a time. These comparisons can involve any two networks, so we can also include spatial replicates of the same system, or even entirely different systems, as we map their functioning relativistically. The best way I have found to do this is with network alignment.

Network alignment is a class of methods designed to turn two networks (or matrices, or tables; Figure 6.1) into a single number. This number, the alignment score, is usually a nonnegative member of the real numbers $\mathbb{R}$, being no less than zero but having no upper bound. An alignment score of zero means the two networks are identical, though not usually as a mathematical isomorphism (Fortin, 1996). Large alignment scores mean the two networks are somehow different. What "somehow" means varies tremendously, and matters tremendously. These methods are trying to measure the distance between two networks. If that distance is not Euclidean, what is it?

Here I have used my own network alignment. It is a free R package called `netcom` (Langendorf, 2017, R Core Team, 2017). There are many other network alignments (see Clark and Kalita, 2014, for a comparative review), but `netcom` is particularly relevant to our goal of measuring systemic change because it was designed to capture differences in how networks function as opposed to patterns in their layout. It works by comparing the dynamics of diffusion originating from each node in a pair of networks. Note however that `netcom` alignments are not a mathematical distance metric. The resulting state space of distances between networks may be distorted in non-Euclidean ways, such as triangles between three networks having sides with impossible lengths (e.g., a hypotenuse longer than the sum of the other two sides).

Consider network alignment as trying to compare two hypothetical cities of houses connected by roads. The approach implemented here is to pairwise compare each house with those in the other city by creating a house-specific signature. This is accomplished by quantifying the predictability of the location of a person at various times after they left their house, assuming they move randomly. This predictability across all houses captures much of the way each city is organized and functions. `netcom` aligns networks using this conceptual rationale, with nodes as houses, edges as roads, and random diffusion representing people leaving their houses and walking around the city to other houses.

6.4 Visualization

Network alignment produces a giant distance matrix. Let's call this matrix D for distances, as in (6.2) in the second step of the recipe at the end of this chapter. D is a square matrix where each element is a number, denoted by its location in row r and column c. This number is the distance between the two networks r and c. The diagonal of D will always be all zeros because the distance between a network and itself is zero (they are the same thing). In the case of `netcom`, D is also symmetric across its diagonal, because the distance between the two networks r and c is the same regardless of which network you start measuring from. Just note that not all network alignments are commutative.

Distance matrices like D are a powerful kind of data. For our purposes, they contain the information we need to plot the behavior of the system being

128   *Structural Comparisons of Complex Systems*

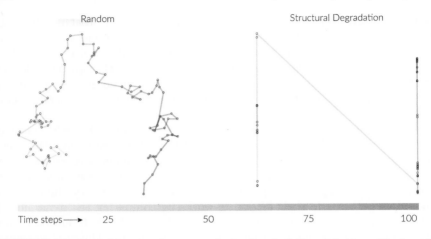

FIGURE 6.2: Two dynamical systems being tracked through time. Each point in each panel is a network representation of their respective systems. Closer points are times when the system functioned more similarly as measured by the network aligner `netcom` (Langendorf, 2017).

studied with network alignment. We can do this using a class of methods called ordination, which turn high-dimensional data into a smaller number of dimensions, typically two. This is tremendously powerful. It allows us to plot an arbitrary number of networks in fewer dimensions using their pairwise distances in the alignment matrix D. In these plots, closer points are more similar, just as you would expect. Note though that ordination is almost never perfect, distorting some of the distances to fit into the smaller number of dimensions, but it lets us visualize changes between networks, allowing plots of systemic behavior.

Figure 6.2 shows example visualizations of system behavior. Both panels show a single network changing through 100 time steps. The one on the left is changing randomly, moving around in the two-dimensional ordination space reminiscent of a particle undergoing Brownian motion. The system on the right is a community with a rich-get-richer structure called preferential attachment (Newman, 2001) that is being randomly scrambled at each time step. This structural degradation eventually tips the system into an alternate functional state.

6.5   Example: the Chesapeake Bay

The Chesapeake Bay is a wonderful example of a complex dynamical ecosystem that we would like to monitor for signs of ecological deterioration. Not

Example: the Chesapeake Bay

only is it an important protected natural resource, but "nineteen physical, chemical and biological characteristics are monitored [up to] 20 times a year in the Bay's mainstem and many tributaries" (Huang et al, 2018, Testa et al, 2019). Can we use this data to understand the Bay's dynamics? How are different parts of it changing? Which are most at risk of degrading?

Figure 6.3 shows the behavior of the Bay at a single water quality monitoring station, TF1.6. The left panel shows the dynamics of eight common measures of water quality recorded at the surface near this station from 1985 to 2015. The right panel shows the dynamics of these data altogether as a system inferred with network alignment. Just as in Figure 6.2, closer points are more similar instances of the Bay as it functions at that water quality monitoring station.

Notice the way the monthly deviations became more extreme over time (darker colors are more recent observations). This is evidence that the Bay near the TF1.6 station is becoming unstable, despite each individual measure of water quality appearing stable (left panel of Figure 6.3). Had we not considered the dynamics of the Bay systemically, with network alignment, we would not have noticed this increasing instability in its functioning near station TF1.6. This is because the instability is not in any individual measure, but in the relationships between them. We cannot know if this instability portends functional deterioration or productive growth, but as a hypothesis generator network alignment has identified a station in need of more attention. Either way, not all stations appear to be increasingly unstable. Figure 6.4 shows two other stations that are alongside two that are becoming more stable.

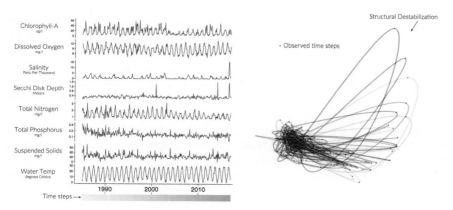

FIGURE 6.3: The dynamics of water quality monitoring station TF1.6. **Left:** Eight monthly measures of surface water quality recorded at observation station TF1.6 from 1985 to 2015. This "Tidal Fresh" station is upstream of the main part of the Chesapeake Bay (see Figure 6.5), near to where freshwater sources discharge into the Bay. **Right:** Points are observations. Closer points are dates when that part of the Bay functioned more similarly. Time progresses from lighter to darker colors, identically in both panels.

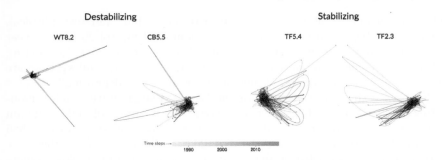

FIGURE 6.4: Monitoring stations in the Chesapeake Bay with destabilizing (left) and stabilizing (right) dynamics.

This kind of inference can generate tremendous quantities of data because the number of unique pairs of networks grows proportional to the square of the number of data points. For this chapter I aligned 1.14 billion pairs of networks, consisting of 360 months of data at each of the 133 monitoring stations. The smallest list form of this much data occupies 26 gigabytes. Altogether these distances describe dynamics across the entire Chesapeake Bay at a high resolution. Figure 6.5 is an example of this, plotting the change in variability of all 133 water quality monitoring stations from 1985 through 2014.

The Chesapeake Bay appears less stable (largest circles) closer to land, possibly responding more acutely to sediment and nutrient inputs from freshwater discharges than the larger open parts of the Bay farther south where the water comes from many of these freshwater sources. However, some of the variability in the less stable upper parts of the bay seem to be stabilizing (bluer circles). An example of this is the water stemming from stations up north by Washington D.C., which travels south near Fort Hunt and Alexandria. Why is the water quality stabilizing there but destabilizing in the more northern parts of the bay, despite both being variable? Why is the water near Newport and Norfolk similarly stabilizing despite higher variability? And, why is the bay destabilizing more on the western side of its most northern parts? Future work is needed to answer these questions, and contextualize previous descriptions of the Bay's dynamics and their drivers (Lefcheck et al, 2018, Testa et al, 2018, 2019, Zhang et al, 2018). In this way, using structural comparisons to measure the behavior of complex systems can help us identify where and how to intervene.

6.6 Critical considerations

The value of measuring systemic change is that it tracks dynamics not entirely captured by any individual constituent component. How then can we know

Critical considerations 131

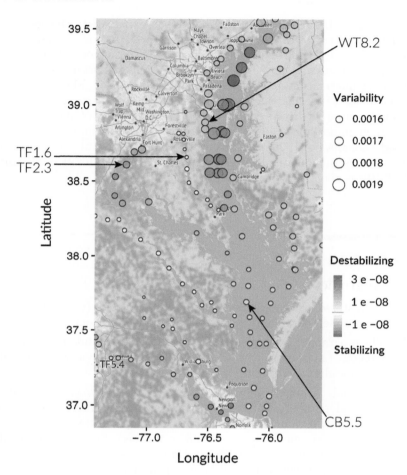

FIGURE 6.5: Chesapeake Bay water quality monitoring stations. The size of each station is proportional to the standard deviation of the dynamics at that station from 1985 through 2014. The color is the change of this variation in the station's dynamics across these 30 years.

if changes we see in a systemic variable are real? If none of the component variables have changed, is it justifiable to intervene? I have not found an entirely satisfying answer. We will have to validate these kinds of systemic measures well enough that we can trust their inference in novel systems. In the meantime, given that we can infer them without additional observations, why not combine systemic measures with what we are already monitoring? One of the great lessons from the growth in machine learning is that ensemble methods are the best predictors (Dietterich, 2000).

Prediction is becoming more important than explanation, thanks to that machine learning growth but also a growing need for quick management decisions. Even so, good explanations remain better at out-of-sample prediction (Meinshausen et al, 2016). To this end, it is important to be careful in ascribing mechanisms to dynamics in alignment space. Measuring a system's behavior as in this chapter is meant to be hypothesis generating. As an example, putative drivers can be regressed against axes of alignment space to test their importance the way axes from Principal Component Analyses are used (Zonana et al, 2019). More work is also underway to improve the network reconstruction step. Research in causal inference, for example Runge et al (2019), is one of the best examples of this.

6.7 Recipe

6.7.1 Ingredients

1. Data stored as a table where columns are variables (the first can be dates/time points) and rows are observations of them.
2. The programming language R (R Core Team, 2017) and the package netcom (Langendorf, 2017). You can of course use any method of network alignment in any language you like.
3. (optional) A supercomputer to run everything in parallel. I recommend parallel computing if your system has more than 1000 variables. The number of variables in your system (columns in the data) matters more than the number of observations (rows), but if you have more than 1000 observations of a system with even 100 variables, parallelization will be indispensable.

6.7.2 Step 1/3: Data

There is a caveat to this entire chapter: you need systemic data in the first place. Remember that the data types in Figure 6.1 are all of interactions. Unfortunately, most data are not. Most databases are filled with the values of variables through space and time, not the interactions between them. This is not accidental. Interactions are far harder to measure.

Causal inference is perhaps the most promising kind of approach to this problem of inferring interactions from observational time series data. I recommend Runge et al (2019) as an introduction to the science of causality. (Also, see Chapter 7 discussing causality analysis of climate and ecosystem time series.) However, these methods are challenging and, I think, not to be squeezed in here.

Instead, I used weighted correlations between each variable to infer the series of Chesapeake Bay networks, one for each observation, using the R package Hmisc (Harrell Jr et al, 2019). The edges in each network are correlation coefficients, but with every other observation weighted based on how similar the variables are to the focal observation. There is actually a precedent for this kind of weighting method being used to generate a time series of networks (Deyle et al, 2016). The resulting networks certainly contain many edges that are type I errors (also known as "false positive"), but likely few type II (also known as "false negative"). Moreover, the type I edges are probably indirect interactions or variables with a common driver. Including them in the network is unlikely to indicate an entirely different kind of systemic functioning. Below is an example of R code that creates a list of correlation networks.

```
# This code assumes you have a table/dataframe/tibble named data
# where columns are variables and rows are observations
variables <- colnames(data)
networks <- replicate(nrow(data),
                      matrix(0,
                             nrow = length(variables),
                             ncol = length(variables),
                             dimnames = list(variables,
                                             variables)),
                      simplify = FALSE)
theta <- 10

for (observation in 1:nrow(data)) {
    distances <- Rfast::dista(data[observation,],
                              data,
                              type = "euclidean")
    weights <- exp(-theta * distances) / mean(distances)
    net <- stats::cov.wt(data,
                         wt = as.numeric(weights),
                         cor = TRUE)
    networks[[observation]] <- net$cor
}
```

6.7.3 Step 2/3: Network alignment

All network alignments were calculated using the *align* function in the R package netcom (Langendorf, 2017) with the *align* function. By looping through each pair of networks we can compute a matrix of alignments like D in (6.2) which is defined after the following code:

```
D <- matrix(NA,
            nrow = length(networks),
            ncol = length(networks))

for (row in 1:nrow(D)) {
```

```
        for (col in 1:ncol(D)) {
            if (col > row) {
                D <- netcom::align(networks[[row]],
                                   networks[[col]],
                                   base = 2,
                                   characterization = "entropy",
                                   normalization = FALSE)
                D[row, col] = network_alignment$score
                D[col, row] = network_alignment$score
            }
        }
    }
}
```

If you are curious, the mechanics of this network alignment algorithm, which are conceptually akin to flow algorithms and Laplacian dynamics (Latham II, 2006), can be analytically expressed as a Markov chain (matrix A) raised to successive powers which are the durations of diffusion. `netcom` then uses the normalized entropy in (6.1), where the denominator is the entropy H (Shannon, 2001) of a set of 1's with length N_x equal to the number of nodes in network x, to compare the predictability of diffusion emanating from each node n in each network x at each time step t spreading across all the j nodes in the network:

$$S_{x_{n,t}} = \frac{-\sum_{j=1}^{N_x} A_{x_{n,j}}^{(t)} \ln\left(A_{x_{n,j}}^{(t)}\right)}{H(\mathbf{1}^{N_x})}. \tag{6.1}$$

A distance matrix D gets created with the numerically integrated differences between every pair of nodes' entropy-over-time curves where rows (a) are nodes in one network and columns (b) are nodes in the other network:

$$D_{ab} = \sqrt{\sum_{t \in T} \left(S_{x_{1_a,t}} - S_{x_{2_b,t}}\right)^2}. \tag{6.2}$$

The Hungarian algorithm (Kuhn, 1955) is then used to find the optimal way to pair each node in each network with at most one node in the other network.

6.7.4 Step 3/3: Visualization

Plots like Figures 6.3 and 6.4 showing the dynamics of systemic data involve ordination to reduce the pairwise distances between any number of observations to as few as three visible dimensions. This can be accomplished with the *metaMDS* function in the R package `vegan` (Oksanen et al, 2019).

```
ordination <- vegan::metaMDS(D, k = 2)
```

You can then plot the systemic dynamics using the R package `ggplot2` (Wickham, 2016).

```
ggplot(ordination) + geom_path(aes(x = MDS1, y = MDS2))
```

6.8 Final thought

Intervention ought to be a dynamic process with real-time inference based on continuously updating data. Pairwise comparing the structure of a system as it changes through time (or space) can make us more effective managers. In this era of change, efficiency matters. Too many complex systems are changing too quickly for us to support them equally. The goal then should be to get better at identifying behaviors of systems in need of our help.

References

Auditor-General (2007) The conservation and protection of national threatened species and ecological communities. Tech. Rep. 31 of 2006–07, Australian National Audit Office, Canberra, Australia

Clark C, Kalita J (2014) A comparison of algorithms for the pairwise alignment of biological networks. Bioinformatics 30(16):2351–2359

Clements FE (1905) Research Methods in Ecology. University Publishing Company, Lincoln, NE

Deyle ER, May RM, Munch SB, Sugihara G (2016) Tracking and forecasting ecosystem interactions in real time. Proceedings of the Royal Society B: Biological Sciences 283(1822):20152258

Dietterich TG (2000) Ensemble methods in machine learning. In: International Workshop on Multiple Classifier Systems, Springer, Berlin, Heidelberg, 1–15

Fortin S (1996) The graph isomorphism problem. Tech. Rep. TR96-20, The University of Alberta, Edmonton, AB, Canada

Gleason HA (1927) Further views on the succession-concept. Ecology 8(3):299–326

Harrell Jr FE, Dupont C, et al (2019) Hmisc: Harrell Miscellaneous. URL https://CRAN.R-project.org/package=Hmisc, R package version 4.3-0

Huang X, Iliev IR, Lyubchich V, Gel YR (2018) Riding down the bay: Space-time clustering of ecological trends. Environmetrics 29(5-6):e2455

Kuhn HW (1955) The Hungarian method for the assignment problem. Naval Research Logistics Quarterly 2(1-2):83–97

Langendorf RE (2017) netcom: Dynamic Network Alignment. URL https://CRAN.R-project.org/package=netcom, R package version 1.0.4

Langendorf RE, Doak DF (2019) Can community structure causally determine dynamics of constituent species? A test using a host-parasite community. The American Naturalist 194(3):E66–E80

Latham II LG (2006) Network flow analysis algorithms. Ecological Modelling 192(3-4):586–600

Lefcheck JS, Orth RJ, Dennison WC, Wilcox DJ, Murphy RR, Keisman J, Gurbisz C, Hannam M, Landry JB, Moore KA, Patrick CJ, Testa JM, Weller DE, Batiuk RA (2018) Long-term nutrient reductions lead to the unprecedented recovery of a temperate coastal region. Proceedings of the National Academy of Sciences 115(14):3658–3662

Meinshausen N, Hauser A, Mooij JM, Peters J, Versteeg P, Bühlmann P (2016) Methods for causal inference from gene perturbation experiments and validation. Proceedings of the National Academy of Sciences 113(27):7361–7368

Montoya JM, Raffaelli D (2010) Climate change, biotic interactions and ecosystem services. Philosophical Transactions of the Royal Society B: Biological Sciences 365(1549):2013–2018

Newman ME (2001) Clustering and preferential attachment in growing networks. Physical Review E 64(2):025102

Odum EP (1964) The new ecology. BioScience 14(7):14–16

Oksanen J, Blanchet FG, Friendly M, Kindt R, Legendre P, McGlinn D, Minchin PR, O'Hara RB, Simpson GL, Solymos P, Stevens MHH, Szoecs E, Wagner H (2019) vegan: Community Ecology Package. URL https://CRAN.R-project.org/package=vegan, R package version 2.5-6

R Core Team (2017) R: A Language and Environment for Statistical Computing. R Foundation for Statistical Computing, Vienna, Austria, URL https://www.R-project.org/

Runge J, Bathiany S, Bollt E, Camps-Valls G, Coumou D, Deyle E, Glymour C, Kretschmer M, Mahecha MD, Muñoz-Marí J, van Nes EH, Peters J, Quax R, Reichstein M, Scheffer M, Schölkopf B, Spirtes P, Sugihara G, Sun J, Zhang K, Zscheischler J (2019) Inferring causation from time series in Earth system sciences. Nature Communications 10(1):2553

Scheffer M, Carpenter SR, Lenton TM, Bascompte J, Brock W, Dakos V, Van De Koppel J, Van De Leemput IA, Levin SA, Van Nes EH, Pascual M, Vandermeer J (2012) Anticipating critical transitions. Science 338(6105):344–348

Shannon CE (2001) A mathematical theory of communication. ACM SIGMOBILE Mobile Computing and Communications Review 5(1):3–55

Simberloff DS, Wilson EO (1969) Experimental zoogeography of islands: the colonization of empty islands. Ecology 50(2):278–296

Testa JM, Murphy RR, Brady DC, Kemp WM (2018) Nutrient-and climate-induced shifts in the phenology of linked biogeochemical cycles in a temperate estuary. Frontiers in Marine Science 5:114

Testa JM, Lyubchich V, Zhang Q (2019) Patterns and trends in Secchi disk depth over three decades in the Chesapeake Bay estuarine complex. Estuaries and Coasts 42(4):927–943

Tylianakis JM, Laliberté E, Nielsen A, Bascompte J (2010) Conservation of species interaction networks. Biological Conservation 143(10):2270–2279

Ulanowicz RE (2012) Growth and Development: Ecosystems Phenomenology. Springer, New York

Wickham H (2016) ggplot2: Elegant Graphics for Data Analysis. Springer-Verlag, New York

Zhang Q, Tango PJ, Murphy RR, Forsyth MK, Tian R, Keisman J, Trentacoste EM (2018) Chesapeake Bay dissolved oxygen criterion attainment deficit: three decades of temporal and spatial patterns. Frontiers in Marine Science 5:422

Zonana DM, Gee JM, Bridge ES, Breed MD, Doak DF (2019) Assessing behavioral associations in a hybrid zone through social network analysis: Complex assortative behaviors structure associations in a hybrid quail population. The American Naturalist 193(6):852–865

7

Causality Analysis of Climate and Ecosystem Time Series

Mohammad Gorji Sefidmazgi
Charlotte, NC, USA

Ali Gorji Sefidmazgi
Rasht, Guilan, Iran

CONTENTS

7.1	Introduction	139
7.2	Methods of causality detection	141
	7.2.1 Granger causality	141
	7.2.2 Nonlinear state space methods	143
	7.2.3 Causal graphical models	145
7.3	Simulations	149
	7.3.1 Simulated data	150
	7.3.2 Arctic and the midlatitude jet stream	152
	7.3.3 Sardine–anchovy and sea surface temperature	155
7.4	Conclusions	157
References	....	159

7.1 Introduction

Identifying causal relationships among multiple variables and direction/strength of these causal links are key challenges in the analysis of complex dynamical systems. Statistical correlation and regression analysis have been important tools in understanding the relationships in social and environmental systems. However, these tools are not adequate for finding stimulus–response mechanisms. A well-known statement is that *correlation does not imply causation*. For example, correlation between variables A and B might be created in three scenarios of causal relationships, that is, A is a cause of B, B is a cause of A, or a third variable C is the cause of both A and B. If two variables are causally related (for example, A causes B: $A \to B$), a change in A must produce a change in B. Unlike symmetry in correlation, the causal relation

$A \to B$ does not imply $B \to A$. Therefore, a statistical correlation is necessary but not sufficient to make a claim of causality.

Interventional studies make it possible to discover causal links by changing the state of a variable and observing its effect on the system. Unlike medical or social systems, such an experiment is not possible for real environmental systems. But physical models of climate system such as *general circulation model (GCM)* can be used for such an experiment (see a brief overview of such models in Chapter 1). However, GCMs are simplified representations of real-world systems and are affected by both numerical and physical modeling errors. Any causal link extracted from GCMs might be inaccurate due to these uncertainties (Hannart et al, 2016). Thus, the main focus of causality analysis is on the observational type of methods based on the data-driven approaches. Since most of environmental data are in the form of time series, causality analysis for time series is an important problem in this area.

The causality problem can be defined as detecting the cause-effect relationship between two variables. Generally, two types of bivariate causal structure can be found in real-world systems. In *recursive schemes*, the response variable of a system, A, acts as a stimulus variable of a system, B, that follows A in a chain. Here, we say that A is the cause of B or $A \to B$ (Figure 7.1(a)). In a *feedback loop* structure, there is also a regulation between B and A (Figure 7.1(b)). In this case, the causal link represented by $A \leftrightarrow B$ is bidirectional and there is an interdependence between A and B (Barbieri, 2013). Such a bivariate analysis might lead to incorrect conclusions, because additional confounding factors that might exist in complex systems are not taken into account in the causality analysis. This bivariate definition should be extended to a multivariate case by considering additional variables.

A common approach of bivariate causality detection is Granger method (Granger, 1969) which is based on prediction improvement in regression models between two time series. Pearl (1988) proposed the use of graphical models to represent probabilistic independence relationships between variables. The Granger method was also incorporated into graphical models for multivariate time series regression models known as graphical Granger models (Arnold et al, 2007). A *causal network* between a set of features $X_1, \ldots, X_p$ is defined as a directed graph over the features, in which each edge represents the causal effect. Lack of an edge between a pair of features does imply that the two features are conditionally independent, given some subset of the other features. For the case of time series, each edge might be labeled with a natural number called the *lag* of the edge representing the time delay between cause and effect features. A lag of k between $X_i \to X_j$ means that $X_i(t-k)$ has a causal effect on $X_j(t)$ (Figure 7.1(c)). For the time series generated from complex dynamical systems, the goal is to find causal links and their associated time lags. These lags might be in the range of days or months for different climate variables.

Causal discovery methods have already been applied extensively in many fields such as social sciences, econometric, engineering, biomedical, and

Methods of causality detection

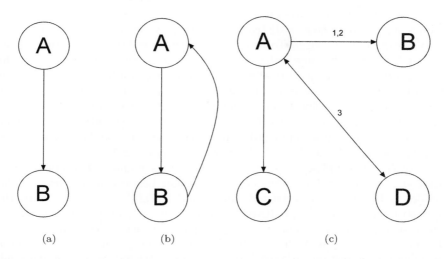

FIGURE 7.1: Different structures for causal links: (a) recursive scheme, (b) feedback loop, and (c) causal network with lags between cause and effect shown on the edges.

bioinformatics. The goal of this chapter is to review some common approaches of causality detection in the areas of climate and environmental science. Here, we focused on three classes of methods to demonstrate their application in the area and compare their performance on multiple generated and real-world time series. While there are multiple other causality methods available in the literature, we focused on three methods that are widely used for environmental analysis and their source codes are available.

The chapter is structured as follows. We review the causality detection methods based on the Granger approach, nonlinear state space models, and graphical models in Section 7.2. In Section 7.3, we test these algorithms with a generated data set and two real-world data sets coming from climate and ecological studies. The methods are then compared and other challenges are discussed in Section 7.4.

7.2 Methods of causality detection

7.2.1 Granger causality

A common technique for analyzing causality in time series is *Granger causality (GC)*, which was originally developed for econometric studies. Generally speaking, a cause occurs prior to its effect. Formally, for two time series, x

and y, generated from a system, it is defined that x Granger causes y if future values of y can be better predicted using the past values of x and y rather than only the past values of y. To test for Granger causality, a regression model is fitted between the time series and the corresponding coefficients about the $x \to y$ interaction are statistically tested. Granger causality and its variations are vastly used in environmental data analysis, e.g., to analyze the effect of anthropogenic and natural factors on global warming (Attanasio, 2012, Kodra et al, 2011, Triacca et al, 2013), effect of climate on vegetation (Kong et al, 2018, Papagiannopoulou et al, 2017, Reygadas et al, 2020) and different species population (Rincón et al, 2019, Solvang and Subbey, 2019).

Consider two univariate stationary time series x and y. If there is a statistically significant improvement of prediction between a restricted linear model (7.1) and an unrestricted linear model (7.2), x is GC of y. In the unrestricted model, y is predicted by using only its past values, whereas in the restricted model, y is predicted by its past values and past values of x. It is common to apply a Student's t-test on coefficients c_i (where $i = 1, \ldots, s$) or likelihood ratio test on variance of residuals for restricted/unrestricted models to reject the null hypothesis of y does not GC x.

$$y(t) = \beta + a_1 y(t-1) + a_2 y(t-2) + \ldots + a_s y(t-s) \\ + c_1 x(t-1) + c_2 x(t-2) + \ldots + c_p x(t-p) + \epsilon(t) \quad (7.1)$$

$$y(t) = \gamma + b_1 y(t-1) + b_2 y(t-2) + \ldots + b_s y(t-s) + \epsilon(t) \quad (7.2)$$

The linear Granger causality analysis was also extended to P-dimensional multivariate time series, where a linear *vector autoregressive model (VAR)* is used for modeling purposes:

$$X(t) = \sum_{l=1}^{L} A^{(l)\top} X(t-l) + \epsilon(t) \quad (7.3)$$

Here, $A^{(l)}$ is the matrix of coefficients that models the effect of the time series with l lags. Usually the minimum value for l is 1. In the case of *instantaneous (contemporaneous) causation*, $l = 0$. The instantaneous causation occurs when the length of the measurement interval is too long so that the cause/effect action happens in less time than the length of a single time interval. If all of the l VAR coefficient matrices are lower triangular, then x fails to GC y. This can be tested using Wald or likelihood ration tests.

The assumption of linearity in a VAR-based Granger causality test significantly simplifies the modeling task, but it can be impractical in many real applications. Thus, extended methods using kernel regression (Kong et al, 2018, Marinazzo et al, 2011, Wu et al, 2011) and nonparametric methods (Diks and Panchenko, 2006, Hu and Liang, 2014, Pagnotta et al, 2018) have been developed in literature.

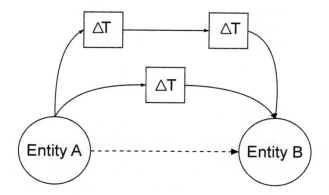

FIGURE 7.2: Different delays might exist between two variables in a causal network.

Another challenge of Granger causality is existence of confounding variables, i.e., additional variables that are driving the modeled variables. The challenge is that not all influential confounders are observed in the real-world data sets. For example, in a bivariate case of x and y, there might be another variable z, where both $z \to x$ and $z \to y$. Here, the Granger method might state that x causes y, while z actually drives both x and y. Similarly, Granger causality does not account for indirect effects or mediating variables that generate additional lags. A variable x may indirectly stimulate y via a third process z, i.e., $x \to z \to y$. Here, the Granger method states that x is a cause of y without including the necessary link z. The cause-effect interaction among two entities might happen in multiple delays (Figure 7.2). For example, if two causal links exist in a system as $x \to y$ and $x \to z \to y$, multiple lags should be considered in the Granger method. This is a known problem in biological and neural causality analyses where intermediate factors can introduce different delays into the regulation of target variables (Wibral et al, 2013, Zoppoli et al, 2010).

Implementation of the Granger method can be found in R with `lmtest` and `MTS`, python with `statsmodels` (Seabold and Perktold, 2010), and Matlab with `MVGC` toolboxes (Barnett and Seth, 2014).

7.2.2 Nonlinear state space methods

A state space model is a representation for dynamical systems based on vectors of inputs, outputs, and states of the system which together form a first order difference equation:

$$\begin{aligned} X(t+1) &= f(X(t), U(t)); \\ Y(t) &= g(X(t), U(t)), \end{aligned} \quad (7.4)$$

where f and g are nonlinear functions, and X, Y, and U are vectors of states, outputs and inputs of the dynamical system. For a *linear time-invariant (LTI)* system, the state space representation can be simplified as:

$$X(t+1) = AX(t) + BU(t);$$
$$Y(t) = CX(t) + DU(t), \quad (7.5)$$

where A, B, C, and D are model matrices.

Granger causality is based on the time dependency between cause and effect, and is critically dependent on the assumption that cause and effect are separable. Unlike linear stochastic systems, the separability might not be satisfied for nonlinear deterministic systems. It means that the system cannot be separated into subsystems and rather behaves as a whole. Additionally, ecosystems are typically subject to forcing by external driving variables (such as temperature, precipitation, etc.) that might lead to correlations between non-interacting variables, making the causality detection more complex. Another issue is that the Granger causality is useful for detecting interactions between strongly coupled variables in nonlinear systems, not the commonly weak coupling in ecological systems (Harnack et al, 2017, Sugihara et al, 2012, Yang et al, 2018).

The causality detection method based on *convergent cross mapping (CCM)* has been developed by Sugihara et al (2012) to address these issues. The CCM method has been successfully applied in environmental causality detection, such as analyzing the effect of galactic cosmic rays on global temperature (Tsonis et al, 2018), temperature/precipitation on butterfly abundance (Kawatsu et al, 2019), soil moisture on precipitation amount (Wang et al, 2018), and feedback between greenhouse gases and global temperature (Van Nes et al, 2015). Several variations of the CCM method are reported by Mønster et al (2017), and the effects of weak and strong couplings on the results are discussed.

The CCM method considers the time series as output of a nonlinear state space system. This method is based on Taken's theorem specifying that a high-dimensional state space system can be represented by lagged values of corresponding time series instead of its unknown or unobserved variables. Consider $X \in \{X_1, X_2\}$ are the states of the nonlinear system. Then, E time-lagged values of X are used as coordinate axes to create a *shadow attractor manifold*, M_X. The lagged values of X are $\{X(t-\tau), X(t-2\tau), \ldots, X(t-(E-1)\tau)\}$, where τ is the positive time lag value and E is the length of time segment (library size). In dynamical systems theory, time-series variables are causally linked if they share a common attractor manifold, M. Thus if $X_1 \to X_2$, the local neighborhoods on the respective lagged reconstructions, M_{X_1} and M_{X_2}, map to each other since X_1 and X_2 are essentially alternative observations of the common attractor manifold, M. Also, if X_1 is cause of X_2, information about states of X_1 can be recovered from X_2, but not vice versa. In fact, the manifold M_{X_2} can be reconstructed from lagged values of X_2 and then used to estimate past values of X_1. In noise-free situations as $L \to \infty$, the estimated

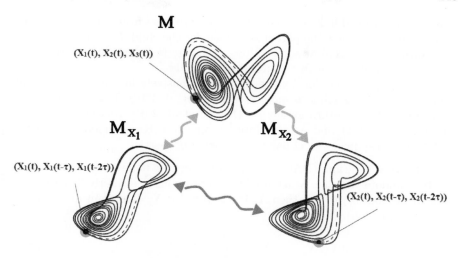

FIGURE 7.3: Two shadow manifolds, M_{X_1} and M_{X_2}, are reconstructed for the original manifold, M. The points that are nearby on M (e.g., within the purple circle) will correspond temporally to points that are nearby on M_{X_1} (brown circle) and M_{X_2} (green circle) (Sugihara et al, 2012).

value of X_2 i.e., $\hat{X}_1|M_{X_2}$ converges to true values. In practical application with process disturbances and measurement noise, the estimation precision will be limited.

To study the causality of $X_1 \rightarrow X_2$, the shadow manifolds, M_{X_1} and M_{X_2}, are reconstructed. Then, a vector on M_{X_2} is selected, and its $E+1$ nearby points on M_{X_2} are found. The time indices of these points on M_{X_2} are used to identify the corresponding points in M_{X_1} (Figure 7.3). Then, a locally weighted mean is calculated to find the $\hat{X}_1|M_{X_2}$. The weights are found based on the distance between selected point in M_{X_2} and its $E+1$ neighbors. If the causality $X_1 \rightarrow X_2$, exists, the $\hat{X}_1|M_{X_2}$ should converge to $X_1(t)$ as value of L increases. The predictability is measured by error metrics such as mean absolute error and root mean square error (MAE and RMSE), or the correlation between observed and predicted values (ρ). This procedure is repeated over many random subsamples of the time series and the final result is the aggregation of these values over different L values (Sugihara et al, 2012).

Implementation of the CCM method can be found in R with rEDM package (Sugihara et al, 2012), and in Python with skccm library. Pu et al (2019) has presented an implementation of CCM with Apache Spark.

7.2.3 Causal graphical models

A graphical model represents a set of distributions where each node is a random variable. An edge connecting two nodes shows the lack of conditional independencies between those nodes. A directed graphical causal model represents the causal links between the nodes. An edge from a parent node to a child node shows that the parent is a cause for the child. It means that if all other variables are fixed at some values, a change in value of the parent will make change in value (or distribution) of the child.

Causal graphical models have been used extensively in the environmental science for studying climate indices (Barnes et al, 2019, Ebert-Uphoff and Deng, 2012), temperature anomalies (Harari et al, 2019, Runge et al, 2014, Zerenner et al, 2014), and Arctic winter circulations (Kretschmer et al, 2016).

A causal graphical model has the following properties:

- Directed acyclic graph (DAG): consists of a set of n nodes, each node represents a random variable, which might be continuous or discrete. If there is an edge from node X_i to X_j, then X_i is a parent for X_j. The joint distribution of the graph can be defined as:

$$p(X_1, X_2, \ldots, X_n) = \prod_{i=1}^{n} p(X_i | X_{parents(i)}). \qquad (7.6)$$

If a node does not have parents, it is defined as an *exogenous* variable; otherwise it is an *endogenous* variable. The graph does not have cycles, since a causal loop like $X_1 \to X_2 \to X_1$ is not acceptable.

- d-separation: is a relation between three disjoint sets of nodes in a directed graph. If a set of nodes, Z, blocks all connections of a certain type between X and Y in a graph G, then X and Y are d-separated by Z in G. For example, in the causal link of $X \to Y \to Z$, Y blocks the only directed path connecting X and Z, so X and Z are d-separated by Y in this DAG. In a statistical notation, for all of the distributions, D, that the G can represent, if X and Z are d-separated by Y, then X and Z are independent conditional on Y in D, or

$$X \perp\!\!\!\perp Z | Y, \qquad (7.7)$$

$$p(Z|X, Y) = p(Z|Y). \qquad (7.8)$$

Note that several DAGs might represent a d-separation relation. For example, in (7.7), all of the following relationships are possible:

$$\begin{aligned} X \to Y \to Z \\ X \leftarrow Y \leftarrow Z \\ X \leftarrow Y \to Z \end{aligned} \qquad (7.9)$$

- Causal Markov assumption: states that a variable, X, is independent of every other variable (except X's effects) conditional on all of its direct causes. This means that all the relevant probabilistic information about a variable can be obtained from its direct causes (and itself). For a node X_i

$$X_i \perp\!\!\!\perp X_{non-childs(i)} | X_{parents(i)}, \qquad (7.10)$$

where *non-childs(i)* are nodes which X_i is not their parents.

- Sufficiency: refers to the absence of hidden (or latent confounder) variables, means that we have measured all the common causes of the measured variables.
- Faithfulness: means that when multiple causal paths exist from one node to another, the combined effect is not exactly equal to zero, i.e., two causal links do not cancel out each other's effects.

There are several approaches to extract the model structure from data by estimating the statistical parameters of networks. One of common techniques is called *PC* (named after its inventors Peter Spirtes and Clark Glymour) (Spirtes et al, 2001). It conducts numerous conditional independence tests to find the structure of the underlying causal network. The PC algorithm is based on assumption of independent and identically distributed (i.i.d.) samples, Markov condition, and the faithfulness. Under these conditions and when there is no latent confounder, two variables are directly causally related (with an edge in between) if, and only if, there does not exist any subset of the remaining variables conditioning on which they are independent. The algorithm removes an edge if a conditional independence is found (i.e., by not rejecting the null hypothesis of independence at some significance level by tests such as Fisher's Z test). The PC algorithm has the following steps:

1. Start with a complete undirected graph among the nodes.
2. Remove edges between the variables that are unconditionally independent.
3. For each pair of variables (X, Y) having an edge between them, and for each variable Z with an edge connected to either of (X, Y), eliminate the edge between X and Y, if $X \perp\!\!\!\perp Y | Z$.
4. For each pair of variables (X, Y) having an edge between them, and for each pair of variables (Z, W) with edges both connected to X or both connected to Y, eliminate the edge between X and Y if $X \perp\!\!\!\perp Y | \{Z, W\}$ (means that X and Y are independent conditional on Z and W).

    Continue checking the independencies until no adjacent pairs (X, Y) exist such that there is a subset of variables whose variables are adjacent to X or all adjacent to Y.

5. For each set of variables (X, Y, Z) where X and Y are adjacent, Y and Z are adjacent, and X and Z are not adjacent, set the direction of edges by creating a v-structure as $X \to Y \leftarrow Z$.
6. For each set of variables (X, Y, Z) where $X \to Y - Z$, and X and Z are not and adjacent, set the direction of edge as $Y \to Z$ (Glymour et al, 2019).

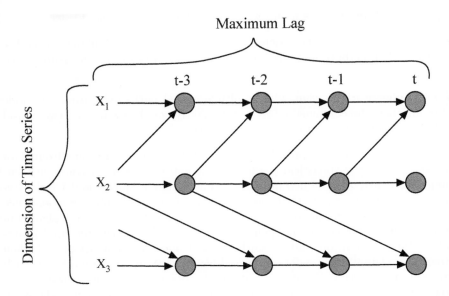

FIGURE 7.4: A sample recovered DAG for a three-dimensional time series. In this case there are two causal links between $X_2(t-1) \rightarrow X_1(t)$ and $X_2(t-2) \rightarrow X_3(t)$. Also three self-regulating links exist for three dimensions with one lag.

The original PC algorithm does not consider the order of data. For the case of time series, a modified algorithm should be used. For this goal, additional nodes are created for the DAG nodes at different time lags (Figure 7.4). Since an event in the future cannot have an effect on an event in the past, any node with a time index should only be pointing toward nodes with the same time index or later (Ebert-Uphoff and Deng, 2012, Runge, 2018). For a time series $X(t)$, the nodes in DAG represent the $X(t)$ at different time lags. The parents of $X(t)$ denoted as $\mathcal{P}(X(t))$ should be selected from the set of $X^-(t) = \{X(t-1), X(t-2), \dots\}$. A link exists between $X_i(t-\tau)$ and $X_j(t)$ if $X_i(t-\tau)$ is not conditionally independent of $X_i(t-\tau)$ given the past of all variables:

$$X_i(t-\tau) \not\!\perp\!\!\!\perp X_j(t) | X^-(t) \setminus X_i(t-\tau), \qquad (7.11)$$

where $i, j \in \{1, \dots, dimension(X)\}$, and $\not\!\perp\!\!\!\perp$ denotes the absence of conditional independence. Here, $X^-(t) \setminus X_i(t-\tau)$ means the X^- set after removing $X_i(t-\tau)$.

Running conditional independence tests on many nodes in a time series graph is problematic due to high dimensionality. Runge et al (2019b) developed the PCMCI approach as an extension that runs the tests on two separate steps. In the first step, PC, a larger value is chosen for p-value (such as 0.2) to run conditional independence tests and select a set of possible causal links.

In the second step, *momentary conditional independence (MCI)* removes the extra links using a smaller *p*-value.

- Let $\hat{\mathcal{P}}(X_j(t))$ be the parents of a node $X_j(t)$ in a time series DAG. The time series DAG consists of $X(t)$ at different time lags, and thus the elements of $\mathcal{P}(X_j(t))$ should be selected from $X^-(t)$. In the first step, $\hat{\mathcal{P}}(X_j(t)) = X^-(t)$. Then, the variables without unconditional dependencies are removed from $\hat{\mathcal{P}}(X_j(t))$. In the second step, the variables that are independent conditional on parents (of the first step) with highest dependency (based on their absolute test statistics value) are removed from $\hat{\mathcal{P}}(X_j(t))$. Next, variables are removed that are independent conditionally on the two strongest drivers of the previous step. This procedure is continued until no edge exists to check, and we find $\hat{\mathcal{P}}(X_j(t))$ for all the nodes. This PC step converges to a network with some high probable edges and possibly some false positive edges.

- Next, the MCI test is applied on the output of PC step to remove the false positive edges. For every edge $X_i(t-\tau) \to X_j(t)$, this test is performed:

$$X_i(t-\tau) \not\perp\!\!\!\perp X_j(t) | \hat{\mathcal{P}}(X_j(t)) \setminus \{X_i(t-\tau)\}, \hat{\mathcal{P}}(X_i(t-\tau)). \qquad (7.12)$$

The above equation represents that the independence conditions are tested on the parents of $X_j(t)$ (i.e., $\hat{\mathcal{P}}(X_j(t)) \setminus \{X_i(t-\tau)\}$) and also the time-shifted parents of $X_i(t)$ (i.e., $\hat{\mathcal{P}}(X_i(t-\tau))$). This additional condition helps to account for the effect of autocorrelation in variables and decrease the false positive rate in causality detection (Runge et al, 2019b).

The implementation PC and its variations can be found in Python with `TIGRAMITE` (Runge et al, 2019b) and R with `pcalg` packages.

7.3 Simulations

In this section, the causality in three data sets is studied with the three discussed approaches and their results are compared.

- The Granger causality is implemented by the `MVGC` toolbox in Matlab (Barnett and Seth, 2014). It can fit a VAR model by ordinary least squares (OLS) to the time series while the optimal lag is found by information theory criteria such as the Akaike or Bayesian information criterion (AIC or BIC).

- The CCM method is simulated using the `rEDM` package in R (Sugihara et al, 2012).

- The PCMCI approach is implemented in `TIGRAMITE` package in Python (Runge et al, 2019b), which uses nonparametric conditional independence tests for discrete or continuous time series.

7.3.1 Simulated data

We test performance of the causality methods on the following generated data borrowed from Runge et al (2019a). The true network structure is shown in Figure 7.5(a). This model includes auto-correlation and lagged and contemporaneous causality links. While there is a direct causality $Y \rightarrow Z$, a lagged causality $Y \rightarrow Z \rightarrow W$ also exists:

$$\begin{aligned} X(t) &= aY(t) + E^X(t) \\ Y(t) &= E^Y(t) \\ Z(t) &= bZ(t-1) + cY(t-1) + E^Z(t) \\ W(t) &= dW(t-1) + eZ(t) + E^W(T), \end{aligned} \quad (7.13)$$

where $a = b = c = e = 1$ and $d = 0.1$. Also, E^X, E^Y, E^Z, and E^W are $N(0, 0.1^2)$. The length of data is $T = 500$.

- Granger: The recovered network is shown in Figure 7.5(b). The Granger method can identify the link $Y \rightarrow Z$, but the contemporaneous link, $Y \rightarrow X$, cannot be detected. However, the contemporaneous link of $Z \rightarrow W$ is found since there is an indirect link as $Y(t-1) \rightarrow Z(t) \rightarrow W(t)$. Another spurious link $Y \rightarrow W$ is found due to other detected links of $Y \rightarrow Z$ and $Z \rightarrow W$.

- CCM: The model (7.13) is linear and separable. By removing the noise terms, the states will converge to zero at infinite time, and no manifold will be generated, thus the CCM method cannot be applied. Adding an input $u(t) = 0.1\sin(0.1t)$ ensures the states will have a manifold. However, CCM still finds causal links between all of the nodes. For example in Figure 7.6, both of the correlation values for causal links $Y \rightarrow Z$ and $Z \rightarrow Y$ are converged to 1. This means that the CCM has detected both of the links, while only the $Y \rightarrow Z$ is correct. This result shows that CCM is not a suitable approach for this linear separable equation.

- PCMCI: We applied the PCMCI approach, which uses the partial correlation as a conditional independence test. In the partial correlation testing approach for $X \perp\!\!\!\perp Y | Z$, two OLS regressions are fitted for $X \sim Z$ and $Z \sim X$. Then the dependency of the residuals is tested with the Pearson correlation test. The PCMCI algorithm returns the p-value of these conditional independence tests for contemporaneous and lagged variables and also the values of linear coefficients as below:

```
## Significant links at alpha = 0.05:

    Variable X has 1 link(s):
        (Y 0): pval = 0.00000 | val = 0.703

    Variable Y has 1 link(s):
        (X 0): pval = 0.00000 | val = 0.703
```

Simulations

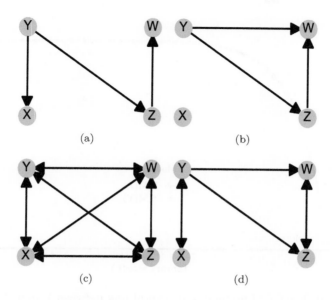

FIGURE 7.5: True causal network (a) and recovered using three methods: (b) Granger method is unable to detect contemporaneous links, and two false links are detected; (c) CCM method found links between all the nodes; (d) PCMCI found the true links and one indirect link. It also found two false positive links for instantaneous links.

```
Variable Z has 3 link(s):
    (Y -1): pval = 0.00000 | val = 0.719
    (Z -1): pval = 0.00000 | val = 0.673
    (W  0): pval = 0.00000 | val = 0.670

Variable W has 3 link(s):
    (Z  0): pval = 0.00000 | val = 0.670
    (Y -1): pval = 0.00000 | val = 0.588
    (Z -1): pval = 0.00000 | val = 0.566
```

The recovered graph is shown in Figure 7.5(d). A spurious link between $Y(t-1) \to Z$ is detected similar to the Granger method. PCMCI finds only two instantaneous links, $Z \to W$ and $Y \to X$, and the directions are not found. For example, the value of coefficients for both directions of $Z - W$ is 0.67. All of the estimated coefficients are positive matching the original coefficients in the data-generating dynamical model. Comparing to the Granger method, PCMCI is able to find the contemporaneous links, but both methods have the indirect link of $Y \to W$.

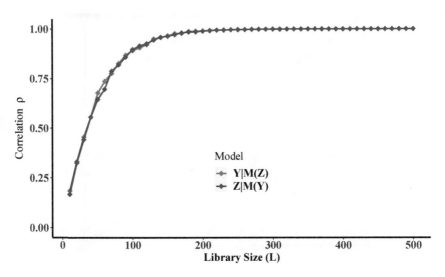

FIGURE 7.6: The CCM method finds causal link between Y and Z, since the correlation between prediction and true values are converging to 1. Here, the detected link $Z \to Y$ is false positive.

7.3.2 Arctic and the midlatitude jet stream

In this section, we investigate the causal links between Arctic temperatures and the jet streams with the data borrowed from Samarasinghe et al (2019). The PC and Granger causality method were tested on this data in Samarasinghe et al (2019) showing that Arctic temperature and jet speed and position are linked together by two robust positive feedback loops that operate on time scales of 5–25 days.

The daily data is extracted from the Community Earth System Model Large Ensemble (CESM-LE; Kay et al, 2015), a fully coupled general circulation model. We use years 402 to 2200 of the pre-industrial control run (all external forcing is fixed at its levels from 1850), resulting in 656,634 days (1798 years) of data that acts as a proxy for a very long observational record. The data is gridded at a 1° horizontal grid spacing, that is, 0.9° in latitude by 1.25° in longitude. The seasonal cycle is removed from the daily data, and the data is then averaged into non-overlapping 5-day chunks to smooth out higher-frequency variability. Afterwards, each time series is standardized, by subtracting its mean and dividing by the standard deviation.

In this analysis, we focus on the winter season of December, January, and February (DJF), roughly dividing the number of data samples for each experiment by four. The winter season is analyzed here because the teleconnection patterns between different regions are the strongest in the winter, and

Simulations

extratropical storm activity itself is greatest in winter. The data is stationary in the long term, as they were generated by a control run with no external forcing, and the impacts of the seasonal cycle are minimized by removing the first four Fourier harmonics of the data. The mean subtraction in the standardization ensures that all variables used in the models have zero means. Here, we focus on the North Pacific (120°E–240°E, covering 97 grid boxes in longitude), and we analyze the circulation using the following three one-dimensional time series, each consisting of 32,381 5-day averages:

- Jet latitude in the North Pacific, $\mathcal{L}$;
- Jet speed in the North Pacific, $\mathcal{S}$;
- 850 hPa Arctic temperature averaged over 70° N – 90° N at all longitudes $\mathcal{T}$.

Jet latitude, $\mathcal{L}$, and jet speed, $\mathcal{S}$, represent the position and strength of the eddy-driven jet, usually used as proxies for the position and strength of the jet streams. They are calculated by determining the maximum position and strength of the zonal component of the winds at 850 hPa over the North Pacific basin (120° E–240° E). First, the 850 hPa zonal winds are averaged over all longitudes in the North Pacific basin to create a zonal-mean profile of the zonal wind. The resulting zonal-mean zonal wind profile is interpolated to a 0.01° latitude grid. A quadratic polynomial is fit around the maximum of this interpolated wind profile. The maximum of this quadratic polynomial is the jet speed, $\mathcal{S}$, whereas its latitudinal position is the jet latitude, $\mathcal{L}$ (Samarasinghe et al, 2019).

The Pearson correlation between $\mathcal{T}$ and $\mathcal{L}$ is −0.10, and the correlation between $\mathcal{T}$ and $\mathcal{S}$ is 0.1. Figure 7.7 shows the scatter plot and histograms of these three variables, where a linear trend for $\mathcal{T}$ versus $\mathcal{S}$ and $\mathcal{L}$ does not exist.

Granger causality

Fitting the VAR to the data and evaluating the *p*-values at different lags shows that there are significant causal links between $\mathcal{T}$ vs. $\mathcal{L}$ and $\mathcal{T}$ vs. $\mathcal{P}$. However, the VAR coefficients have various signs. For example:

$$\mathcal{T} \sim -0.019\mathcal{P}(t-1) + 0.016\mathcal{P}(t-2) \\ + 0.057\mathcal{P}(t-3) + 0.005\mathcal{P}(t-4) + 0.005\mathcal{P}(t-5) \quad (7.14)$$

While the existence and direction of Granger causality is proven, specifying the polarity is difficult. In (7.14), most of the coefficients are positive, and one coefficient with small magnitude is negative. It is not clear whether or not an increase in $\mathcal{P}$ will increase or decrease the values of $\mathcal{T}$.

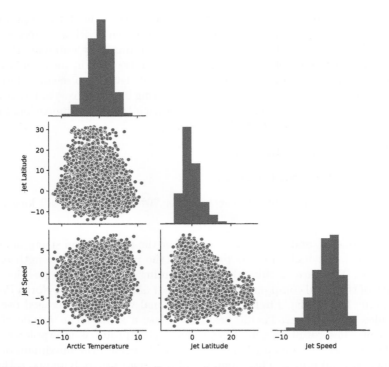

FIGURE 7.7: Scatter plot for three variables of Arctic temperature, jet latitude, and speed for DJF months. No significant correlation or linear trend can be seen for any pair of these variables. However, causality analysis shows some dependencies between them.

CCM

Due to the large length of time series, 32,381, the CCM algorithm cannot be executed in our computer, and the algorithm did not converge when implemented on the Kaggle server.

PCMCI

The PCMCI method provides significant causal links between all three variables $\mathcal{T}$, $\mathcal{L}$, and $\mathcal{P}$. Figure 7.8 shows the detected significant links and the associated time lags.

Most of the coefficients for $\mathcal{S} \to \mathcal{L}$ and $\mathcal{T} \to \mathcal{S}$ are positive. This shows that there is a causal loop (similar to Figure 7.1(b)) between these two variables. For example, a warmer Arctic drives a faster jet, and a faster jet drives a warmer Arctic. On the other hand, most of coefficients for $\mathcal{L} \to \mathcal{T}$ and $\mathcal{T} \to \mathcal{L}$ are negative. These links together form a positive feedback between $\mathcal{T}$ and $\mathcal{L}$. This positive feedback loop between jet latitude and Arctic temperatures

Simulations

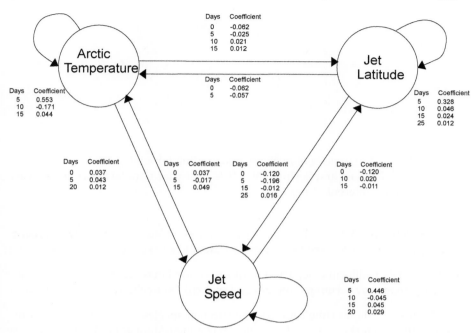

FIGURE 7.8: Recovered causal network for Arctic temperature data along with delays and coefficients. Most of the coefficients for links between Arctic temperature and jet speed are positive. Also, the majority of coefficients of edges between Arctic temperature and jet latitude are negative. This represents two positive feedbacks between these two pairs of variables.

shows that the warmer Arctic drives a southward shift of the jet, which drives further Arctic warming (Samarasinghe et al, 2019). Some detected lags are 0, and our sampling time is 5 days, meaning that the effect of these variables on each other might happen in delays of less than 5 days.

7.3.3 Sardine–anchovy and sea surface temperature

Here, we examine the relationship among Pacific sardine (*Sardinops sagax*) landings, northern anchovy (*Engraulis mordax*) landings, and sea surface temperature (SST) measured at Scripps Pier and Newport Pier in California (Sugihara et al, 2012).

The SST was measured at shore stations: Scripps Pier and Newport Pier.[1] Monthly means were averaged to form yearly time series, and the final time series consisted of 3-year running averages for the SST. The California landings data for Pacific sardine and northern anchovy were taken from two sources:

---

[1] Data available from: http://shorestation.ucsd.edu/active/index_active.html

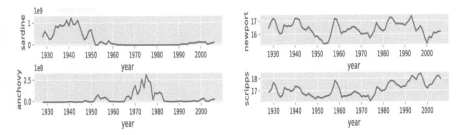

FIGURE 7.9: Time series of anchovy and sardine population, sea surface temperature of Newport and Scripps Pier. It is clear that population of two species have peaks in different times.

- 1928–2002: NOAA Southwest Fisheries Science Center (https://coastwatch.pfeg.noaa.gov/erddap/search/index.html?searchFor=erdCAMarCat)

- 2003–2006: California Department of Fish and Game (https://oceanview.pfeg.noaa.gov/erddap/search/index.html?searchFor=CA_mkt_catch)

Figure 7.9 shows time series of the two fish species, where one population is peaking when the other is low. The environmental question here is whether the species act in direct competition or whether they react differently to common large-scale environmental forcing. Here, we investigate the causal network among these four time series using multiple approaches.

Granger causality

A Granger causality test does not detect any causal link between SST and two fish populations. On the other hand, it detects a link from sardine population to Scripps SST, which is not correct (Figure 7.10(a)).

PCMCI

PCMCI shows that there are causal links between anchovy and SST at Newport and Scripps Piers, but the directions of these links are not identified. On the other hand, no causal link is found between Scripps Pier SST and sardine population (Figure 7.10(b)).

CCM

Figure 7.11(a) shows the result of CCM on the causal links between sardine population and SST. It can be seen that the time series of Scripps Pier SST can be recovered from the manifold created by the sardine time series. A similar pattern exists in Figure 7.11(b) for Newport SST and anchovy population. On the other hand, Figure 7.11(c) does not show a convergence. In conclusion, the recovered causal links are from Scripps Pier SST to sardine population and

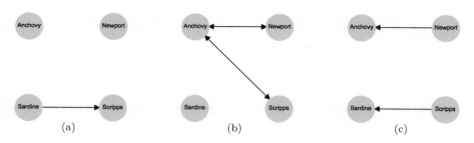

FIGURE 7.10: Recovered causal network for sardine–anchovy time series. (a) the Granger method only detects an incorrect causality from sardine population to Scripps Pier SST; (b) PCMCI finds a links between anchovy and Newport SST, but cannot find the correct direction; (c) CCM finds causal links between Scripps Pier SST to the sardine population and from Newport SST to the anchovy population.

from Newport SST to anchovy population. The recovered network is shown in Figure 7.10(c).

7.4 Conclusions

The majority of studies in climate and environmental science are based on correlation and regression analysis. But finding cause and effect relationships between environmental variables requires utilization of other techniques. In this chapter, Granger, graphical causal models, and nonlinear state space methods of causality detection have been reviewed. Performance of these methods is evaluated on three data sets with different challenges like nonlinearity, contemporaneous links, and spurious links.

The econometric approach of Granger with standard regression approaches was successful in many problems in econometrics and other fields. It requires estimation of lagged autoregressive coefficients, which might lead to high dimensional problems for multiple time series. Adding more variables to the problem also increases its dimensionality. On the other hand, climate time series are usually short (usually the length of a few hundred samples) and thus the Granger method has a low-detection power for high-dimensional time series due to the *curse of dimensionality*. In addition, contemporaneous links generated from slower sampling rates cannot be detected by this method. Application of the Granger method is mostly limited to bivariate cases, which are not suitable to detect indirect links or common drivers.

Compared to linear Granger causality, state-space methods have better performance in identifying nonlinear causal links, but it is difficult to extend

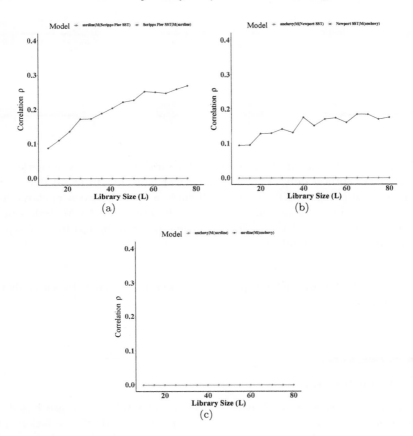

FIGURE 7.11: Recovering the causal link for sardine–anchovy data using CCM: (a) shows existence of a causal link from Scripps Pier SST to the sardine population; (b) shows a similar causal link from Newport SST to the anchovy population; (c) shows that no causal link exists between anchovy to/from the sardine population.

these methods to higher-dimensional problems. The CCM methods can only be used when a manifold (attractor) can be recovered from the data. Additionally, CCM needs tuning of several parameters like embedded delay and library size. CCM has a high computational cost and it is not efficient for long time series.

The PC approach finds the causal graph based on i.i.d. data, faithfulness and sufficiency assumption using conditional independence tests. PC are more suitable than CCM for stochastic time series. Using different types of linear/nonlinear conditional independence tests adds flexibility to the PC algorithm for analyzing different cases. Unlike Granger, PC can detect contemporaneous links. PCMCI, as a variation of PC, performs causality detection in two consecutive steps, which makes it more suitable for high-dimensional problems. In particular situations, PC cannot detect directions of some edges from data and these edges in graph would be undirected. Effects of hidden factors are another challenge for the PC method.

There are still many challenges in recovering the causal relationship from environmental time series. For example, many of these time series are nonstationary and the causal structure or their parameters might change through time. Several other issues also exist such as hidden variables, nonlinearity, and measurement errors. The general problem of estimating the causal generating processes for time series is not close to being solved, but there is progress in understanding the challenges of current methods in different problems (Glymour et al, 2019, Runge et al, 2019a).

Acknowledgments

We are immensely grateful to Dr. Imme Ebert-Uphoff from Colorado State University for sharing with us the data of the Arctic jet stream. We also thank Savini Samarasinghe for providing us additional information about this data set.

We thank Lynn Dewitt from NOAA for providing us access to the Sardine Anchovy data set.

We are also thankful of Martha Audrey Holloman for editing and reviewing of this manuscript.

References

Arnold A, Liu Y, Abe N (2007) Temporal causal modeling with graphical Granger methods. In: Proceedings of the 13th ACM SIGKDD International Conference on Knowledge Discovery and Data Mining, ACM, 66–75

Attanasio A (2012) Testing for linear Granger causality from natural/anthropogenic forcings to global temperature anomalies. Theoretical and Applied Climatology 110(1-2):281–289

Barbieri L (2013) Causality and interdependence analysis in linear econometric models with an application to fertility. Journal of Applied Statistics 40(8):1701–1716

Barnes EA, Samarasinghe SM, Ebert-Uphoff I, Furtado JC (2019) Tropospheric and stratospheric causal pathways between the MJO and NAO. Journal of Geophysical Research: Atmospheres 124:9356–9371

Barnett L, Seth AK (2014) The MVGC multivariate Granger causality toolbox: a new approach to Granger-causal inference. Journal of Neuroscience Methods 223:50–68

Diks C, Panchenko V (2006) A new statistic and practical guidelines for nonparametric Granger causality testing. Journal of Economic Dynamics and Control 30(9-10):1647–1669

Ebert-Uphoff I, Deng Y (2012) Causal discovery for climate research using graphical models. Journal of Climate 25(17):5648–5665

Glymour C, Zhang K, Spirtes P (2019) Review of causal discovery methods based on graphical models. Frontiers in Genetics 10:524

Granger CWJ (1969) Investigating causal relations by econometric models and cross-spectral methods. Econometrica 37:424–438

Hannart A, Pearl J, Otto FEL, Naveau P, Ghil M (2016) Causal counterfactual theory for the attribution of weather and climate-related events. Bulletin of the American Meteorological Society 97(1):99–110

Harari O, Garfinkel CI, Ziskin Ziv S, Morgenstern O, Zeng G, Tilmes S, Kinnison D, Deushi M, Jöckel P, Pozzer A, O'Connor FM, Davis S (2019) Influence of Arctics stratospheric ozone on surface climate in CCMI models. Atmospheric Chemistry and Physics 19(14):9253–9268

Harnack D, Laminski E, Schünemann M, Pawelzik KR (2017) Topological causality in dynamical systems. Physical Review Letters 119:098301

Hu M, Liang H (2014) A copula approach to assessing Granger causality. NeuroImage 100:125–134

Kawatsu K, Yamanaka T, Patoèka J, Liebhold AM (2019) Nonlinear time series analysis unravels underlying mechanisms of interspecific synchrony among foliage-feeding forest Lepidoptera species. Population Ecology 62(1):5–14

Kay JE, Deser C, Phillips A, Mai A, Hannay C, Strand G, Arblaster JM, Bates SC, Danabasoglu G, Edwards J, Holland M, Kushner P, Lamarque JF, Lawrence D, Lindsay K, Middleton A, Munoz E, Neale R, Oleson K, Polvani L, Vertenstein M (2015) The community earth system model (CESM) large ensemble project: a community resource for studying climate change in the presence of internal climate variability. Bulletin of the American Meteorological Society 96(8):1333–1349

Kodra E, Chatterjee S, Ganguly AR (2011) Exploring granger causality between global average observed time series of carbon dioxide and temperature. Theoretical and Applied Climatology 104(3-4):325–335

Kong D, Miao C, Duan Q, Lei X, Li H (2018) Vegetation-climate interactions on the loess plateau: a nonlinear Granger causality analysis. Journal of Geophysical Research: Atmospheres 123(19):11–068

Kretschmer M, Coumou D, Donges JF, Runge J (2016) Using causal effect networks to analyze different Arctic drivers of midlatitude winter circulation. Journal of Climate 29(11):4069–4081

Marinazzo D, Liao W, Chen H, Stramaglia S (2011) Nonlinear connectivity by Granger causality. NeuroImage 58(2):330–338

Mønster D, Fusaroli R, Tylén K, Roepstorff A, Sherson JF (2017) Causal inference from noisy time-series data—testing the convergent cross-mapping algorithm in the presence of noise and external influence. Future Generation Computer Systems 73:52–62

Pagnotta MF, Dhamala M, Plomp G (2018) Benchmarking nonparametric Granger causality: robustness against downsampling and influence of spectral decomposition parameters. NeuroImage 183:478–494

Papagiannopoulou C, Miralles DG, Decubber S, Demuzere M, Verhoest NEC, Dorigo WA, Waegeman W (2017) A nonlinear Granger-causality framework to investigate climate-vegetation dynamics. Geoscientific Model Development 10(5):1945–1960

Pearl J (1988) Probabilistic Reasoning in Intelligent Systems: Networks of Plausible Inference. Morgan Kaufmann, San Mateo, CA

Pu B, Duan L, Osgood ND (2019) Parallelizing convergent cross mapping using Apache Spark. In: Thomson R, Bisgin H, Dancy C, Hyder A (eds) Social, Cultural, and Behavioral Modeling, Springer International Publishing, Cham, Switzerland, 133–142

Reygadas Y, Jensen JLR, Moisen GG, Currit N, Chow ET (2020) Assessing the relationship between vegetation greenness and surface temperature through Granger causality and impulse-response coefficients: a case study in Mexico. International Journal of Remote Sensing 41(10):3761–3783

Rincón MM, Corti R, Elvarsson BT, Ramos F, Ruiz J (2019) Granger-causality analysis of integrated-model outputs, a tool to assess external drivers in fishery. Fisheries Research 213:42–55

Runge J (2018) Causal network reconstruction from time series: from theoretical assumptions to practical estimation. Chaos 28(7):075310

Runge J, Petoukhov V, Kurths J (2014) Quantifying the strength and delay of climatic interactions: the ambiguities of cross correlation and a novel measure based on graphical models. Journal of Climate 27(2):720–739

Runge J, Bathiany S, Bollt E, Camps-Valls G, Coumou D, Deyle E, Glymour C, Kretschmer M, Mahecha MD, Muñoz-Marí J, van Nes EH, Peters J, Quax R, Reichstein M, Scheffer M, Schölkopf B, Spirtes P, Sugihara G, Sun J, Zhang K, Zscheischler J (2019a) Inferring causation from time series in Earth system sciences. Nature Communications 10(1):2553

Runge J, Nowack P, Kretschmer M, Flaxman S, Sejdinovic D (2019b) Detecting and quantifying causal associations in large nonlinear time series datasets. Science Advances 5(11):eaau4996

Samarasinghe SM, McGraw MC, Barnes EA, Ebert-Uphoff I (2019) A study of links between the Arctic and the midlatitude jet stream using Granger and Pearl causality. Environmetrics 30(4):e2540

Seabold S, Perktold J (2010) statsmodels: Econometric and statistical modeling with Python. In: 9th Python in Science Conference, Austin, Texas

Solvang HK, Subbey S (2019) An improved methodology for quantifying causality in complex ecological systems. PLoS ONE 14(1):e0208078

Spirtes P, Glymour C, Scheines R (2001) Causation, Prediction, and Search. MIT Press, Cambridge, MA

Sugihara G, May R, Ye H, Hsieh CH, Deyle E, Fogarty M, Munch S (2012) Detecting causality in complex ecosystems. Science 338(6106):496–500

Triacca U, Attanasio A, Pasini A (2013) Anthropogenic global warming hypothesis: testing its robustness by Granger causality analysis. Environmetrics 24(4):260–268

Tsonis AA, Deyle ER, Ye H, Sugihara G (2018) Convergent cross mapping: theory and an example. In: Tsonis AA (ed) Advances in Nonlinear Geosciences, Springer International Publishing, Cham, Switzerland, 587–600

Van Nes EH, Scheffer M, Brovkin V, Lenton TM, Ye H, Deyle E, Sugihara G (2015) Causal feedbacks in climate change. Nature Climate Change 5(5):445–448

Wang Y, Yang J, Chen Y, De Maeyer P, Li Z, Duan W (2018) Detecting the causal effect of soil moisture on precipitation using convergent cross mapping. Scientific Reports 8(1):1–8

Wibral M, Pampu N, Priesemann V, Siebenhühner F, Seiwert H, Lindner M, Lizier JT, Vicente R (2013) Measuring information-transfer delays. PloS one 8(2):e55809

Wu G, Duan X, Liao W, Gao Q, Chen H (2011) Kernel canonical-correlation Granger causality for multiple time series. Physical Review E 83(4):041921

Yang AC, Peng CK, Huang NE (2018) Causal decomposition in the mutual causation system. Nature Communications 9(1):1–10

Zerenner T, Friederichs P, Lehnertz K, Hense A (2014) A Gaussian graphical model approach to climate networks. Chaos 24(2):023103

Zoppoli P, Morganella S, Ceccarelli M (2010) TimeDelay-ARACNE: reverse engineering of gene networks from time-course data by an information theoretic approach. BMC Bioinformatics 11(1):154

Part II
Socioeconomic Impacts

8

Statistical Issues in Detection of Trends in Losses from Extreme Weather and Climate Events

Richard W. Katz
National Center for Atmospheric Research, Boulder, CO, USA

CONTENTS

8.1	Introduction	165
8.2	Loss distribution	170
	8.2.1 Overall distribution of losses	170
	8.2.2 Distribution of extreme high losses	172
	8.2.3 Reconciling implications for extremes	174
8.3	Bias, uncertainty, and variability in losses	176
	8.3.1 Variability and uncertainty as sources of bias	176
	8.3.2 Effects of adjustments	177
8.4	Detection and attribution of trends in losses	178
	8.4.1 Random sum representation	178
	8.4.2 Trend analyses	179
	8.4.3 Issues in normalization of losses	181
8.5	Summary and discussion	182
References	....	185

8.1 Introduction

Losses from extreme weather and climate events, such as floods or hurricanes, receive considerable attention, especially as a possible indicator of climate variations or change. As an example, Figure 8.1 shows the time series of the annual total economic loss (adjusted for inflation to constant 2017 dollars using the US Consumer Price Index) from US billion-dollar weather and climate disasters for the period 1980–2017 (updated from Smith and Katz, 2013; see www.ncdc.noaa.gov/billions/). The total damage for the last year in the record 2017 stands out, being dominated by damage caused by Hurricane

165

Harvey striking Texas, Hurricane Irma striking Florida, and Hurricane Maria striking Puerto Rico. Another year that stands out is 2005 in which Hurricane Katrina struck Louisiana, constituting the highest loss from a single event (over $160 billion in 2017 dollars). While the plot suggests an apparent long-term increasing trend, more noticeable is the incredible magnitude of fluctuations in total loss from year to year.

The annual total losses shown in Figure 8.1 have two sources of variation: (i) variations in the annual number of disasters (for example, see Chapter 2 on the changes in the records of North Atlantic tropical cyclones); and (ii) variation in the losses from individual events. As such, the annual total loss can be viewed as a "random sum" (Embrechts et al, 1997, Katz, 2002). Figure 8.2 shows the time series of annual frequency of US billion-dollar weather and climate disasters, source (i) of variation in the annual total losses. A marked increasing trend is obvious with by far the highest frequencies occurring near the end of the record, 16 disasters in both the years 2011 and 2017 and 15 disasters in 2016. Figure 8.3 shows the losses from individual events versus the year, source (ii) of variation in the annual total losses. These variations are

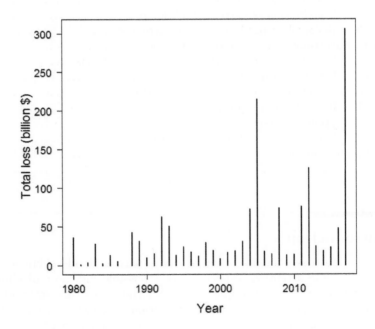

FIGURE 8.1: Annual total economic losses from US billion-dollar weather and climate disasters (adjusted for inflation to constant 2017 dollars) for period 1980–2017.

Introduction

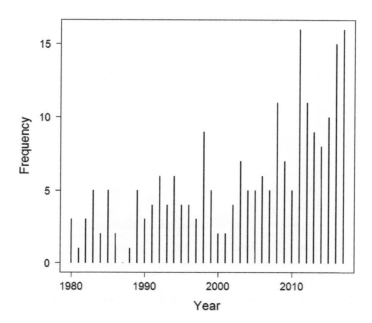

FIGURE 8.2: Annual frequency of US billion-dollar weather and climate disasters for period 1980–2017.

quite erratic, with any increasing trend not necessarily being obvious. Instead, most striking is the highly skewed distribution of losses, with the losses for the vast majority of disasters being at least an order of magnitude smaller than the highest values (of course, by definition all losses in this data set are at least $1 billion US dollars). We will apply extreme value theory to fit a generalized Pareto distribution to extreme high losses (Coles, 2001). Then we will compare this analysis with the traditional approach of fitting a lognormal distribution to all the loss data (e.g., Nordhaus, 2010).

In trend analysis of time series of losses, one complication is isolating the influence of weather and climate extremes. The effects of shifts in societal vulnerability, including higher population and capital that is more valuable, dominate time series of losses. Thus, we cannot attribute any observed trend in losses to climate change alone. For this reason, we will also consider losses from hurricanes alone, normalized for shifts in societal vulnerability.

Hurricanes (technically, a few were tropical cyclones not attaining hurricane status) making landfall along the Gulf and Atlantic coasts of the US are the weather or climate phenomenon causing the most loss among billion-dollar disasters (Smith and Katz, 2013). As such, losses caused by hurricanes have

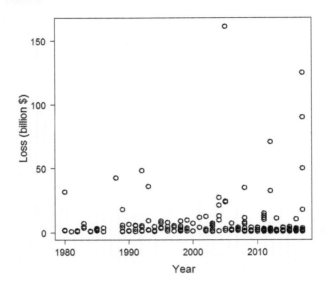

FIGURE 8.3: Losses from individual US billion-dollar weather and climate disasters for period 1980–2017.

received more attention, resulting in higher quality estimates than for other loss data (e.g., for floods). Further, Pielke Jr et al (2008) created a normalized hurricane loss data set for the period 1900–2005, adjusted for both inflation and shifts in societal vulnerability to the year 2005. For purposes of trend analysis, the time series of hurricane losses has the advantage of being considerably longer than the billion-dollar weather and climate disaster data set, although not extending as close to the present. We note that the hurricane loss data set does not constitute simply a subset of the billion-dollar disaster data set. Rather it consists of losses from essentially all hurricanes (i.e., not just those losses exceeding a billion dollars), but only accounts for the effects of high winds (hurricane losses in the billion-dollar disaster data set consist of combined losses caused by both wind and flooding).

In this chapter, we first characterize the statistical distribution of losses caused by extreme weather and climate events, including an attempt to reconcile the common use of the lognormal distribution for all the loss data with a heavy-tailed distribution based on extreme value theory for only extreme high losses (Section 8.2). Next we demonstrate how the uncertainty and variability in loss data can introduce bias in losses (e.g., through the conversion of insured loss to total loss, Section 8.3). In Section 8.4, we perform trend analyses for both losses from billion-dollar weather and climate disasters and hurricane losses alone. Then we demonstrate how normalization techniques for shifts in

Introduction

societal vulnerability can introduce artificial trends. Finally, Section 8.5 consists of a summary and discussion. We relegate details about extreme value theory, focusing on penultimate approximations applied to the lognormal distribution for overall loss data, to the technical box (p. 183). Previous attempts to quantify uncertainties in loss data include Smith and Katz (2013) and Smith and Matthews (2015).

Generalized Pareto Distribution

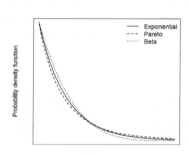

GP distribution

The generalized Pareto (GP) distribution arises as the approximate distribution for the excess over a high threshold. That is, given a random value X and a threshold u, extreme value theory implies that the random variable $Y = X - u$ has an approximate GP distribution for sufficiently high threshold u (Coles, 2001). An expression for the cumulative distribution function, H say, of the GP is

$$H[y; \sigma, \xi] = 1 - \left[1 + \xi \left(\frac{y}{\sigma}\right)\right]^{-1/\xi}, \quad y > 0.$$

The GP distribution has two parameters: (i) a scale parameter $\sigma > 0$ (strictly speaking, σ depends on the threshold u); and (ii) a shape parameter ξ determined by the upper tail of the distribution of the individual observations. Depending on the sign of the shape parameter, the GP distribution has three types (see graphic above showing GP probability density function):

- Pareto type ($\xi > 0$) with a "heavy" tail (i.e., slowly decaying in the form of a power law);
- beta type ($\xi < 0$) with a finite upper tail; and
- exponential type ($\xi = 0$) with a light upper tail, intermediate between the Pareto and beta types.

8.2 Loss distribution

In this section, we describe the general characteristics of the probability distribution of losses from extreme weather and climate events. Because this distribution is highly positively skewed (i.e., only a few disasters account for the vast majority of total losses), it is common to fit a lognormal distribution to overall losses (e.g., Nordhaus, 2010). Because of the special attention to extreme high losses (e.g., by the insurance and reinsurance industries), an alternative approach is to fit a generalized Pareto distribution (Coles, 2001), based on extreme value theory, solely to the events with losses exceeding a high threshold (i.e., only to the upper tail of the distribution).

8.2.1 Overall distribution of losses

First we fit lognormal distributions to the losses from billion-dollar disasters and from hurricanes alone. If a random variable X has a lognormal distribution, then the random variable $Y = \ln X$ is normally distributed, say with mean μ_Y and variance σ_Y^2. That is,

$$Y = \ln X \sim N\left(\mu_Y, \sigma_Y^2\right). \tag{8.1}$$

Here $N\left(\mu_Y, \sigma_Y^2\right)$ denotes a normal distribution with mean μ and variance σ^2. In other words, assuming a lognormal distribution is equivalent to fitting a normal distribution to the log-transformed losses. Other technical details include that, for losses from billion-dollar disasters, we subtract $1 billion from the data before log transforming (to account for the loss always exceeding $1 billion). For losses from hurricanes alone, we exclude events with loss below $0.1 billion (and subtract $0.1 billion from the data before log transforming) to eliminate a bias in the case of relatively low losses (see Katz, 2016, Pielke Jr et al, 2008).

Application to losses from billion-dollar disasters

Table 8.1 includes parameter estimates, along with standard errors, for the fit of a lognormal distribution to the losses from billion-dollar weather and climate disasters (sample size $n = 219$). As a diagnostic, Figure 8.4 shows a quantile-quantile (Q-Q) plot for the fit of a normal distribution to the log-transformed losses. The scatterplot of sample quantiles versus theoretical quantiles falls quite close to a straight line, as expected if the losses actually constituted a sample drawn from a lognormal distribution. There are some apparent systematic departures from a straight line for very high losses, but with the magnitudes of these discrepancies being relatively small.

Loss distribution

TABLE 8.1: Maximum likelihood estimates for parameters of lognormal distribution fit to losses from individual billion-dollar weather and climate disasters for period 1980–2017 and to losses from hurricanes alone for period 1900–2005 (standard error given in parentheses)

Data Set	Parameter	Estimate
(i) Losses from billion-dollar disasters	μ_Y	0.444 (0.106)
($n = 219$)	σ_Y	1.561 (0.075)
(ii) Losses from hurricanes alone	μ_Y	0.081 (0.167)
($n = 160$)	σ_Y	2.115 (0.118)

Application to losses from hurricanes

Table 8.1 also includes parameter estimates, along with standard errors, for the fit of a lognormal distribution to the losses from hurricanes alone (sample size $n = 160$). Figure 8.5 shows the corresponding Q-Q plot for the fit of a normal distribution to the log-transformed losses. Quite similar to Figure 8.4, the

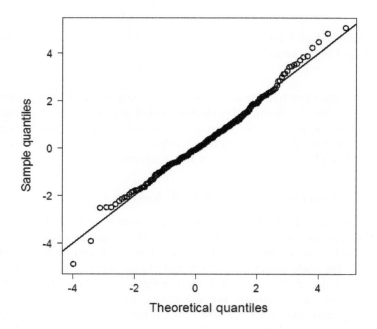

FIGURE 8.4: Q-Q plot for fit of lognormal distribution to losses from individual US billion-dollar weather and climate disasters for period 1980–2017.

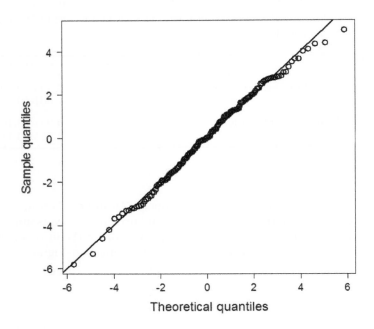

FIGURE 8.5: Q-Q plot for fit of lognormal distribution to losses from hurricanes striking US for period 1900–2005.

pattern falls quite close to a straight line, with some systematic departures for very high losses likewise being only relatively small in magnitude. In summary, for many purposes, practitioners would not hesitate to adopt the lognormal distribution for statistical estimation and inference about losses from billion-dollar weather and climate disasters or from hurricanes alone.

8.2.2 Distribution of extreme high losses

For a random variable X, the corresponding random variable $Y = X - u$ denotes the "excess" over a high threshold u. Based on extreme value theory (Coles, 2001), we assume that this excess has a generalized Pareto (GP) distribution with scale parameter $\sigma > 0$ and shape parameter ξ (see box on p. 169 for more details about the GP distribution). In reality, the GP distribution is only an approximation, becoming more accurate as the threshold u increases. Typically, extreme high losses have a heavy-tailed (or "power law") distribution (i.e., $\xi > 0$; Katz, 2016). In practice, we chose the threshold u by trial and error, with a trade-off between a more accurate GP approximation

Loss distribution

TABLE 8.2: Maximum likelihood estimates for parameters of GP distribution fit to excesses in loss over a high threshold from individual billion-dollar weather and climate disasters for period 1980–2017 and from hurricanes alone for period 1900–2005 (standard error given in parentheses)

Data Set	Parameter	Estimate
(i) Losses from billion-dollar disasters ($n = 219$, $u = \$10.5$ billion)	σ ξ	16.278 (6.329) 0.470 (0.346)
(ii) Losses from hurricanes alone ($n = 31$, $u = \$7.5$ billion)	σ ξ	11.603 (3.677) 0.476 (0.275)

for higher threshold value and more excesses from which to estimate the GP parameters for lower threshold value.

Application to losses from billion-dollar disasters

Table 8.2 includes parameter estimates, along with standard errors, for the fit of a GP distribution to the excesses in loss from individual billion-dollar weather and climate disasters above a high threshold of $u = \$10.5$ billion ($n = 25$ excesses). Although a billion dollars might seem like a high threshold, we need to use a considerably higher threshold in order for the GP approximation to be acceptable. For this data set, it is challenging to select the threshold, with a relative lack of stability in the shape parameter estimates as the threshold varies. We obtained a maximum likelihood estimate of 0.470 for the shape parameter ξ, or apparently a quite heavy tail (e.g., a shape parameter of 0.5 or above would imply infinite variance). As a diagnostic, Figure 8.6 shows a Q-Q plot for the fit of a GP distribution to these excesses in loss from billion-dollar weather and climate disasters. The scatterplot appears reasonably close to a straight line, except perhaps for the highest value.

Application to losses from hurricanes

Table 8.2 also includes parameter estimates, along with standard errors, for the fit of a GP distribution to the excesses in loss from hurricanes alone above a high threshold of $u = \$7.5$ billion ($n = 31$ excesses). Katz (2016) used this same threshold value with its selection being straightforward, unlike the previous billion-dollar disasters example, perhaps because only one type of disaster is involved. This threshold value is only slightly lower than the one used for billion-dollar disasters, after converting from 2005 dollars to 2017 dollars. We obtained a maximum likelihood estimate of 0.476 for the shape parameter ξ, consistent with other analyses of hurricane losses (e.g., Jagger et al, 2011) and quite close to that for billion-dollar disasters. Figure 8.7 shows a Q-Q plot for the fit of a GP distribution to these excesses in loss

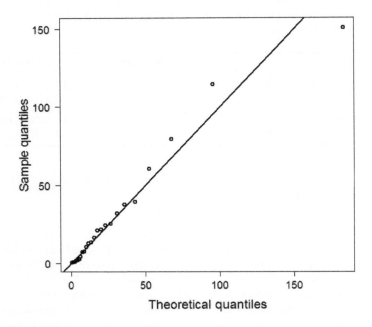

FIGURE 8.6: Q-Q plot for fit of GP distribution to excesses in loss over a threshold of $10.5 billion from individual US billion-dollar weather and climate disasters.

from hurricanes. It is quite close to a straight line even for the highest value, perhaps a bit better in appearance than Figure 8.6 for billion-dollar disasters.

8.2.3 Reconciling implications for extremes

The GP distributions fitted to extreme high losses for billion-dollar weather and climate disasters and for hurricanes alone both have positive estimated shape parameters indicative of heavy tails. Yet, strictly speaking, the upper tail of a lognormal distribution is light in the sense of standard extreme value theory (i.e., shape parameter $\xi = 0$; e.g., Chapter 3 of Embrechts et al, 1997). In this subsection, we attempt to reconcile these seemingly inconsistent results. This reconciliation makes use of penultimate approximations or more refined, second-order extreme value theory as detailed in the box on p. 183.

Modeling all the loss data with a lognormal distribution is common in applications. It is convenient for correlation and regression analyses, as such techniques can be applied directly to log-transformed losses (e.g., to study the effect of the El Niño phenomenon on losses from hurricanes; Katz, 2002).

Loss distribution

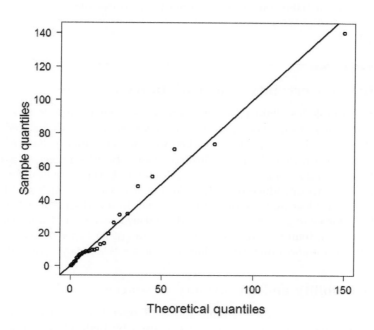

FIGURE 8.7: Q-Q plot for fit of GP distribution to excesses in loss over a threshold of $7.5 billion from US hurricanes.

Penultimate extreme value theory serves as a partial justification for this approach. In particular, for the lognormal parameter values of $\sigma_Y = 1.5$ and 2 (as consistent with the estimates in Table 8.1), the penultimate shape parameter is roughly 0.4 or 0.5 (see Table 8.5). Such values are in close agreement with the values of the shape parameter obtained for the loss data (Table 8.2), despite the "ultimate" extreme value theory approximation for the lognormal of shape parameter $\xi = 0$.

Still one would worry about using the lognormal distribution for losses if the focus is on catastrophic (or "black swan") events, as in the reinsurance industry (Murnane, 2004). In particular, it would be a more robust strategy to estimate return levels of losses for long return periods using the GP distribution, especially when attaching a confidence interval to such estimates (Coles, 2001). A compromise, but less parsimonious approach is to fit a "hybrid" distribution to the loss data; that is, a conventional distribution such as the lognormal to low and moderate values but a GP to high values. Such an approach involves technical details such as constraining the distribution to be continuous at the change point between the two distributions (e.g., Furrer and

Katz, 2008). Frigessi et al (2002) proposed an even more involved "dynamic mixture" of two distributions with an application to loss data.

8.3 Bias, uncertainty, and variability in losses

Routinely available loss data typically need adjustment to produce loss estimates in a desired form. For example, total losses (i.e., both insured and uninsured) caused by hurricanes or other weather or climate disasters are needed in practice rather than only insured losses. Besides reflecting a clear source of uncertainty is loss estimates, less obvious is the potential for such loss adjustments to introduce bias that can be substantial (Smith and Katz, 2013). In treating loss as a random variable, we do not distinguish between variability in losses (e.g., attributable to the natural variation of weather and climate over small temporal and spatial scales) and other types of uncertainty (e.g., involving unknown quantities that are not necessarily even measured).

8.3.1 Variability and uncertainty as sources of bias

Adjustments to losses involve simple forms of operation such as taking a ratio. For example, insured hurricane loss caused by high wind, denoted by $L_{Insured}$, is commonly multiplied by 2 (equivalently, divided by 0.5) to convert to approximate total loss, denoted by L_{Total} (Smith and Katz, 2013). Formally,

$$L_{Total} = L_{Insured}/R. \qquad (8.2)$$

Here R denotes the insurance participation rate R, $0 < R < 1$. Further, R is not really a constant value, but varies both spatially and temporally. We note that similar forms of adjustments arise for other issues, including taking into account shifts in societal vulnerability (Pielke Jr et al, 2008). It might be naively assumed that ignoring any random variations in R, instead always using an average value (e.g., $R = 0.5$), would be relatively harmless. Nevertheless, it turns out that ignoring this variation can actually introduce a substantial bias in the adjusted loss.

Jensen's inequality

Suppose a function f is strictly convex. One condition for convexity is that the second derivative of f is positive. Consider a non-constant random variable X with expected value (i.e., mean of its probability distribution) denoted by $E(X)$. Then Jensen's inequality states that (e.g., Chapter 1 of Berger, 1985)

$$f[E(X)] < E[f(X)]. \qquad (8.3)$$

Bias, uncertainty, and variability in losses

In other words, the order in which averaging is applied makes a systematic difference in the result. We note that Jensen's inequality only specifies the direction of bias, not its magnitude.

Application of Jensen's inequality

If we treat the insurance participation rate R as random variable, then the adjustment (8.2) involves the factor $1/R$. Taking the reciprocal corresponds to a convex function, $f(x) = 1/x$, $0 < x < 1$. So applying Jensen's inequality (8.3), we have

$$1/\mathrm{E}(R) < \mathrm{E}(1/R). \tag{8.4}$$

It follows that the common practice of ignoring the variation in R and substituting $\mathrm{E}(R)$ in place of R in (8.2) introduces a systematic underestimation of total loss. That is,

$$\mathrm{E}(L_{Insured})[1/\mathrm{E}(R)] < \mathrm{E}(L_{Total}). \tag{8.5}$$

8.3.2 Effects of adjustments

In this subsection, we illustrate the magnitude of this underestimation of loss in practice for loss estimation. As a rough approximation to the observed variation in hurricane insurance participation rate, we assume that R has a beta distribution on the interval (0.25, 0.75) with both shape parameters $p = q = 2$ (see Chapter 24 of Johnson and Kotz, 1970). This distribution has expected value (or mean) of $\mathrm{E}(R) = p/(p+q) = 0.5$, with about a 50% chance of R falling between 0.4 and 0.6 (Figure 8.8).

We want to estimate the bias in using $1/\mathrm{E}(R) = 2$ to adjust the hurricane loss from insured to total. So we conducted a simulation experiment in which 100,000 pseudo random numbers were generated from a beta distribution with $p = q = 2$ for R, and then transformed these numbers into the corresponding values of $1/R$. The estimated mean of the reciprocal of the participation rate, $1/R$, is about 2.12 rather than 2. In other words, ignoring the variation in the participation rate results in an underestimation of the total loss by about 5.5% on average.

For more insight into how this positive bias arises, Figure 8.9 shows a nonparametric density function estimate for the 100,000 simulated values of $1/R$. The nonlinear operation of taking the reciprocal has converted a distribution symmetric about 0.5 on the interval (0.25, 0.75) into a positively skewed distribution on the interval (4/3, 4).

The introduction of bias occurs for other loss adjustments in an analogous manner. Even the well-intentioned practice of rounding off uncertain factors (e.g., the factor two for inflating hurricane loss) creates additional bias. See Smith and Katz (2013) for an example of the bias introduced by rounding off the inflation factors in the case of insured losses from flooding caused by hurricanes.

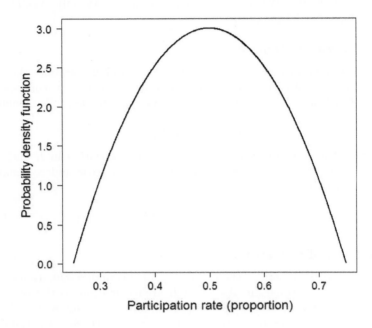

FIGURE 8.8: Beta probability density function with parameters $p = q = 2$ on interval (0.25, 0.75) for insurance participation rate.

8.4 Detection and attribution of trends in losses

Some researchers have argued that hurricanes should become increasingly destructive as part of global warming (Emanuel, 2005). In this section, we make use of the random sum representation of annual total loss, conducting trend analyses of the individual components, both the annual frequency of events and the losses from individual events. Then we illustrate by means of a simulation experiment why methods for adjusting losses for shifts in societal vulnerability may actually introduce additional biases.

8.4.1 Random sum representation

As mentioned in the Introduction, annual total loss is a random sum. In this case, it is generally more informative to model trends in the two component processes of a random sum: (i) the frequency of events and (ii) the individual loss associated with each event.

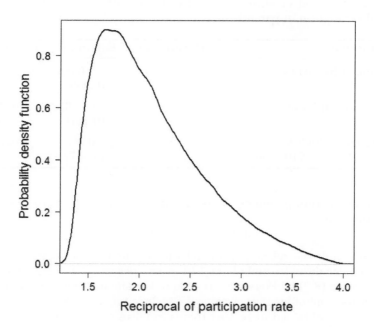

FIGURE 8.9: Estimated probability density function for reciprocal of participation rate.

Let the random variable $N(t)$ $(= 0, 1, \ldots)$ denote the number of events in year t, $t = 1, 2, \ldots$. Conditional on $N(t) > 0$, let X_k denote the loss from the kth event in year t, $k = 1, \ldots, N(t)$. Then the total annual loss in year t, say $S(t)$, can be expressed as

$$S(t) = X_1 + X_2 + \cdots + X_{N(t)}. \tag{8.6}$$

By the so-called "law of small numbers," it is natural to assume that the annual frequency of events $N(t)$ has a Poisson distribution, say with rate parameter $E[N(t)] = \lambda > 0$. In Section 8.2, we assumed a lognormal distribution for overall loss X_k and a GP distribution for extreme high loss, $X_k > u$. We next examine each of these three distributions for possible trends.

8.4.2 Trend analyses

Annual frequency of events

We allow the rate parameter of the Poisson distribution for the annual frequency of events to vary over time, now denoted by $\lambda(t)$ for year t, $t = 1, 2, \ldots$.

TABLE 8.3: Trend analyses of annual frequency of billion-dollar weather and climate disasters and of losses from individual events for period 1980–2017 (standard error given in parentheses)

Component	Parameter	Estimate	P-value
(i) Annual frequency ($n = 38$)	λ_1	0.0485 (0.0067)	$< 10^{-13}$
(ii) Individual losses ($n = 219$)	μ_1	0.0693 (0.1076)	0.520
(iii) Extreme high losses ($n = 25$, $u = \$10.5$ billion)	σ_1	0.0058 (0.0277)	0.837

To constrain the rate parameter to be positive, it is convenient to assume a trend of the form

$$\ln \lambda(t) = \lambda_0 + \lambda_1 t. \tag{8.7}$$

Without a trend, the estimated annual rate is about 5.76 events per year for billion-dollar disasters and about 1.51 events per year for hurricanes. The results of fitting (8.7) by Poisson regression to the annual frequency of billion-dollar disasters and of hurricanes alone are included in Table 8.3(i) and 8.4(i), respectively. We obtained increasing trends in mean annual frequency, about 5.0% per year for all disasters and about 1.0% per year for hurricanes, both highly statistically significant (see P-values based on likelihood ratio test in Table 8.3(i) and Table 8.4(i)). It is well known that the state of El Niño affects the frequency of damaging hurricanes (e.g., Katz, 2002). If the state of El Niño is included as a second variable on the right-hand side of (8.7), we obtain a quite similar trend estimate (still highly statistically significant).

Losses from individual events

Consistent with a lognormal distribution, we allow the mean of the log-transformed loss from individual events, now denoted by $\mu_Y(t)$ for year t, to vary linearly over time. That is,

$$\mu_Y(t) = \mu_0 + \mu_1 t. \tag{8.8}$$

The results of fitting (8.8) by standard linear regression to log-transformed losses from individual billion-dollar disasters and from hurricanes alone are included in Table 8.3(ii) and Table 8.4(ii), respectively. We obtained an increasing trend in terms of median loss for all disasters of about 7.2% per year and a decreasing trend in median loss for hurricanes of about 5.5% per year, but neither slope estimate is close to statistically significant (see P-values based on t-test in Table 8.3(ii) and Table 8.4(ii)).

TABLE 8.4: Trend analyses of annual frequency of hurricanes alone and of losses from individual events for period 1900–2005 (standard error given in parentheses)

Component	Parameter	Estimate	P-value
(i) Annual frequency ($n = 106$)	λ_1	0.0096 (0.0027)	< 0.001
(ii) Individual losses ($n = 160$)	μ_1	−0.0567 (0.0445)	0.204
(iii) Extreme high losses ($n = 31$, $u = \$7.5$ billion)	σ_1	−0.0132 (0.0076)	0.094

Extreme high losses

We allow the scale parameter of the GP distribution for excess loss above a high threshold to vary over time, now denoted by $\sigma(t)$ for year t. To constrain the scale parameter to be positive, it is convenient to assume a trend of the form

$$\ln \sigma(t) = \sigma_0 + \sigma_1 t. \qquad (8.9)$$

Such a trend in the scale parameter is proportional to a trend of the same form in the mean excess (i.e., expected value of GP distribution). The results of fitting (8.9) by maximum likelihood to excess loss above a high threshold extracted from all disasters and from hurricanes alone are included in Table 8.3(iii) and Table 8.4(iii), respectively. We obtained an increasing trend in mean excess loss from all disasters of about 0.6% per year (far from statistically significant), but a decreasing trend of about 1.3% per year with borderline statistical significance for excess loss from hurricanes (see P-values based on likelihood ratio test in Table 8.3(iii) and Table 8.4(iii)).

8.4.3 Issues in normalization of losses

In the trend analyses, we obtained apparent decreasing trends in overall loss and extreme high loss from hurricanes, although not necessarily statistically significant. Such results are inconsistent with the expectation that hurricanes are becoming more damaging as part of global warming. Still recall that the hurricane losses were normalized in an attempt to remove the effects of shifts in societal vulnerability. In this subsection, we will more closely examine the methods for normalizing losses to identify possible sources of bias.

In Section 8.3.2, we showed how ignoring the variation in insurance participation rates (as in current practice) can introduce a negative bias when converting insured loss to total loss. Now suppose that the random variation in participation rates is increasing over time. With increased variability, the negative bias should increase (in absolute magnitude) as well. We implement

TABLE 8.5: Estimated mean of reciprocal of insurance participation rate along with proportional bias based on 100,000 simulated values from beta distribution with parameters $p = q = 2$ on various subintervals of interval $(0, 1)$

Range of distribution	$E(1/R)$	Bias (%)
(0.25, 0.75)	2.117	−5.5
(0.20, 0.60)	2.171	−7.9
(0.15, 0.85)	2.253	−11.2
(0.10, 0.90)	2.367	−15.5
(0.05, 0.95)	2.539	−21.2

such an increase in variability by gradually increasing the width of the subinterval of the interval $(0, 1)$ on which the beta distribution is defined (i.e., from $(0.25, 0.75)$ to $(0.05, 0.95)$). The same parameter values of $p = q = 2$ are retained for the beta distribution, so that $E(R) = 0.5$.

Again based on simulating 100,000 values from each beta distribution, Table 8.5 lists the estimated mean of the reciprocal of the participation rate, along with the proportionate bias (i.e., comparing the estimate of $E(1/R)$ with $1/E(R) = 2$). As anticipated, the underestimation gradually increases in absolute magnitude from about 5.5% to about 21%.

Of course, such a shift in the variability of the distribution of insurance participation rates may well not be plausible. Yet if we consider the normalization of losses for population increases instead, these simulation results seem relevant. Population adjustments involve a multiplicative factor made at the county level, analogous to that for insurance participation rates (see (8.2) and Pielke Jr et al, 2008). Not only has population increased considerably over the years, but greater urbanization would imply that the spatial variation in population has increased as well. The results in Table 8.5 suggest that normalization of losses for population shifts over time, effectively ignoring changes in spatial patterns of population at finer scales than counties, could well induce an artificial decreasing trend in normalized losses. Although speculative, perhaps such a trend could be of sufficient magnitude to counteract a real increasing trend in losses attributable to climate change.

8.5 Summary and discussion

This chapter focuses on issues arising in the statistical analysis of losses from extreme weather and climate events, especially for the purpose of the detection and attribution of trends. Making use of the statistical theory of extreme values, we attempt to reconcile the different approaches to modeling the probability distribution of losses, using the lognormal distribution fit to all the loss data versus using the GP distribution fit to only extreme high losses. Despite

Summary and discussion

showing that the two approaches are both capable of producing an apparent heavy tail, we still recommend use of the GP distribution when the interest is in catastrophic disasters.

Variability and uncertainty in loss estimates are important not only for their own sake, but because they can introduce bias into adjusted losses. We show how the standard adjustment technique for converting insured loss to total loss (i.e., both insured and uninsured) can result in a substantial underestimation on average. The normalization of losses to remove shifts in societal vulnerabilities raises analogous issues. In particular, a common technique to correct for shifts in population over time can actually introduce an artificial decreasing trend, if the spatial variation in population has increased because of urbanization. Such an effect could well hide any real trend in losses due to climate change. Although alternative normalization methods have been proposed (e.g., Estrada et al, 2015), they still appear to have serious limitations and are not ready to be adopted in practice.

With the new paradigm behind the recent rise of the field of data science, one could conceive of making breakthroughs through statistical analysis of individual claim data (as in Lyubchich and Gel, 2017). On the one hand, such an approach could potentially produce much useful information about loss and its relationship to weather and climate. On the other hand, challenges would remain such as dealing with inconsistencies in loss estimation (e.g., due to changes in government insurance programs for crops and for floods; Smith and Katz, 2013).

Acknowledgments

I thank Adam Smith for providing US billion-dollar weather and climate disaster data and for advice on the contents of this chapter. The statistical analysis made use of the `ismev` package in the open source statistical programming language R (www.r-project.org). The National Center for Atmospheric Research is sponsored by the National Science Foundation of the US.

Penultimate Approximation in Case of Lognormal Parent Distribution

Rather than the GP approximation for the distribution of the excess over a high threshold, it is more convenient to consider the equivalent generalized extreme value (GEV) approximation for the distribution of the maximum of a sequence of random variables. Katz (2016) described a method for obtaining an expression for the shape parameter of the GEV in a penultimate approximation to the distribution of the maximum. It is based on the "hazard rate" $h_F(x)$ of the "parent" cumulative distribution function (cdf) F; that is,

$$h_F(x) = \frac{F'(x)}{[1 - F(x)]}, \tag{8.10}$$

where F' (i.e., the derivative of F) denotes the corresponding probability density function.

The limiting distribution of the maximum of lognormal random variables, suitably normalized, converges to the Gumbel, a GEV with shape parameter $\xi = 0$ (equivalent to the exponential type of GP; Chapter 3 of Embrechts et al, 1997). Instead, the penultimate approximation consists of a GEV distribution with shape parameter ξ_n, depending on the block size n (i.e., the length of the sequence of random variables from which the maximum value is extracted), given by

$$\xi_n \approx (1/h_F)'(x)\Big|_{x=u(n)} \qquad (8.11)$$

Here $u(n)$ is the "characteristic largest value," or $(1 - 1/n)$th quantile of the cdf F; that is,

$$u(n) = F^{-1}(1 - 1/n) \qquad (8.12)$$

For the lognormal distribution (1), with parameter ξ_y (without loss in generality, set $\mu_Y = 0$), (8.11) and (8.12) yield

$$\xi_n \approx \left[\sigma_Y (2\ln n)^{1/2} - 1\right] / (2\ln n) \qquad (8.13)$$

(e.g., Wadsworth et al, 2010). We note that $\xi_n > 0$, but ξ_n necessarily decreases to zero as the block size $n \to \infty$ (to obtain the Gumbel type with $\xi = 0$ as the ultimate approximation). See Chapter 3 for more examples of using GEV distributions.

Because (8.13) is still an approximation, we conducted a limited simulation study of how well it works in practice. Table 8.6 shows the results of estimating the shape parameter through direct fit of the GEV to maxima based on simulated sequences from the lognormal distribution, with $\sigma_Y = 1.5$ and 2 to mimic the values obtained for loss data (Table 8.1) and block size $n = 50, 100, 200$ (40,000 maxima for each pair of values of n and σ_Y). The shape parameter estimates for the fitted GEV distributions tend to be somewhat farther above zero than those based on the penultimate approximation (8.13). Thus, while the penultimate approximation remains imperfect, it is clearly preferable to assuming a shape parameter of $\xi = 0$ as in the ultimate approximation.

It is not completely clear how best to convert the block size n in the GEV approximation into a high threshold in the GP approximation. One way is to make use of the relationship (8.12) for the characteristic largest value as does Katz (2016). Nevertheless, the results are not very sensitive to how this conversion is made, because the penultimate approximation (8.13) has a logarithmic dependence on the block size.

TABLE 8.6 Estimates of shape parameter ξ for GEV distribution fit to maxima of block size n simulated from lognormal distribution (with parameters $\mu_Y = 0$ and σ_Y), along with shape parameter (denoted by ξ_n) based on penultimate approximation (8.13) (standard error given in parentheses)

n	σ_Y	ξ_n	Estimated ξ
50	1.5	0.408	0.450 (0.005)
50	2.0	0.587	0.654 (0.005)
100	1.5	0.386	0.434 (0.005)
100	2.0	0.550	0.609 (0.005)
200	1.5	0.366	0.410 (0.005)
200	2.0	0.520	0.574 (0.005)

References

Berger JO (1985) Statistical Decision Theory and Bayesian Analysis, 2nd edn. Springer Series in Statistics, Springer Science & Business Media, New York

Coles S (2001) An Introduction to Statistical Modeling of Extreme Values. Springer, London

Emanuel K (2005) Increasing destructiveness of tropical cyclones over the past 30 years. Nature 436(7051):686–688

Embrechts P, Klüppelberg C, Mikosch T (1997) Modelling Extremal Events: for Insurance and Finance. Springer-Verlag, Berlin

Estrada F, Botzen WJW, Tol RSJ (2015) Economic losses from US hurricanes consistent with an influence from climate change. Nature Geoscience 8(11):880–884

Frigessi A, Haug O, Rue H (2002) A dynamic mixture model for unsupervised tail estimation without threshold selection. Extremes 5(3):219–235

Furrer EM, Katz RW (2008) Improving the simulation of extreme precipitation events by stochastic weather generators. Water Resources Research 44(12):W12439

Jagger TH, Elsner JB, Burch RK (2011) Climate and solar signals in property damage losses from hurricanes affecting the United States. Natural Hazards 58(1):541–557

Johnson NL, Kotz S (1970) Distributions in Statistics: Continuous Univariate Distributions, vol 2. John Wiley, New York

Katz RW (2002) Stochastic modeling of hurricane damage. Journal of Applied Meteorology 41(7):754–762

Katz RW (2016) Economic impact of extreme events: An approach based on extreme value theory. In: Chavez M, Ghil M, Urrutia-Fucugauchi J (eds) Extreme Events: Observations, Modeling, and Economics. American Geophysical Union Monograph 214, Wiley, Hoboken, NJ, 207–217

Lyubchich V, Gel YR (2017) Can we weather proof our insurance? Environmetrics 28(2):e2433

Murnane RJ (2004) Climate research and reinsurance. Bulletin of the American Meteorological Society 85(5):697–707

Nordhaus WD (2010) The economics of hurricanes and implications of global warming. Climate Change Economics 1(01):1–20

Pielke Jr RA, Gratz J, Landsea CW, Collins D, Saunders MA, Musulin R (2008) Normalized hurricane damage in the United States: 1900–2005. Natural Hazards Review 9(1):29–42

Smith AB, Katz RW (2013) US billion-dollar weather and climate disasters: data sources, trends, accuracy and biases. Natural Hazards 67(2):387–410

Smith AB, Matthews JL (2015) Quantifying uncertainty and variable sensitivity within the US billion-dollar weather and climate disaster cost estimates. Natural Hazards 77(3):1829–1851

Wadsworth JL, Tawn JA, Jonathan P (2010) Accounting for choice of measurement scale in extreme value modeling. The Annals of Applied Statistics 4(3):1558–1578

9

Event Attribution: Linking Specific Extreme Events to Human-Caused Climate Change

Stephanie Herring

National Oceanic and Atmospheric Administration, Boulder, CO, USA

CONTENTS

9.1	Why is this chapter in this book?	187
9.2	Background on event attribution	188
9.3	Event attribution methodologies	188
9.4	Impact attribution	192
9.5	FAR = 1 or "Not possible without climate change"	194
9.6	Communicating event attribution studies	195
9.7	Summary	197
References		197

9.1 Why is this chapter in this book?

The overall aim of this book is to provide an overview of the current state of assessing and quantifying climate change and its socioeconomic and environmental impacts through a lens of statistical and data sciences. One component of this discussion is to assess the methodologies for quantifying impacts of climate change on specific socioeconomic and environmental outcomes that occur as a result of extreme events. However, before one can begin to examine the implications climate change is having on society through extreme events, it is essential to first determine whether the climate change impact on the extreme event in question can be quantified. Quantitatively connecting the impact of anthropogenic climate change on extreme events is the domain of the field of climate change event attribution, which examines whether climate change played a role in altering the risk of a specific event through a probabilistic approach.

The field of event attribution will be the focus of this chapter with a review of the current state of attribution science, methodological approaches, communication of results, and a few recent developments in the field as well as future areas of research.

9.2 Background on event attribution

Examining the impact of human-caused climate change on extreme events is a relatively new focus within climate change science, with the idea initially proposed in 2003 (Allen, 2003) and the first extreme heat event attribution paper published in 2004 (Stott et al, 2004) looking at the 2003 European heat wave. Since that time the interest in this area of research has continued to grow, and methodologies have been refined and improved (see the Bulletin of the American Meteorological Society's special annual supplement, Explaining Extreme Events from a Climate Perspective, e.g., Herring et al, 2019). All manner of event types have been investigated including temperature and precipitation extremes, marine heat waves, drought, storm surge, sea level rise, coastal inundation, sea surface temperature, forest fires, snowpack drought, snow storms, tropical cyclones, Arctic and Antarctic sea ice, and sunshine, to name a few.

9.3 Event attribution methodologies

An important component of this book is that it advances a quantitative rather than a merely qualitative analysis into climate change impacts. This is becoming increasingly possible from a science perspective, and increasingly important from an application perspective, in particular for adaptation and resiliency efforts. Knowing that extreme precipitation is changing is certainly of interest, but if, for example, a community is designing a new storm drainage system then they also need to know by how much precipitation is expected to change for their region. Extreme event attribution is focused largely on this question of how much. The results of event attribution studies are not binary yes or no results. Instead, they are focused on investigating whether the influence of climate change can be quantified and the confidence in the results assessed.

A detailed analysis of event attribution methodologies was recently published by the US National Academy of Sciences (NAS, 2016), and it explores in greater detail different approaches as well as their strengths and weaknesses for certain applications. In general, most event attribution analysis employ the widely accepted technique of calculating the fraction of attributable risk (FAR) for the event, a statistical approach borrowed from epidemiology and

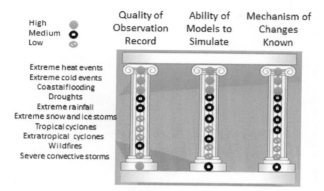

FIGURE 9.1: The three scientific pillars of attribution upon which attribution assessments are built are the quality of the observational record, the ability of the models to simulate the event, and whether how human cause climate change will impact the event are known. The strength of these pillars varies across different extreme event types.

public health. FAR is defined by the equation:

$$\text{FAR} = 1 - P_0/P_1.$$

P_1 is the probability of a climatic event (such as a heat wave) occurring in the presence of anthropogenic climate change. This is the world we live in today and the event's probability is established by models that can often be validated against observations. P_0 is the probability of the event occurring if anthropogenic climate change had not been present in the world, or to some other baseline "pre-industrial" climate. This alternative world is based on model runs of a "control" world that only include natural forcing mechanisms and ignore the changes to atmospheric composition driven by human greenhouse gas emissions. By comparing the probability of the event in the world that is with a world that might have been, the change in event probability can be quantified.

Confidence in the attribution results depends on three primary elements: (1) the strength of the observational record, (2) the ability of the models to capture the extreme event, and (3) the understanding of the physical mechanisms that lead to changes in extremes as a result of climate change. The quality of these three elements varies significantly for different event types (Figures 9.1 and 9.2).

Attribution methodology has come a long way since its inception fifteen years ago with the Stott et al (2004) paper. As stated in the US Government's Climate Science Special Report from 2017, "the science of event attribution is rapidly advancing through improved understanding of the mechanisms that

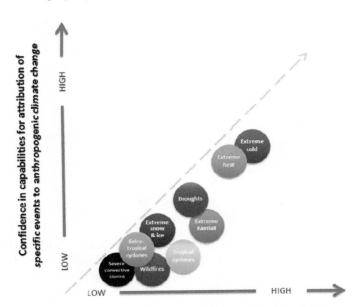

FIGURE 9.2: Schematic depiction of the assessment of the state of attribution science for different event types.

produce extreme events and the marked progress in development of methods that are used for event attribution (high confidence)" (USGCRP, 2017). However, in all cases it is important to be aware of two important factors that can impact how results should be interpreted.

First, event definition is critical to understand. How has an "event" been defined in space and time can influence whether a role for climate change is, or is not, found, and the extent of the influence. For example, after Hurricane Harvey there were two analyses that looked at the extreme precipitation caused by Hurricane Harvey. First, Van Oldenborgh et al (2017) concluded, "that global warming made the precipitation about 15% (8%–19%) more intense, or equivalently made such an event three (1.5–5) times more likely." Risser and Wehner (2017) found that, "human-induced climate change likely increased the chances of the observed precipitation accumulations during Hurricane Harvey in the most affected areas of Houston by a factor of at least 3.5. Further, precipitation accumulations in these areas were likely increased by at least 18.8% (best estimate of 37.7%)..." Note that in both papers, the authors provide a "most likely" estimate (15% and 37.7%, respectively), as well as the full range of probabilities that are likely. "At least" values represent the lower bound of the extent to which climate change played a role. Although both papers conclude that human caused climate change made the precipitation from Hurricane Harvey worse, there are differences in the extent of the influence. While these may seem minor, these differences could potentially be very important to decision makers, such as city planners rebuilding after an extreme in an effort to enhance resilience to future flooding risk. So what drove these differences? In part, differences could be driven by the fact that the two papers examine different "events." The Van Oldenborgh et al (2017) analysis covered a region that extended along the coast of several states (27.5°N–31.0 °N, 85.0°W–97.5°W, see Fig. 2 in their paper, panels b and c). This region included Houston, TX, and Corpus Christi, TX, two of the epicenters for human impacts of the event. However, it also extends significantly to the east along the Gulf Coast. In contrast, Risser and Wehner (2017) used Global Historical Climatology Network (GHCN) stations within a much smaller region of the event, focused more directly over Houston, TX (see Fig. 1 of their paper). They also examined different periods. Van Oldenborgh et al (2017) took the three-day average for Saturday August 26 to Monday August 28. Risser and Wehner (2017) looked at the period from 25 to 31 August 2017. Although both papers used data measurements from GHCN stations, they used different periods over different regions. So rather than seeing these as contradictory results, the differences in the quantitative assessments are a result of event definition.

Second, methodological choices can, in some cases, lead to important differences in event attribution results. For example, a study of the air pollution episode in Europe in December 2016 (Vautard et al, 2018) found different results depending on the type of climate model used. With a multimodel ensemble, a significant human-induced effect was found on the stagnant winter time conditions that prevailed over northwestern Europe during that month, but this was not found with two single-model ensembles. A second example is the record 2016 heat in Asia, which was found not to be possible without human-caused climate change, and the authors concluded the fraction of attributable risk (FAR) to climate change was effectively 1. This result is based on the atmospheric general circulation model (AGCM) simulations using the observed sea surface temperatures (SST). Thus, it is suggested that "the observed heat anomaly have zero probability of occurrence with the certain, observed, SST variability pattern." However, it is not clear how the FAR would be impacted if the uncertainty of the natural variability of SST were considered.

Given that attribution results are potentially sensitive to event definition and methodological choices it is important to clearly communicate this information within each study and, when possible, also to explore such methodological sensitivities in the study itself. Even so, there is an ongoing debate in the scientific community about the effects of methodological choices and optimal strategies for attribution of extreme events. In general, there are several best practices that have broad agreements.

First, regarding models, when possible multiple models should be used. Also the model should be verified by assessing the ability of the models to effectively capture the extreme event type in a particular region against the observational record. This will establish whether the model is suitable for the intended purpose. Time constraints can also play a factor in selecting the appropriate approach. If a rapid turnaround time is desired, the analysis may have to rely primarily on observational based approaches. Modeling approaches that are highly conditioned can be completed more quickly, and unconditional approaches may be based only on available simulations that have already been completed. Further work is needed to fully understand the effects such choices are having, and this is an ongoing area of research and discussion within the event attribution community. In general, multiple studies looking at the same event using independently validated approaches will yield the most robust scientific understanding. Multiple studies can help distinguish between results that are robust from those that are more sensitive to framing and approach.

Second, it is important to explore multiple physical drivers of an event as the physical drivers investigated can influence whether a link to climate change is identified. For example, drought can be caused by a combination of many factors that can include precipitation, temperature, soil moisture, and water usage levels to name a few. The value of looking at multiple drivers is illustrated in two studies of the Northwest Plains Drought of 2017. Two independent studies reached the same conclusion, which was that precipitation patterns had not changed significantly in that region (Hoell et al, 2019, Wang et al, 2019). However, climate change played a role in the drought by exacerbating heat and evapotranspiration. By exploring multiple drivers of the event (i.e., precipitation patterns, temperature changes, and evapotranspiration), a more complete understanding of the event emerged.

9.4 Impact attribution

In the past several years there have also been an increasing number of impact attribution papers that draw a line connecting climate change to the altered risk of an extreme event and the subsequent impact of the event. Impact attribution is increasingly being recognized as the next major area of advancement for attribution science to enhance the field's ability to connect to indices relevant to people (Otto, 2016).

The first paper to do this for human health was published in 2016 when attribution scientists partnered with public health officials to assess the role climate change played in increased mortality from a specific event—the 2003 European heat wave (Mitchell et al, 2016). Their results concluded that in the summer of 2003, "out of the estimated ∼315 and ∼735 summer deaths directly attributed to the heat wave event in Greater London and Central Paris, respectively, 64 (±3) deaths were attributable to anthropogenic climate change in London, and 506 (±51) in Paris." For the first time a methodology had been established for connecting the increased intensity of a heat wave due to climate change to the mortality of a specific heat extreme heat event. Clearly, multiple approaches could be taken to address these questions, and the paper by Mitchell et al (2016) lays out just one. Also, just as with any event attribution analysis, it would be premature to regard this result—that 506 (±51) deaths in Paris in summer 2003 are attributable to anthropogenic climate change—as the last word on the matter. Unquantified uncertainties need to be further explored owing to different observational, modeling, and methodological strategies for both climate attribution and health sciences. And the confidence with which a linkage can be made between anthropogenic emissions and impacts is different for other event types (Figures 9.1 and 9.2). As noted earlier, there are three pillars of sound attribution that drive the confidence with which an attribution statement can be made about any particular extreme event. Since the ability to make robust attribution statements about heat events is quite high, this linkage between a heat wave and the public health impacts is stronger. For other extreme event types, such as tornadoes, it would be very challenging to link climate change to the extreme event and subsequently any socioeconomic impacts.

Drawing connections to environmental impacts is also an area where research is beginning to emerge. For example, in a study of the 2016 extreme Great Barrier Reef bleaching event Lewis and Mallela (2018) concluded that the risk of the extreme event was increased through anomalously high sea surface temperature and the accumulation of thermal stress caused by human-caused climate change. They used a multistep approach that included selecting a variety of variables that are known to impact coral reef bleaching beyond thermal stress from elevated ocean temperatures, including:

1. Precipitation anomalies, which are linked to cloud cover, temperatures, and runoff;
2. Cloudiness anomalies as increased cloud cover potentially reduces UV exposure and ameliorates thermal stress;
3. Chlorophyll-a concentrations which provide an estimate of the live phytoplankton biomass in the surface layer as a nutrient indicator; and
4. Concentration of particulate organic carbon as an indicator of water quality.

Lewis and Mallela (2018) then examined how climate change has impacted these variables. In this way they are able to examine a broad range of variables that influence coral bleaching and assess the relative contribution of increasing ocean temperatures caused by human activity. This type of broader context is an important component of impact attribution, as it addresses various confounding factors that might be influencing a socioeconomic or environmental impact beyond climate change.

In addition to Lewis and Mallela (2018), Jacox et al (2018), and Brainard et al (2018) both examined how high ocean temperatures caused in part by human-caused climate change impacted living marine resources like coral bleaching, reduced fish stocks, and a decrease in seabird counts in the California current and the equatorial Pacific, respectively. On land, Sippel et al (2018) found that human-caused climate change is causing warmer winters on the Iberian Peninsula and, when coupled with a wet spring, drove higher ecosystem productivity in the region in 2016. There has also been work done in Alaska looking at how increased ocean (e.g., Walsh et al, 2018) and atmospheric temperatures (e.g., Thoman et al, 2020) have impacted wildlife as well as coastal communities.

These papers represent early approaches to impact attribution. The largest challenges to impact attribution, however, are not always in conducting a robust attribution analysis on the extreme event. They often arise when trying to create a direct line between the extreme event and the impact being measured. For example, to understand how many more people were impacted by a heat wave due to climate change induced warming, the research must first be able to answer how many people would have been impacted if climate change had not played a role. In the case of the heat waves in the developed world, there is often epidemiological data about previous heat waves and their health impacts that can serve as a framework to understand the health impacts of each additional degree increase in temperature. For other socioeconomic impacts, the linkage between the changing environment and the variable being measured can be quite complicated, and introduce significant levels of uncertainty into the analysis.

9.5   FAR = 1 or "Not possible without climate change"

When the Climate Science Special Report (CSSR; USGCRP, 2017) was published in 2017 it stated that, "To our knowledge, no extreme weather event observed to date has been found to have zero probability of occurrence in a preindustrial climate, according to climate model simulations. Therefore, the causes of attributed extreme events are a combination of natural variations in the climate system compounded (or alleviated) by the anthropogenic change to the climate system. . . . In the future, as the climate change signal gets stronger compared to natural variability, humans may experience weather events which are essentially impossible to simulate in a preindustrial climate." However, in the report "Explaining extreme events of 2016 from a climate perspective" (Herring et al, 2018), which was released shortly afterwards in the winter of 2017, the researchers examining three different events concluded that they were not possible in a pre-industrial climate. In a paper analyzing the 2016 global heat record Knutson et al (2018) concluded that the record global warmth "was only possible due to substantial centennial-scale human-caused warming." In a second study that investigated the record heat over Asia, it was found that the extreme warmth across Asia in 2016 "would not have been possible without climate change" (Imada et al, 2018). And finally, researchers studying a large, persistent area of anomalously warm ocean water off the coast of Alaska found "no instances of 2016-like anomalies in the preindustrial climate" for sea surface temperatures in the Bering Sea (Walsh et al, 2018). These three papers suggest the possibility that "the future" the CSSR refers to may already be here. In addition, because of the small sample size of extreme events that have been looked at to date in the peer reviewed literature it is possible that other temperature-related extreme events occurring in prior years may also have been impossible to achieve without human-induced climate change. In other words, perhaps the future has been with us for a while and these studies are simply the first to detect a reality we have already been living with. Retrospective studies would be needed to explore this possibility.

These results are significant because climate scientists have been predicting that, based on the ongoing global warming of Earth's climate, the influence of human-caused climate change would at some point become sufficiently strong and emergent to push an extreme event beyond the bounds of natural variability alone. It was also anticipated that we would likely first see this result for heat events where the human-caused influences are most strongly observed. It is striking how quickly we are now starting to see such results. However, their dependence on model-based estimates of natural variability in the absence of human-induced change will require ongoing validation of the time-of-emergence for extreme event magnitudes at local scales.

All three papers use the FAR methodology outlined earlier in this chapter, and concluded that the FAR = 1, meaning that the event was only possible in a world with human-emitted greenhouse gases. While human factors were found to have altered the risk of the event, it should be noted that other climate drivers can also affect the probability of these extremes and may have contributed to the likelihood of the event occurring. Each of these papers applied large model ensembles (e.g., CMIP5 for both the global heat and Alaska marine heat wave analyses and the atmospheric general circulation model; MIROC5 for the Asia heat study) to determine the FAR for these events.

9.6 Communicating event attribution studies

What does it mean to say that an event was not possible without human-caused climate change? How should this result be interpreted, and what does it mean for the associated impacts of the event on society and the environment? Climate scientists have long repeated the mantra that "all events are due in part to natural variability," and this remains true even for events not possible without climate change. Every weather and climate event is built on a foundation of naturally occurring meteorological drivers such as atmospheric circulation patterns, sea surface temperature, ENSO cycles, etc. These drivers are present in both the world we live in, and a world without anthropogenic climate change. What the FAR = 1 results say is that without climate change the event could not have surpassed the temperature threshold that it did. So 2016 likely would have been a warm year globally and for Asia even without climate forcings, however, only with the influence of anthropogenic climate change were these events able to surpass the temperature thresholds that they did. If FAR does equal 1 and an event cannot be replicated in models without human forcings, natural variations can still be a significant player in the event. Natural variability is a factor in extreme events whether FAR = 1 or not.

Why is this an important distinction in how results are interpreted? Because it may impact what component of human impacts can be attributed to anthropogenic climate change. Even if it is determined, for example, that a 100°F (37.8°C) day was not possible without climate change, it does not mean that all impacts associated with that hot day can be connected to climate change. It may have been possible for the day to reach 90°F (32.2°C) on natural variability alone, for example, and if so any health or economic impacts from a 90°F day could not be fully attributed to climate change.

Communicating event attribution results is also important when assigning responsibility for climate change–related impacts of an event. Damage assessments for hurricanes is an example of where clearly communicating what aspect of the event is attributable to climate change is important. Climate science predicts that hurricanes will become more intense in the future, and certain recent trends are consistent with what would be expected in a warming world. For example, "the severity of the 2017 Atlantic hurricane season was consistent with a combination of natural and human-caused variability on decadal and longer time scales" (USGCRP, 2018). However, event attribution analysis connecting a specific hurricane to these predicted trends has not been done, and the evidence connecting recent events to these longer-term trends remains limited. Yet there is strong evidence that the precipitation (e.g., Risser and Wehner, 2017, Van Oldenborgh et al, 2017) and storm surge caused by hurricanes (e.g., Sweet et al, 2017) has been made worse by human-caused climate change. In addition, new evidence is emerging that the propensity of hurricanes to stall may be increasing due to human caused climate change (Kossin, 2018). These distinctions are important when quantifying the impact of climate change on hurricane-related damages. Damage caused from high winds would be very difficult to attribute to human-caused climate change. However, assigning damages caused by storm surge and increased precipitation to climate change is possible. Thus, clearly communicating the attribution of an event such as a hurricane involves parsing out all the variables, including the scientific confidence in the hurricane itself, the trajectory of the hurricane, the precipitation, and storm surge associated with the hurricane. This creates a level of complexity that can be challenging.

Climate change attribution science is a rapidly evolving field of study, and this introduces additional complexity in communicating the latest science. Prior to the emergence of event attribution science it was commonly expressed that, "we can never attribute any individual event to climate change." Some scientists even said it was "impossible." Of course, today we know that event attribution is absolutely possible using a probabilistic approach. And prior to 2019 the mantra among scientists was that all events to date have been possible without climate change; however, with the publication of the three papers mentioned above and others, the role of climate change on certain extremes will also need to be communicated in new ways. In addition, if retrospective studies reveal $FAR = 1$ for previous events the research community will have to acknowledge that the influence of climate change on certain extremes has been underestimated to date. Some such studies are currently in progress (based on personal communication) and depending on their results the scientific community may again need to rewrite the script on communicating attribution science. In such a rapidly changing scientific environment the communication challenges are only enhanced.

9.7 Summary

When an extreme event hits, it is normal to ask questions to try and put that event in context. For example, "How unusual was this event?" "Should we plan for more events like this in the future?" "Is this the new normal?" The focus of event attribution is answering questions such as these. Given current and future predicted greenhouse gas emissions, the influence of human-caused climate change on all weather events, including extremes, will continue to increase. The expectation is that the changes in extreme events will become stronger, more pronounced, and easier to identify with improved scientific methodologies. In addition, the tools that researchers have to examine extreme events will continue to improve, from the observational record, the quality of the models, and advancements in the understanding of physical processes. The research community will have increased confidence in attribution results, enhancing their value in a decision support context.

References

Allen M (2003) Liability for climate change. Nature 421(6926):891–892

Brainard RE, Oliver T, McPhaden MJ, Cohen A, Venegas R, Heenan A, Vargas-Ángel B, Rotjan R, Mangubhai S, Flint E, Hunter SA (2018) Ecological impacts of the 2015/16 El Niño in the central equatorial Pacific. Bulletin of the American Meteorological Society 99(1):S21–S26

Herring SC, Christidis N, Hoell A, Kossin JP, Schreck III CJ, Stott PA (2018) Explaining extreme events of 2016 from a climate perspective. Bulletin of the American Meteorological Society 99(1):S1–S157

Herring SC, Christidis N, Hoell A, Hoerling MP, Stott PA (2019) Explaining extreme events of 2017 from a climate perspective. Bulletin of the American Meteorological Society 100(1):S1–S117

Hoell A, Perlwitz J, Dewes C, Wolter K, Rangwala I, Quan XW, Eischeid J (2019) Anthropogenic contributions to the intensity of the 2017 United States northern great plains drought. Bulletin of the American Meteorological Society 100(1):S19–S24

Imada Y, Shiogama H, Takahashi C, Watanabe M, Mori M, Kamae Y, Maeda S (2018) Climate change increased the likelihood of the 2016 heat extremes in Asia. Bulletin of the American Meteorological Society 99(1):S97–S101

Jacox MG, Alexander MA, Mantua NJ, Scott JD, Hervieux G, Webb RS, Werner FE (2018) Forcing of multiyear extreme ocean temperatures that impacted California current living marine resources in 2016. Bulletin of the American Meteorological Society 99(1):S27–S33

Knutson TR, Kam J, Zeng F, Wittenberg AT (2018) CMIP5 model-based assessment of anthropogenic influence on record global warmth during 2016. Bulletin of the American Meteorological Society 99(1):S11–S15

Kossin JP (2018) A global slowdown of tropical-cyclone translation speed. Nature 558:104–107

Lewis SC, Mallela J (2018) A multifactor risk analysis of the record 2016 Great Barrier Reef bleaching. Bulletin of the American Meteorological Society 99(1):S144–S149

Mitchell D, Heaviside C, Vardoulakis S, Huntingford C, Masato G, Guillod BP, Frumhoff P, Bowery A, Wallom D, Allen M (2016) Attributing human mortality during extreme heat waves to anthropogenic climate change. Environmental Research Letters 11(7):074006

NAS (2016) National Academies of Sciences, Engineering, and Medicine. Attribution of Extreme Weather Events in the Context of Climate Change. National Academies Press, Washington, DC

Otto FEL (2016) Extreme events: the art of attribution. Nature Climate Change 6(4):342–343

Risser MD, Wehner MF (2017) Attributable human-induced changes in the likelihood and magnitude of the observed extreme precipitation during hurricane Harvey. Geophysical Research Letters 44:12457–12464

Sippel S, El-Madany TS, Migliavacca M, Mahecha MD, Carrara A, Flach M, Kaminski T, Otto FEL, Thonicke K, Vossbeck M, Reichstein M (2018) Warm winter, wet spring, and an extreme response in ecosystem functioning on the Iberian Peninsula. Bulletin of the American Meteorological Society 99(1):S80–S85

Stott PA, Stone DA, Allen MR (2004) Human contribution to the European heatwave of 2003. Nature 432(7017):610–614

Sweet W, Zervas C, Gill S, Park J (2017) Hurricane Sandy inundation probabilities today and tomorrow. Bulletin of the American Meteorological Society 94(9):S17–S20

Thoman RL, Bhatt US, Bieniek PA, Brettschneider BR, Brubaker M, Danielson SL, Labe Z, Lader R, Meier WN, Sheffield G, Walsh JE (2020) The record low Bering Sea ice extent in 2018: context, impacts, and an assessment of the role of anthropogenic climate change. Bulletin of the American Meteorological Society 101(1):S53–S58

USGCRP (2017) Climate science special report. In: Wuebbles DJ, Fahey DW, Hibbard KA, Dokken DJ, Stewart BC, Maycock TK (eds) Fourth National Climate Assessment, vol 1, U.S. Global Change Research Program, Washington, DC

USGCRP (2018) Impacts, risks, and adaptation in the United States. In: Reidmiller DR, Avery CW, Easterling DR, Kunkel KE, Lewis KLM, Maycock TK, Stewart BC (eds) Fourth National Climate Assessment, vol 2, U.S. Global Change Research Program, Washington, DC

Van Oldenborgh GJ, Van Der Wiel K, Sebastian A, Singh R, Arrighi J, Otto F, Haustein K, Li S, Vecchi G, Cullen H (2017) Attribution of extreme rainfall from hurricane Harvey, August 2017. Environmental Research Letters 12(12):124009

Vautard R, Colette A, Van Meijgaard E, Meleux F, Jan van Oldenborgh G, Otto F, Tobin I, Yiou P (2018) Attribution of wintertime anticyclonic stagnation contributing to air pollution in Western Europe. Bulletin of the American Meteorological Society 99(1):S70–S75

Walsh JE, Thoman RL, Bhatt US, Bieniek PA, Brettschneider B, Brubaker M, Danielson S, Lader R, Fetterer F, Holderied K, Iken K, Mahoney A, McCammon M, Partain J (2018) The high latitude marine heat wave of 2016 and its impacts on Alaska. Bulletin of the American Meteorological Society 99(1):S39–S43

Wang H, Schubert SD, Koster RD, Chang Y (2019) Attribution of the 2017 Northern High Plains drought. Bulletin of the American Meteorological Society 100(1):S25–S29

10

Financing Weather and Climate Risks in the United States

Roger S. Pulwarty
Physical Sciences Laboratory, National Oceanic and Atmospheric Administration, Boulder, CO, USA

David R. Easterling
National Centers for Environmental Information, National Oceanic and Atmospheric Administration, Asheville, NC, USA

Jeffery Adkins
Office of the Chief Economist, National Oceanic and Atmospheric Administration, Silver Spring, MD, USA

Adam B. Smith
National Centers for Environmental Information, National Oceanic and Atmospheric Administration, Asheville, NC, USA

CONTENTS

10.1	Disasters in the United States—the recent record	201
10.2	Climate and extremes	203
10.3	Assessing economic impacts	206
10.4	Insurance and risk financing	211
10.5	Data and analytical challenges	219
10.6	Implementation challenges	222
10.7	Financing mitigation and resilience	223
10.8	Pathways and conclusion	226
References		229

10.1 Disasters in the United States—the recent record

During 1980–2019, the United States has sustained 258 separate billion-dollar weather and climate-related disasters with over $1.75 trillion in insured losses and more than 13,000 fatalities. Hurricane Hugo, which made landfall in

Charleston, South Carolina, on September 22, 1989, was the first natural disaster in the United States costing more than $1 billion of insured losses (Insurance Information Institute, 2000). The National Center for Environmental Information, part of the National Oceanic and Atmospheric Administration (NOAA), records the number of natural disasters that cause at least a billion dollars in losses in the United States "billion-dollar" disasters. The frequency of 'billion-dollar' disasters (adjusted for inflation) has been increasing since the 1980s. In fact, the United States experienced more than twice the number of billion-dollar weather and climate disasters during the 2010s (119) as compared with the 2000s (59)—even after adjusting for inflation (Smith, 2020). Costs of over $300 billion occurred in 2017, with Hurricane Harvey alone costing an estimated $125 billion (2017 dollars). Hurricane Katrina (2005) remains the costliest storm in US history with over $161 billion in losses. Much uncertainty remains about the final cost estimation of these storms. In addition, the cumulative cost of small, but more frequently occurring extreme weather-related events is not insignificant. The average cost of direct flood damages in the United States averages $4 billion annually, despite the construction and maintenance of 8500 miles of levees, nearly 100 shore protection projects, and almost 400 flood control reservoirs (USACE, 2013). The cost of constructing, operating, and maintaining these structures is high.

Weather-related losses accounted for 88% of all property losses paid by insurers during this period. All other property losses, including those associated with earthquakes and terrorist events, accounted for much of the remainder. Weather-related damages are also responsible for many indirect and nonmarket impacts that are not entirely accounted for, if at all, in economic terms, such as environmental damage. Important segments of the US economy are particularly vulnerable to coastal hazards like hurricanes and rising sea levels.

Important segments of the US economy are particularly vulnerable to coastal hazards like hurricanes and rising sea levels. In 2010, 2.8 million employees generated over $250 billion in gross domestic product in jobs that directly depend on the resources of the oceans and Great Lakes; these figures represent a diverse array of economic activities ranging from offshore oil and gas exploration and production to commercial fishing and tourism (NOAA, 2013a). The total level of economic activity that is vulnerable to damage from coastal storms is much higher; counties immediately adjacent to the coasts employ 50 million people and generate 45% of the nation's gross domestic product (NOAA, 2013b).

The main drivers of the increasing losses from natural disasters are two socioeconomic factors that directly influence the level of economic damage: degree of urbanization and value at risk. At the same time, government regulators are asked to balance the need to protect consumers from high insurance rates with the need to keep insurance companies from going out of business entirely. This chapter will describe the drivers, impacts, and financial services that have been employed at the national level in the United States.

The Midwest floods of 2019 and 2017–2018 wildfires in California: a changing landscape

The wettest spring and summer on record for much of the United States occurred in 2019. The United States Department of Agriculture (USDA) estimated that the 19 million acres of insured farmland went unplanted, which is the largest since USDA's "prevented-plant" acreage record keeping began in 2007. Also, 70% of those lands were located in Midwestern states. For two of most important US crops—corn and soybeans—this represented 13% and 6% of total acreage, respectively. In addition, 5 million acres were planted in unfavorable conditions. In the words of one expert "it turned out to be a really bad bet." Major additional costs were incurred for propane heat costs for corn that had to be dried before being put into silos. The prevented-plant payout may be $3.6 billion this year, nine times more than last year and shattering the previous record of $2.2 billion in 2011 (Schnitkey, 2019). Fortunately, areas outside of those most heavily affected and stored corn were able to make up the difference for this year. Subsidized trade assistance, disaster assistance, and federal crop insurance made up nearly 40% of farm income in 2019, or $33 billion out of $88 billion total (American Farm Bureau Federation, 2019). According to the USDA, rains were not just intense but falling at inopportune times for harvesting and the use of heavy equipment, instead of the middle of the growing season when it would be of most use (Todey, 2019). Additionally, farm bankruptcy filings by September 2019 were 24% higher than the previous year.

In addition to the extended California drought of 2011–2016, California's wildfires have grown so costly and damaging that insurance companies have increasingly been canceling people's policies in fire-prone regions of the state. The state recently passed a law barring insurers from leaving the state due to events that have been exacerbated by climate change. Recent research shows that the wildfires of 2017 and 2018 alone wiped out a full quarter-century of the insurance industry's profits. The 2018 Camp Fire was the costliest disaster anywhere in the world that year, according to the insurer Munich Re. As it faces the wildfire emergency, California is expanding its 51-year-old FAIR Plan. The insurer-backed program is meant to be a temporary option for stranded consumers but is getting more heavily used in communities prone to wildfires. The policies, which are bare bones and can be even more expensive than traditional insurance, almost tripled in 2018 from three years earlier in the 10 counties with the most homes at high risk of wildfire damage. The danger of insurers being overwhelmed by worsening natural disasters is very real.

10.2 Climate and extremes

Weather and climate extremes have always been a part of the climate system and present serious challenges to society. The climate of the United

States is strongly connected to the changing global climate. Climate stresses place great political and financial burden on federal and local governments as they assume broader exposures and are pressured to serve as insurers of last resort. Changes in climate are expected to lead to changes in the occurrence of extreme events (Easterling et al, 2000). However, this does not imply a one-to-one relationship between hazards' occurrences and the degree of impacts (Changnon et al, 2000). Climate extremes can result from natural variability, forcing due to increasing greenhouse gases, or more likely some combination of the two. For example, some of the more robust climate change signals related to extremes in both the observed record and in model simulations for the future are increases in the number of unusually warm days and nights, decrease in the number of unusually cold days and nights, and an increase in heavy precipitation events (Seneviratne et al, 2017). Other changes include a likely increase in the intensity of hurricanes in the North Atlantic since about 1970 (Knutson et al, 2020).

The US Global Change Program's Climate Science Special Report (Wuebbles et al, 2017) summarizes the past, present, and projected climate of the United States as follows:

- Global annually averaged surface air temperature has increased by about 1.8°F (1.0°C) over the last 115 years (1901–2016). This period is now the warmest in the history of modern civilization. The last few years have also seen record-breaking, climate-related weather extremes, and the last three years have been the warmest years on record for the globe. These trends are expected to continue over climate time-scales.

- Changes in the characteristics of extreme events are particularly important for human safety, infrastructure, agriculture, water quality and quantity, and natural ecosystems. Heavy rainfall is increasing in intensity and frequency across the United States and globally and is expected to continue to increase. The largest observed changes in the United States have occurred in the Northeast.

- In addition to warming, many other aspects of global climate are changing, primarily in response to human activities. For example, global average sea level has risen by about 7–8 inches (18–20 cm) since 1900, with almost half (about 3 inches) of that rise occurring since 1993. Human-caused climate change has made a substantial contribution to this rise since 1900, contributing to a rate of rise that is greater than during any preceding century in at least 2,800 years. Global sea level rise has already affected the United States; the incidence of daily tidal flooding is accelerating in more than 25 Atlantic and Gulf Coast cities.

- Global average sea levels are expected to continue to rise—by at least several inches in the next 15 years and by 1–4 feet (0.3–1.2 m) by 2100. Sea level rise will be higher than the global average on the East and Gulf Coasts of the United States.

- Heat waves have become more frequent in the United States since the 1960s, while extreme cold temperatures and cold waves are less frequent. Annual average temperature over the contiguous United States has increased by 1.8°F (1.0°C) for the period 1901–2016; over the next few decades (2021–2050), annual average temperatures are expected to rise by about 2.5°F for the United States, relative to the recent past (average during 1976–2005), under all plausible future climate scenarios.

- The incidence of large forest fires in the western United States and Alaska has increased since the early 1980s and is projected to further increase in those regions as the climate changes, with profound changes to regional ecosystems.

- Annual trends toward earlier spring melt and reduced snowpack are already affecting water resources in the western United States and these trends are expected to continue. Under higher scenarios, and assuming no change to current water resources management, chronic, long-duration hydrological drought is increasingly possible before the end of this century.

- The magnitude of climate change beyond the next few decades will depend primarily on the amount of greenhouse gases (especially carbon dioxide) emitted globally. Without major reductions in emissions, the increase in annual average global temperature relative to preindustrial times could reach 9°F (5°C) or more by the end of this century. With significant reductions in emissions, the increase in annual average global temperature could be limited to 3.6°F (2°C) or less.

Many of these extremes can be directly linked to large human and monetary costs to society conditioned by human factors (Changnon et al, 2000). Unanticipated changes in the nature, scale, or location of hazards are among the most important threats to the insurance system (Mills et al, 2005). The key components of calculating climate-sensitive economic risks include the development of

- The stochastic module: weather and climatic events and their statistical distributions (historical data, scientific analyses and expert opinions)—characteristics of intensity and their distributions.

- The exposure module: elements at risk.

- The damage function: calculation of potential crucial damage for different intensities and experiences. These drive the financial or loss quantification module to determine the cost of catastrophic risk.

- The recurrence interval (T) is number of years in the record (N) divided by the number of events (n). When there is a magnitude associated with the data (such as discharge with a flood) the recurrence interval is $T = (n+1)/m$, where n is the number of years of the record and m is the magnitude ranking.

Certain risks are more amenable to insurance or risk pooling than others (Cutler and Zeckhauser, 2004). A "tail risk" describes the potential recurrence extremely rare and destructive weather event. The name comes from the standard, bell-curve-shaped probability distribution, where rare events occur at the far ends—the "tails"—of the distribution. Damages from natural disasters are fat tailed and dependent. A fat-tailed distribution is one in which the probability of an extreme event falls more slowly, and the most extreme event can be many multiples of the second most extreme (Cooke et al, 2014). Climate change can increase the frequency of these tail risks (so they become "fat tails"), and it increases the likelihood that normally separate "tail events" will occur simultaneously. Over 20 years ago, Applied Insurance Research, a leading catastrophe modeling firm, postulated that a 3% increase in hurricane wind speed would result in 15% increases in infrastructure damages (Clark, 1997). AIR Worldwide, recently reported that insured losses should also be expected to double roughly every 10 years because of increases in construction costs, increases in the number of structures, and changes in their characteristics. Two available national-scale studies that examine the economic effects of climate change across US sectors suggested that potential economic effects could be significant and unevenly distributed across sectors and regions. For example, for 2020 through 2039, one study estimated between $4 billion and $6 billion in annual coastal property damages from sea level rise and more frequent and intense storms (GAO, 2017). Also, under this study, the Southeast likely faces greater effects than other regions because of coastal property damages.

Nationally, considering riverine and coastal floods together, the average increase in the Special Flood Hazard Areas (SFHAs) by the year 2100 is projected to be about 40% or 45%. According to Zillow Research, "almost 1.9 million homes—worth a combined $916 billion—are at risk of being underwater by 2100" (Bretz, 2017). While wealthier homeowners may have more to lose in dollars, this scenario could be especially catastrophic for owners of the lowest-valued homes, because lower-income Americans spend a disproportionately larger share of their earnings on mortgage payments.

10.3 Assessing economic impacts

The cost of disaster preparedness, response, and recovery efforts displaces spending for infrastructure improvement, business expansion, and education and other human services (Kousky, 2014, NRC, 1999). Methods used to estimate the potential economic effects of climate change in the United States—using linked climate science and economics models – are based on still developing research. The methods and the studies that use them produce imprecise

Assessing economic impacts

results because of modeling and other limitations but can convey insight into potential climate damages across sectors in the United States.

Hazards can cause significant and often long-lasting disruptions of normal life and even disease and death. They also damage and destroy irreplaceable historical, cultural, and ecological assets (Heinz Center, 2000). Funding the response and recovery efforts associated with large-scale disasters can increase the cost of borrowing across the economy at large. It can also affect the strength of a nation's currency and foreign trade balances, and undermine efforts to alleviate poverty and promote economic development (Benson and Clay, 2004). Howe and Cochrane (1993) provide a useful framework for classifying the economic effects of natural hazards. Of the five major classes that these authors propose, the discussion so far encompasses only two: (1) lost production and (2) damages to structures, infrastructure, and other human-built capital.

Assessing the effects of natural disasters is a difficult but necessary task. However, there are several factors that make such assessments difficult. "Disasters affect the economic system in multiple ways, and defining the 'cost' of a disaster is tricky" (Hallegatte and Przyluski, 2010). The effects of weather events are diverse. Properties are damaged, public services are disrupted, and the direct and indirect effects are experienced across the economy, the environment, and society at large. The total cost of disasters increases with the duration of the effects (Rose, 2004). The specific needs for information on the cost of weather events differ depending on who is framing the question (Hallegatte and Przyluski, 2010). No single federal agency has the responsibility to account for all of the direct effects associated with natural disasters, and no private entity does so. Agencies such as USDA, NOAA, and the Federal Emergency Management Agency (FEMA) collect data and perform analyses necessary to support their own missions and objectives from riverine flooding to crop damages. Thus, this work does not, even collectively, account for the full range of effects (Booz Allen Hamilton, 2013). Private federal agencies collect information that is needed to support their various objectives as well. Communities who are considering investments to mitigate the effects of weather hazards want to know about the potential damages to all the homes, businesses, infrastructure, and business activity in that community rather than at the regional or national level. Finally, because of these disparate data needs, there is no single source of information on the total cost of weather events. In most cases, the most robust source of information is the data collected and maintained by the government insurers and the private insurance industry. Primary insurers, for example, provide claim information to the Insurance Services Office/Property Claims Services (PCS), who then provides the data to others for a number of uses.

Despite these difficulties, it is still necessary to understand the economic effects of natural disasters. One contributing factor to this difficulty is the lack of agreement on how to classify disaster costs. Typologies used in peer-reviewed literature sometimes lump all social and economic costs into a single class or divide them into two or three classes (e.g., Lindell and Prater, 2003, Meyer et al, 2013, Rose, 2004). Direct effects can be estimated by starting where the data are best documented—insured losses—and developing multipliers to account for uninsured losses. These multipliers account for uninsured and underinsured property, deductibles, and insurance caps. Total direct effects, which include both insured and uninsured losses, can then be used as inputs into econometric models that account for the ways that natural disasters affect parts of the economy that suffered no physical harm. Uneven standard data collection has led to many gaps and overlaps, further complicating the task of integrating data from primary sources (Booz Allen Hamilton, 2013). Taxes paid on inputs to recovery efforts, for example, represent financial costs but are transfers of wealth and not true economic costs (Rose, 2004).

The basic measure for assessing the catastrophe exposure of a house, city or any portfolio of assets is called the exceedance probability (EP) curve. An EP curve is basically the mathematical tool used to summarize, for a given location/infrastructure/hazard, all the possible events that can happen and the probability associated with them. More precisely, the EP curve indicates the probability p that at least \$X (or lives) is lost in a given year for a given location and type of risk. A typical EP curve can be constructed where the likelihood that losses will exceed L_i is given by p_i, that is, the horizontal axis shows the magnitude of the loss in US dollars, and the vertical axis depicts the annual probability that losses will exceed this level.

Direct effects

Perhaps the broadest accounting of the direct effects associated with natural disasters is performed by NOAA's National Centers for Environmental Information (NCEI) in its quarterly assessment of US billion-dollar disasters (Smith, 2020, Smith and Katz, 2013). This analysis quantifies the loss from numerous weather and climate disasters including: tropical cyclones, floods, drought and heat waves, severe local storms (i.e., tornado, hail, and straight-line wind damage), wildfires, crop freeze events, and winter storms. These loss estimates reflect direct effects of weather and climate events (i.e., not including indirect effects) and constitute total losses (i.e., both insured and uninsured). The insured and uninsured direct loss components include: physical damage to residential, commercial and government/municipal buildings, material assets within a building, time element losses (i.e., businesses interruption), vehicles, boats, offshore energy platforms, public infrastructure (i.e., roads, bridges, and buildings), and agricultural assets (i.e., crops, livestock, and timber).

NCEI draws from numerous public and private sector loss data sets (Smith and Matthews, 2015), however much of the data is derived from three primary data sources of data on insured losses:

- Insurance Services Office Property Claims Services (PCS),

Assessing economic impacts 209

- FEMA National Flood Insurance Program (NFIP),
- USDA Risk Management Agency.

NCEI then develops multipliers that are applied to insured losses to estimate uninsured losses. This approach used by NCEI to estimate losses is broader, but similar to that used by others in the federal government and also global reinsurance companies (i.e., Munich Reinsurance and Swiss Reinsurance). Also, these multipliers can be quite large, yielding uninsured loss estimates that are four times greater than insured losses in some cases. The results are also refined using information from other sources, such as Presidential Disaster Declarations, the United States Department of Agriculture National Agricultural Statistics Service (USDA NASS), and state emergency management agency reports. NOAA also produces independent assessments of the direct effects of disasters including weather-related damages at its National Hurricane Center (NHC) and Weather Forecast Offices (WFO) and economic impact analyses at the National Marine Fisheries Service for fisheries, commercial, and recreational fishing industries in areas declared a federal fisheries disaster.

Another federal loss tool is HAZUS, an application developed by FEMA that enables governments at the federal, state, and local levels to identify the potential impacts of earthquakes, floods, and hurricanes. Based on a standardized methodology, HAZUS contains models that enable users to assess the physical, economic and social impacts of disasters and corresponding loss estimates. The United States Geological Survey (USGS) uses the Science Application for Risk Reduction (SAFRR) to facilitate scenario development to assist in disaster preparedness, response, and resilience.

Calculating higher-order effects

Higher-order effects are sometimes called indirect effects. In econometric modeling, however, indirect effects include only part of the higher-order effects. The use of the term "higher-order effects" avoids the confusion of using the same term in two different ways. Higher-order effects of disasters include those that spill over from the area of impact to areas that suffered no physical harm. Their magnitude is directly associated with the amount of time it takes the affected area to recover (Hallegatte and Przyluski, 2010, Meyer et al, 2013, Rose, 2004).

Induced effects are even more remotely connected to the physical damage of a disaster. They occur, for example, when workers whose wages have been reduced by the direct or indirect effects of a storm may not eat out as often or may delay the purchase of a new car. In this case, the induced effects are those felt by the restaurants and car dealerships (NRC, 1999).

Two commonly used models for measuring these spillover effects are the Input-Output models (I-O) and the Computable General Equilibrium (CGE) models (Meyer et al, 2013). Both rely on detailed tables with purchases and sales that represent the interdependencies between the various segments of the economy (Rose, 2004). Both models account for two higher-order effects of natural disasters—the indirect supply-side and demand-side effects on firms with economic linkages to damaged firms and the effects induced across the economy at large. These indirect and induced effects are often expressed in terms of multipliers that are applied to the direct effects of a disaster.

CGE models, on the other hand, capture the ability of firms to adapt production processes in response to the shortages of inputs, bankrupt customers, and price changes that commonly accompany large-scale natural disasters. They also account for increasing and decreasing returns to scale. Because they do not account for firms' ability to respond to shortages and price increases, I-O models tend to overstate the effects of disasters. While they address many of the shortcomings of I-O models, CGE models tend to understate the effects of disasters (Hallegatte and Przyluski, 2010). In the real world, prices do not change immediately, firms are slow to find new sources of inputs and new customers, and limits exist in their ability to substitute one input for another. The tendencies of I-O models to overstate the effects of disasters and those of CGE models to understate them can be at least partially overcome by more sophisticated use of the models. In any case, the true value of higher-order effects probably lies somewhere between the values generated by I-O and CGE models (Hallegatte and Przyluski, 2010).

Nonmarket effects

The impacts of a disaster broadly include both market-based and non-market effects (NRC, 1999). For instance, the temporal and spatial complexity of drought events makes it one of the most difficult natural hazards on which to fully assess impacts, as these filter through the economy, communities, and the environment long after precipitation has returned to normal or average conditions (see Pulwarty and Verdin, 2013). Many of the direct and high-order effects of disasters are not well-represented in the market data. These effects fall into four classes: household production; damage to historical assets; human injury, sickness, and death; mitigation costs.

The latter issue of the cost of mitigating disaster losses has not been considered to the same extent as relief and recovery. The current levels of loss reflect historical and ongoing investments by governments, businesses, and individuals to reduce the harmful effects of disasters. This includes government expenditures on a wide range of civil works projects such as floodwalls, levees, flood control reservoirs, and shore protection projects (GAO, 2018, USACE, 2013). Expenditures to conserve and restore natural vegetation and buffers like wetlands and dunes can reduce the damages from storm surge and coastal erosion. Modifications to structures, such as the use of hurricane straps and the elevation of structures, are funded by businesses and home-owners, sometimes in response to the government regulations, such as those associated with the NFIP. Federal, state, and local governments support hazard mitigation and evacuation planning and implement early warning systems that aim to mitigate the harmful effects of natural hazards. Natural hazards bring large costs suddenly, which makes planning and actions designed to reduce their impact very important. However, funding for such measures is rarely a high priority with governments and the voters who hold politicians accountable for disaster relief but not for disaster preparedness and mitigation (ABI, 2005, Healy and Malhotra, 2009).

10.4 Insurance and risk financing

Insurance facilitates the transfer of risk from individuals and governments to insurance companies and capital markets, thereby alleviating extended hardship after a disaster and disruption to development programs due to unforeseen expenditure on rehabilitation. Other types of risk pooling mechanisms, such as public-private systems for reducing and sharing disaster losses, international support for micro-insurance schemes, weather hedges, and assistance to governments in financing risk to critical public infrastructure have been cited as a means to address the financial costs of extreme weather events (Linnerooth-Bayer and Vari, 2006). Insurance organizations manage very large portfolios of investments and are concerned with those factors that affect the value of these investments and in particular where investment returns might be affected by the largest catastrophe losses.

A wide range of financial arrangements have been developed to address the high cost of disaster losses. A number of financial steps can be undertaken before disasters occur (*ex ante*). These measures fall into four general classes: mitigation expenditures, savings, contingency financing, and risk transfer mechanisms (Ghesquiere and Mahul, 2010). The mitigation costs discussed above are funded at all levels of society. A large share of disaster costs is financed through different forms of savings that were set aside before the disaster. Household and business savings are generally small in comparison to the cost of a disaster, but they can be quickly accessed and used at the discretion of the owner. Contingency financing is a formal arrangement with lenders that specifies the terms of a loan that can be used to respond to and recover from future disasters. Funds are pre-authorized and can be disbursed quickly. Households, businesses, and governments can also transfer the risk of disasters to third parties.

The most common risk transfer instruments by far are the many forms of insurance offered by governments and private insurance companies (OECD, 2015). The goals of the major federal insurance programs are fundamentally different from those of private insurers. Under certain circumstances, the private sector may determine that a risk is uninsurable. For example, while homeowner insurance policies typically cover damage and losses from fire and other perils, they usually do not cover flood damage because private insurance companies are largely unwilling to bear the financial risks associated with its potentially catastrophic impact. In other instances, the private sector may be willing to insure a risk, but at rates that are not affordable to many property owners. Without insurance, affected property owners must rely on their own resources or seek out disaster assistance from local, state, and federal sources. In situations where the private sector will not insure a particular type of risk, the public sector may create markets to ensure the availability of insurance.

The two major federal insurance programs—NFIP and the Federal Crop Insurance Corporation (FCIC)—pay about 5% of insured costs. Although the performance of both NFIP and FCIC is sensitive to weather, the two programs insure fundamentally different risks and operate in very different ways. This is discussed further below.

The National Flood Insurance Program (NFIP) and the Federal Crop Insurance Corporation (FCIC)

The US government sponsors two weather-related disaster insurance programs: The National Flood Insurance Program (NFIP) and the Federal Crop Insurance Corporation (FCIC). Insurance for other weather- and climate-related disasters, such as damage from storms, is available from the private sector. The US federal government also provides disaster relief in the form of grants from one-time funding appropriations on an individual event basis. Claims vary significantly from year to year—largely due to the effects of catastrophic weather events such as hurricanes, floods, and droughts. The growth in population in hazard-prone areas, and consequent real estate development and increasing real estate values, have generally increased insurers' exposure to weather-related events and help to explain their increased losses. Due to these and other factors, the federal insurance programs' liabilities have grown significantly, leaving the federal government increasingly vulnerable to the financial impacts of extreme events.

Whereas private insurers stress the financial success of their business operations, the statutes governing the NFIP and FCIC promote affordable coverage and broad participation by individuals at risk. Both programs manage risk within their statutory guidelines, unlike the private sector, and neither program is required to limit its catastrophic risk strictly within the programs' ability to pay claims on an annual basis. The statutes governing the NFIP and FCIC promote broad participation over financial self-sufficiency in two ways: (1) by offering discounted or subsidized premiums to encourage participation and (2) by making additional funds available during high-loss years. Primary insurers transfer portions of their risk to reinsurers, e.g., Munich Reinsurance and Swiss Reinsurance (two of the largest globally). Governments and reinsurers can also spread disaster risks to private capital markets through instruments such as catastrophic bonds, weather derivatives, catastrophe equity puts, exchange-traded catastrophe options, and indemnity contracts. Primary insurers and reinsurers can also transfer portions of the risks to private capital markets through "sidecars," in which premiums are transferred to buyers who provide funds for payouts in the event of a disaster (Freeman et al, 2003, Milken Institute, 2008).

At the federal level, the Congress established the NFIP and the FCIC to provide coverage where voluntary markets do not exist. In the United States, federal funding for disaster events may only be provided when the president declares a major disaster or state of emergency. In these situations, the Budget Control Act supports a cap adjustment exclusively for disaster relief, providing a budget vehicle for disaster requirements and facilitating a shift from a reliance on supplemental appropriations.

Flood insurance was offered by the US private sector beginning in 1896. As a result of major losses during the 1927 Mississippi floods insurance companies withdrew coverage of property in highly flood-prone areas. Flooding during Hurricane Betsy (1965), revealed that few homes were insured against flood, prompting federal disaster relief and congressional support for creating the NFIP (Knowles and Kunreuther, 2014). In 100-year flood plains of the United States, only roughly half of homes are insured against floods, and even fewer outside these areas carry flood insurance (Adams-Schoen and Thomas, 2015, Dixon et al, 2006, Prevost, 2013).

Residential flood insurance has been provided mainly by the federally-run National Flood Insurance Program (NFIP) since its creation in 1968. The NFIP was developed due to the position by private insurance companies following the Mississippi floods of 1927, and maintained through the 1960s, that this peril was uninsurable. The Congress established the NFIP in 1968, partly to provide an alternative to disaster assistance for flood damage. Participating communities (over 20,000) are required to adopt and enforce flood plain management regulations, thereby reducing the risks of flooding and the costs of repairing flood damage. FEMA, within the Department of Homeland Security, is responsible for, among other things, oversight and management of the NFIP. Under the program, the federal government assumes the liability for covered losses and sets rates and coverage limitations.

The National Flood Insurance Program began as a way to extend government insurance to homeowners in communities that tend to flood. Over 5.5 million property owners hold federal flood insurance policies, 80% of whom pay market rates. Every property with a mortgage in a designated flood plain must have flood insurance, and the federal government insures a vast majority of them. In Florida, which has the most federal flood insurance policies in the country, over 260,000 (or 13%) of them are subsidized. Approved by Congress in July 2012 as part of a wide-ranging transportation bill, the Biggert–Waters Act was intended to regain control of an increasingly unsustainable National Flood Insurance Program. The subsidies within that program, in the view of critics, encouraged development in risky areas and led to costly claims after catastrophic events, payouts that were borne largely by those paying market rates.

Following severe financial problems caused by the insufficient collection of premiums, a reform was passed in 2012 calling on FEMA, and other agencies, to make a number of changes to the way the NFIP is run. Key provisions of the legislation require the NFIP to raise rates for many policyholders to reflect true flood risk, make the program more financially stable, and change how Flood Insurance Rate Map updates impact policyholders. However, price increases have led to affordability challenges for some homeowners prompting further legislation aimed at limiting price increases and improving affordability. Homeowners with mortgages from federally regulated lenders on property in communities identified as being in high flood risk areas are required to purchase flood insurance on their dwellings. Optional, lower-cost flood insurance is also available under the NFIP for properties in areas of lower flood risk. NFIP offers coverage for both the property and its contents, which may be purchased separately. NFIP claims totaled about 11% of all-weather related insurance claims.

The Federal Crop Insurance Corporation (FCIC) is financed primarily through general fund appropriations and farmer-paid premiums. In addition to the premiums paid by producers, FCIC receives an annual appropriation to cover necessary costs for the program's premium subsidies, excess losses, delivery expenses, and other authorized expenses.

The Congress established the FCIC in 1938 to help reduce the impact of the Great Depression and the weather effects of the dust bowl. In 1980, the Congress expanded the program to provide an alternative to disaster assistance for farmers that suffer financial losses when crops are damaged by droughts, floods, or other natural disasters. Participation is voluntary, but the federal government encourages it by subsidizing their insurance premiums. USDA's Risk Management Agency is responsible for administering the crop insurance program, including issuing new insurance products and expanding existing insurance products to new geographic regions. RMA administers the program in partnership with private insurance companies, which share a percentage of the risk of loss or the opportunity for gain associated with each insurance policy written.

The FCIC insures commodities on a crop-by-crop and county-by-county basis based on farmer demand for coverage and the level of risk associated with the crop in a given region. Over 100 crops are covered by the program. Major crops, such as grains, are covered in almost every county where they are grown, and specialty crops, such as fruit, are covered only in some areas. Participating farmers can purchase different types of crop insurance, including yield and revenue insurance, and at different levels. For yield insurance, participating farmers select the percentage of yield of a covered crop to be insured and the percentage of the commodity price received as payment if the producer's losses exceed the selected threshold. Revenue insurance pays if actual revenue falls short of an assigned target level regardless of whether the shortfall was due to low yield or low commodity market prices.

Insurance and risk financing

Three causes of loss—drought, excess moisture, and hail—account for more than three-quarters of crop insurance claims. In particular, drought accounted for more than 40% of all insured crop losses. Excess moisture totaled 28%, followed by hail at 10%. The remaining claims were spread among 27 different causes of loss, including frost and tornadoes.

Since 1980, the FCIC has covered about 14% of all weather-related claims. RMA's risk assessment/rate-setting methodology is complex because the risk of growing a particular crop varies by county, farm, and farmer. Each year, RMA follows a multistep process to establish rates for each crop included in the program. The process involves establishing base rates for each county crop combination and adjusting these basic rates for a number of factors, such as coverage. For each crop, RMA extracts data on counties' crop experiences from its historical database. The data elements for each crop, crop year, and county include (1) the dollar amount of the insurance coverage sold, (2) the dollar amount of the claims paid, and (3) the average coverage level.

The historical data are adjusted to the 65% coverage level (the most commonly purchased level of coverage) so that liability and claims data at different coverage levels can be combined to develop rates. Using the adjusted data, FCIC computes the loss-cost ratio for each crop in each county. The loss-cost ratio is calculated by dividing the total claim payments by the total insurance in force; the result is stated as a percentage. To reduce the impact a single year will have on the average loss-cost ratio of each county, RMA caps the adjusted average loss-cost ratio for any single year at 80% of all years. To establish the base rate for each county, the average for all the years since 1975 is calculated using the capped loss-cost ratios and a weighting process to minimize the differences in rates among counties. Rates are further adjusted by: a disaster reserve factor, a surcharge for catastrophic coverage for each crop based on pooled losses at the state level, a prevented planting factor, farm divisions, crop type, and differences in both average yield and coverage levels.

The RMA is required to set crop insurance premiums at actuarially sufficient rates, defined as a long-run loss-ratio target of no more than 1.075. From its initial expansion in 1981 through 1994, the crop insurance program had an average loss ratio of 1.47, with a loss ratio averaging 2.15 in recent years.

Generally, producers can purchase crop insurance to insure up to 85% of their normal harvest (yield), based on production history. FCIC losses average about $1.7 billion per year. Data obtained from both the NFIP and FCIC programs indicate the federal government has grown markedly more exposed to weather-related losses regardless of the cause.

Other federal financing

In the United States, a Capital Fund, monitored by the Department of Housing and Urban Development, serves to assist government departments and housing authorities to pay for reconstruction costs of public housing when their insurance coverage has been exhausted or there is no other federal assistance available. The Fund can be used for damage from a presidentially declared disaster or, in some instances, a non-presidentially declared disaster for damage arising from an extraordinary event (earthquake, flood, tornado or hurricane). A public housing authority may apply for assistance from the Fund by providing the requisite documentation with a cost estimate.

The Small Business Administration offers low interest loans to homeowners, renters, businesses of all sizes, and private nonprofit organizations to repair or replace damaged structures, personal property, inventories, and equipment. Government at all levels also have the authority to borrow funds and to levee the taxes that are needed to repay them. Borrowing, whether through *ex ante* or *ex post* arrangements, must be repaid in the future by diverting funds from future productive investments or consumption (Kunreuther, 2006, SBA, 2013).

State-level insurance and risk financing

Several states have established Fair Access to Insurance Requirements (FAIR) plans, which pool resources from insurers doing business in the state to make property insurance available to property owners who cannot obtain coverage in the private insurance market, or cannot do so at an affordable rate. In addition, six southern states have established windstorm insurance pools that pool resources from private insurers to make insurance available to property owners who cannot obtain it in the private insurance market (OECD, 2015). Such pools exist in a number of hurricane-prone states, including wind pools in North Carolina, South Carolina, and Alabama, and insurance associations such as the Louisiana Citizens Property Insurance Corporation Citizens Property Insurance Corporation (Florida), and the Texas Windstorm Insurance Association.

The Florida CPIC is a not-for-profit, tax-exempt, government entity created in 2002 to provide insurance protection against storms (hurricanes) to Florida policyholders that are unable to find property insurance coverage in the private market. The scheme is funded by policyholder premiums and can assess levies against policyholders in the case of any deficit. The CPIC has made use of capital markets to transfer some of the risks they face through the issuance of catastrophe bonds.

In Massachusetts (US), the Fair Access to Insurance Requirements (FAIR), are generally mandated by the state and administered by the insurers (Mills et al, 2005). Most insurers are required to be members of these so-called "Residual Market Mechanisms," which aim to make insurance available to those who have been unable to gain it through the voluntary market, and involve various combinations of public (State) financing and allocation of premiums and liabilities to all insurers in a given market (Mills et al, 2005).

Private risk financing and catastrophe bonds

Insurance organizations manage very large portfolios of investments and are concerned with those factors that affect the value of these investments and in particular where investment returns might be affected by the largest catastrophe losses. Public-private partnerships can also encourage investment in protective measures prior to a disaster, deal with affordability problems and provide coverage for catastrophic risks. Insurance premiums based on risk provide signals to residents and businesses as to the hazards they face and enable insurers to lower premiums for properties where steps have been taken to reduce risk. To address issues of equity and fairness, homeowners who cannot afford insurance could be given vouchers tied to loans for investing in loss reduction measures. The National Flood Insurance Program provides an opportunity to implement a public-private partnership that could eventually be extended to other extreme events.

Furthermore, recent research on insurers' activities to address climate change outlines several other actions that private-sector companies are taking, such as developing specialized policies and new products, evaluating risks to company stock investments, and disclosing to shareholders information about company-specific risks due to climate change. The industry relies on sophisticated risk modeling systems called "cat models" (short for "catastrophe models") to inform their underwriting process. The first advanced cat models were developed in the 1980s, but did not become widely used by insurers until the 1990s (Clark, 1997).

Major insurance losses from Hurricane Andrew (1992) brought the realization that traditional actuarial science based on historical data was unable to properly calculate risk exposure for infrequent and extreme events. The cat models used today are more forward-looking and incorporate cutting-edge meteorological science. These models are an integral part of the modern insurance business, and as a result, the insurance industry is aligned with climate science in a way few other industries are. Aviva Insurance, for example, employs "detailed topographical data to assess varying flood risks for coastal houses" (Kahn et al, 2017, Scolari and Pfister, 2018). This small-scale assessment technique allows Aviva to determine which buildings are the most susceptible to natural disasters, and thus which buildings are the most expensive to insure. Aviva can fine-tune its insurance pricing to reflect the true cost of living in weather-risky/flood-prone areas (GAO, 2017). Risk Management Solutions (RMS) created 20 versions of their storm surge model to reflect gradual sea-level rise and found that sea-level rise alone has the potential to double the economic losses of hurricanes by 2100. RMS also generated hundreds of hurricane frequency models based on the "representative concentration pathways" developed by the Intergovernmental Panel on Climate Change (IPCC).

Catastrophe bonds ("cat bonds") are an increasingly popular insurance alternative for financing "tail risks." Cat bonds succeed where conventional insurance fails by spreading risks farther. Traditional insurance can only spread risks across the insurance market itself, which has significant capacity, but not enough to capture the full breadth of risks. When a major disaster strikes, the insurance market may be too small to absorb the economic losses. Cat bonds, on the other hand, expand the market for risk: they allow private investors to take on economic risk. Cat bonds therefore transfer risks to the broader capital markets—markets which allow for greater risks and absorb more losses. This increased market capacity allows the insurance industry to continue providing insurance to cities and communities, even as the losses associated with climate change continue to increase (Scolari and Pfister, 2018).

Case study: catastrophe bonds protect New York City metro from storm surge threats (OECD, 2015)

Seven months after the one of the most costly hurricanes in history (Hurricane Sandy, 2012), Mayor Bloomberg proposed investing $19.5 billion to make his city much more resilient to future extreme weather events. More than one-quarter of these resources will come from federal funds included in the Disaster Relief Appropriations Act, which provides aid to New York, New Jersey, and other affected states to help them recover from Superstorm Sandy. New Jersey is also investing significant portions of its Superstorm Sandy federal aid in resilience efforts, particularly along the Jersey Shore. These investments will make New York and New Jersey homes, businesses, infrastructure, and coastal areas more resistant to damage from future storms, sea level rise, and other climate change impacts.

Hurricane Sandy (2012) caused storm surges creating major disruptions on New York City's public transportation infrastructure. The storm caused an estimated $4–5 billion in damages to Metropolitan Transportation Authority (MTA) assets. At the time, MTA was only insured up to $1 billion. After the storm, MTA's insurance rates doubled, forcing the municipality to pursue a new risk management strategy. MTA issued a three-year, $200 million cat bond in 2013 to supplement its regular insurance coverage. MTA employed Risk Management Solutions (RMS) to construct a cat model for hurricanes and MTA infrastructure. The cat model generated a storm surge threshold to trigger the cat bond: 8.5 feet (2.6 m) in some critical areas, such as the Battery, and 15.5 feet (4.7 m) in other areas. Existing tidal gauges operated by the United States Geological Survey (USGS) and NOAA provided storm surge monitoring. If another Sandy-scale hurricane had struck New York before August 2016, investors would have lost their $200 million investment, a significant risk, but the odds were in the favor of investors. NOAA's HURISK program, which predicts the return path of storms, estimated that a hurricane like Sandy would strike New York City only once every 175 years. The 20 investors in the MTA cat bonds received a 13.5% return on their investment in 2016, a profit of $27 million. Also see Chapter 13 for a Consolidated Edison of New York (Con Edison) case study.

10.5 Data and analytical challenges

The difficulties faced in accounting for weather-related losses were the subject of the National Academies' work on the impacts of natural disasters (NAS, 1999). Reporting on how best to account for the costs of natural disasters, including weather-related events, NAS found that there was no system in place in either the public or the private sectors to consistently capture information about the economic impact. Specifically, the NAS report found no widely accepted framework, formula, or method for estimating these losses. Moreover, NAS found no comprehensive clearinghouse for the disaster loss information that is currently collected. An OECD (2015) survey on challenges assessing losses/damages—function in creating a comprehensive approach, including

- Insured and uninsured losses;
- Insurance coverage;
- Government spending after a disaster.

Niehörster et al (2013) and Meyer et al (2013) outline the following key issues and recommendations for addressing data gaps:

- Cost assessments are often incomplete and biased. In order to obtain a complete picture of the costs of natural hazards, not only direct costs but also costs due to business interruption, indirect and intangible/nonmarket costs, as well as the costs of risk mitigation should be considered.

- Although improvements have been made over the last few decades, considerable uncertainties still exist in all parts of cost assessments. In any appraisal it is therefore important to identify the main sources of uncertainty at an early stage and try to reduce or handle them. Any residual uncertainties in cost estimates should be documented and communicated to decision makers.

- One of the main sources of uncertainty in the estimation of the costs of natural hazards is the lack of sufficient, comparable, and reliable data. A framework for supporting data collection should be established at the federal level, both for object-specific *ex post* damage data (event analysis) and risk mitigation costs.

- In general, there is a need for a better understanding of the processes leading to damage so that they can be modeled appropriately. With regard to direct damages, multiparameter damage models are needed that better capture the variety of damage influencing parameters, including resistance parameters.

There remain challenges with the underlying model assumptions as well as with the historical data (Niehörster et al, 2013), which lead to alternative and maybe equally likely views and have caused substantial intra-model and inter-model differences. This uncertainty is irreducible, but does not imply that the existing models are not useful or scientifically sound. It rather reflects the limits of the scientific understanding and the ability to predict extreme events in a chaotic system.

More research is needed to understand and to model how markets function outside the state of equilibrium and at different scales. This applies particularly to the dynamics of return to equilibrium after a hazardous event, the associated social and institutional interactions and how agent expectations are formed in situations of high uncertainty. With regard to the costs of risk mitigation, special emphasis should be given to a better estimation of the costs of non-structural measures (Meyer et al, 2013). There is a strong need for appropriate tools, guidance, and knowledge transfer to support decision makers when integrating cost assessment figures into their decision-making process. Such tools or frameworks should communicate and consider uncertainties in cost figures and ensure the transparency of the decision rules. Importantly, the insured loss totals do not account for all economic damage associated with weather-related events, even for hard structures. Specifically, data are not available for several categories of economic losses, including uninsured, underinsured, and self-insured losses. FEMA estimates that one-half to two-thirds of structures in flood plains do not have flood insurance because the uninsured owners either are unaware that homeowners insurance does not cover flood damage, or they do not perceive a serious flood risk. Furthermore, industry analysts estimate that 58% of homeowners in the United States are underinsured—that is, they carry a policy below the replacement value of their property—by an average of 21%. Finally, some individuals and businesses have the means to "self-insure" their assets by assuming the full risk of any damage including business interruption costs.

Damage to the natural environment and ecosystem services

Any discussion of the economic implications of disasters that fails to account for non-market values is an underestimation. Clean air and water, healthy ecosystems, and the preservation of human life, safety, health, and well-being are often treated as having a value of zero despite the fact that society demonstrates a willingness to pay for them in the form of anti-pollution measures, habitat conservation and restoration projects, home protection services, organic food, and memberships to health clubs. Ecosystem-based disaster risk management often realizes highly attractive cost-benefit ratios in many cases greatly exceeding the benefits of retrofitting (UNDRR, 2011). The protection, restoration, and enhancement of ecosystems, including forests, wetlands and mangroves, has two important benefits for DRM. Healthy ecosystems serve as natural protective barriers and buffers against many physical hazards, and they increase resilience by strengthening livelihoods and increasing the availability and quality of goods and resources. Although their value is difficult to measure in economic terms, estimates indicate that regulatory services that mitigate hazards may form the largest proportion of the total economic value of ecosystem services. For example, in the United States of America, coastal wetlands absorb wave energy and act as "horizontal levees," providing $23.2 billion per year in protection from storms.

The values associated with these outcomes do not show up well in the market data and, as a consequence, are likely to be undervalued in an analysis that considers only financial inputs. While some of the damage to the natural environment is reflected in market losses. Damages to a forest used for recreational purposes might result in reduced revenues at campgrounds and retail establishments connected with that recreational use (e.g., sales of hiking equipment). But the natural environment consists of many interrelated ecosystems that provide additional goods and services that fall into four broad classes (Millennium Ecosystem Assessment, 2005):

- Provisioning services (providing goods like food, water, fuel, and inputs to the production of medicine, chemicals, fabric, and timber);

- Regulating services (providing services like maintaining air quality, regulating flooding, controlling erosion, and water purification);

- Cultural services (non-material benefits like the contribution of ecosystems to cultural identity, knowledge, aesthetics, recreation, ecotourism, and a sense of place);

- Supporting services (basic life-support services like soil formation, climate regulation, photosynthesis, water cycling).

The Global Commission on Adaptation (GCA, 2019) has quantified the benefits of several nature-based approaches:

- Investing US$250-500 per hectare in better dryland farming practices could increase cereal yields by 70%–140% bringing net economic benefits of billions;

- Mangroves forests already prevent more than $80 billion in damages—and protect 18 million people—from coastal flooding. In addition, the fisheries, forestry, and recreation they support are worth US$40–50 billion per year—the benefits of mangrove preservation and restoration are up to 10 times the costs;

- Investments that enable more efficient use of water brings benefits that are two to four times the costs, with global net economic benefits of over US$100 billion a year.

See Chapters 5 and 15 discussing other ecosystem-level impacts of climate change.

10.6 Implementation challenges

On the demand side, limited financial awareness and low levels of financial literacy are key challenges in terms of building understanding of insurance as a tool for financial protection and therefore demand for insurance (see Kousky and Kunreuther, 2017, Kousky and Shabman, 2017, Michel-Kerjan, 2012, NAS, 1999). This is exacerbated by the lack of an insurance culture and/or by a population that perceives insurance to be too expensive or is skeptical regarding the operations of insurance companies, including the certainty of claims payment (which hampers penetration even in some economies where disaster insurance is compulsory). Product complexity, for example in the case of innovative index-based or parametric insurance products, can also be an impediment to demand and highlights the need for knowledge transfer and communication. In addition, moral hazard, where individuals or business may be unwilling to pay for insurance given that they expect full compensation for losses from government, was identified by many economies as an important impediment to demand for insurance.

Individuals often fail to purchase insurance against low-probability high-loss events even when it is offered at favorable premiums. Low-probability, high-consequence events are subject to the availability bias, where the judged likelihood of an event depends on its salience (Tversky and Kahneman, 1973). While this may occur because of the relative benefits and costs of alternatives, the tradeoffs may not be explicit. Kunreuther et al (2001) and Kunreuther and Michel-Kerjan (2009) show that the search costs involved in collecting and analyzing relevant information to clarify tradeoffs can be enough to discourage individuals from undertaking such assessments, and thus from purchasing coverage even when the premium is affordable.

An analysis of NFIP policies show that the median tenure of flood insurance was between two and four years, whereas the average length of time in a residence was seven years (Michel-Kerjan et al, 2012). Reasons for the lack of mitigation include property owners underestimating both the risk of a future disaster and the potential benefits of mitigation, and others may not have access to capital to cover the up-front costs (Kunreuther et al, 2013). Field research is needed to untangle which contributing factors are most important and whether policy changes could help counter the tendency to underinvest in insurance and mitigation (Kousky, 2019).

Most consequences of climate change affect more than one line of insurance. For example, extreme heat episodes have caused simultaneous insurance losses ranging from loss of life, to wildfire-driven property loss, to crop damages, to electric power plant shutdowns, to associated business interruptions. Similarly, a given customer class experiences many hazards, e.g., the energy sector experiences service disruptions from lightning strikes on the power grid, outages from lighting strikes or wildfires, and property damages from hurricanes that damage underwater pipelines. In situations where damage is difficult to attribute, also referred to as the problem of proximity, parties may contest at court the extent of a policy's coverage (Cook and Dowlatabadi, 2011).

A fundamental problem within many economic impact studies lies in the unlikely assumption that there are no other influences on the macro-economy during the period analyzed for each disaster. This suggests not only assumptions about stable external and domestic political and economic conditions, but also that no other natural disasters, e.g., earthquakes, occur. In 2017, 22 of 29 Caribbean SIDS were impacted: 4 were affected by 1 storm, 13 by two storms, 5 by three storms. Major impacts can also result from the occurrence of extra-regional disasters, i.e., highly susceptible to impacts in other parts of the world. For instance, the portion of catastrophic risk held within the Caribbean region is 15%–20% (Vermeiren, 2000). During the early and mid-1990s there were no major insurance-loss catastrophes in the Caribbean, yet by the late 1990s premiums more than doubled. This resulted from the so-called reinsurance "crisis" of 1993–1994 (after Hurricane Andrew and the Northridge, California earthquake). Primary insurers imposed a 2% deductible clause. Base property rates on insured value for Eastern Caribbean countries compared with Florida post-Andrew showed that they were at least 50% higher for the Caribbean. Policyholders deliberately begin to underinsure or not insure at all (Vermeiren, 2000).

Entire classes of events that may be expected to worsen under climate change are virtually invisible in the existing data (Mills et al, 2005). In particular, the insurance industry's Property Claims Services (PCS) database is not all-inclusive in terms of types of losses, and excludes from the definition of "catastrophe" an unknown number of "small" events (i.e., those with under $25 million in insured losses). Among the types of events often excluded in the United States are power outages (estimated to result in a cost of $80 billion per year) and lightning strikes (Mills et al, 2005).

According to the Insurance Information Institute (2000), a leading source of information about the insurance industry, primary insurance companies have also raised prices in coastal states to cover rising reinsurance costs. As private insurers limit their exposure, catastrophic risk is transferred to policyholders and the public sector (Cook and Dowlatabadi, 2011).

10.7 Financing mitigation and resilience

The Presidential Policy Directive 8, or PPD-8, for national preparedness defines "mitigation" as:
"Those capabilities necessary to reduce loss of life and property by lessening the impact of disasters. Mitigation capabilities include ... community-wide risk reduction projects; efforts to improve the resilience of critical

Overall Hazard Benefit-Cost Ratio	Federally-funded 6:1	Beyond 2015-I code requirement 4:1
Riverine Flood	7:1	5:1
Hurricane Surge	Too few grants	7:1
Wind	5:1	5:1
Wildland-Urban Interface	3:1	4:1

FIGURE 10.1: Benefit-cost ratio for upfront investment in infrastructure risk mitigation for selected hazard and mitigation measures for 23 years of Federal Grants and International Building, Residential and Wildland-Urban Interface Codes. Adapted from MMC (2017).

infrastructure and key resource lifelines; risk reduction for specific vulnerabilities from natural hazards or acts of terrorism; and initiatives to reduce future risks after a disaster has occurred. Mitigation means adapting buildings, infrastructure, and natural systems that will allow communities to better withstand high winds and rain, ocean storm surge, unusually high temperatures, wild fires, and drought."

The technologies needed to accomplish this goal vary in cost and complexity. New York and New Jersey are buying out homeowners with severely damaged homes located in flood-prone areas using federal funds provided under the Disaster Relief Act. Unlike New York City and New Jersey, many communities lack the financial resources to become more resilient to future extreme weather events. Many communities lack the resources to invest in projects that would protect their structures and inhabitants from major storms.

More than a decade ago, the National Institute of Building Sciences released a study, Natural Hazard Mitigation Saves: An Independent Study to Assess the Future Savings from Mitigation Activities, which found society saves $4 for every $1 spent on mitigation by the FEMA. More recently, the FEMA Multihazard Council (MMC, 2017) released a detailed report outlining the benefits of proactive mitigation for infrastructure risks for a number of weather-related hazards (see Figure 10.1).

A Center for American Progress study estimated for 2011–2013 federal taxpayers spent nearly $6 for disaster recovery for every $1 spent to increase general community resilience over the past three years. The value of upfront or proactive mitigation is clear but still only constitute 10%–12% of disaster-related spending nationally and globally.

Both insurers and reinsurers must also predict the frequency and severity of insured losses with some reliability to best manage financial risk. In some cases, these losses may be fairly predictable. For example, the incidence of most automobile insurance claims is predictable, and losses generally do not occur to large numbers of policyholders at the same time. However, some infrequent weather-related events—for example, hurricanes—are so severe that they pose unique challenges for insurers and reinsurers. Commonly referred to as catastrophic or extreme events, the unpredictability and sheer size of these events— both in terms of spatial scale and number of insured parties affected—have the potential to overwhelm insurers' and reinsurers' capacity to pay claims. Catastrophic events may affect many households, businesses, and public infrastructure across large areas, resulting in substantial losses that deplete insurers' and reinsurers' capital. Given the higher levels of capital that reinsurers must hold to address catastrophic events, reinsurers generally charge higher premiums and restrict coverage for such events. Further, in the wake of catastrophic events, reinsurers and insurers may sharply increase premiums to rebuild capital reserves and may significantly restrict insurance and reinsurance coverage to limit exposure to similar events in the future.

While both major private and federal insurers are exposed to increases in the frequency or severity of weather-related events associated with climate change, the two sectors are responding in different ways. Many major private insurers are incorporating some near-term elements of climate change into their risk management practices using computer-based catastrophe models, One consequence is that, as these insurers limit their own catastrophic risk exposure, by transferring some of risk to policyholders and the public sector. In addition, some private insurers are approaching climate change at a strategic level by publishing reports outlining the potential industry-wide impacts and strategies to proactively address the issue. Federal insurance programs, need to develop the kind of information needed to understand the programs' long-term exposure to climate change for a variety of reasons including the need to increase participation among eligible parties. Consequently, neither program has had reason to develop information on their long-term exposure to the fiscal risks associated with climate change.

The American Insurance Association (AIA) emphasizes the shortcomings of estimating future catastrophic risk by extrapolating solely from historical losses and endorses catastrophe models as a more rigorous approach. Catastrophe models incorporate the underlying trends and factors in weather phenomena and current demographic, financial, and scientific data to estimate losses associated with various weather-related events. According to an industry representative, catastrophe models assess a wider range of possible events than the historical loss record alone. These models simulate losses from thousands of potential catastrophic weather-related events that insurers use to better assess and control their exposure and inform pricing and capital management decisions.

10.8 Pathways and conclusion

Disasters can have a profound effect on local and state government revenues. Michel-Kerjan (2012) poses five questions as pillars of national risk management. What risks do we face and where? What assets and populations are exposed and to what degree? How vulnerable are they? What financial burden do these risks place on individuals, businesses, and the government budget? How best can we invest to reduce risks and strengthen economic and social resilience?

Many governments do not know the answers (Michel-Kerjan, 2012). Production and income taxes decline with production and income (Meyer et al, 2013). The literature is replete with excellent recommendations for improving disaster risk reduction not all of many of which are in practice. The American Insurance Association (American Insurance Association, 2000) made six recommendations for mitigating catastrophic risks and for developing a strategy to identify, prioritize, and guide investments to enhance resilience against future disaster risk including: early warning systems, better land-use planning, improved building codes and catastrophe-resistant reconstruction, improved coordination and planning of national and international relief efforts, assistance in catastrophe contingency planning, and support for pre- and post-event mitigation and response.

The Global Commission on Adaptation (GCA, 2019) has quantified the benefits of several of the above recommendations:

- Early warning systems save lives and assets worth at least ten times their cost. A 24-hour warning of a coming storm or heat wave can cut the ensuing damage by 30%. Investing US$800 million on such systems in developing countries would avoid US$3–16 billion per year in losses alone.

- US$1 trillion in the incremental cost of making infrastructure more resilient in developing countries would generate US$4.2 trillion in benefits.

The GAO (2017) has identified various challenges to resilience building—actions to help prepare and plan for, absorb, recover from, and more successfully adapt to adverse events including those caused by extreme weather. These include challenges for communities in balancing hazard mitigation investments with economic development goals, challenges for individuals in understanding and acting to limit their personal risk, and broad challenges with the clarity of information to inform risk decision-making. These are long-standing policy issues, without easy solutions, that can only be successful though "whole of community" approaches (FEMA, 2019; see Figure 10.2) to develop a holistic risk management culture, facilitating community-, regional-, and state-level loss reduction activities, climate-proofing existing infrastructure investments, and putting in place appropriate zoning and building codes

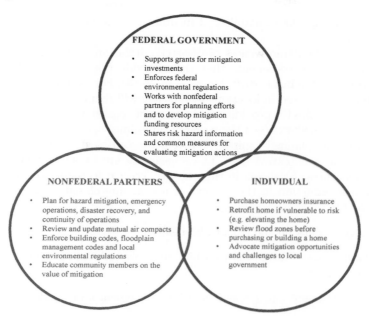

FIGURE 10.2: Examples of Whole of Community roles in mitigation. Source: FEMA (2019).

and enforcing these—all of which will contribute tangibly to managing risks and loss potential.

Integrating climate change considerations into land-use planning is increasingly receiving attention as a proactive strategy. While this area has natural roles for insurers, although the public sector clearly has lead responsibility. One post-Katrina analysis revealed that per-capita economic losses were three-times lower in areas where building codes and comprehensive land-use planning were in use. The NFIP maintains a voluntary community program to incentivize greater investments in flood risk management, some of which are through land use by awarding points for preserving flood plains as open space (Brody and Highfield, 2013). Apart from quantity of development in high-risk locations and housing prices, disaster insurance could impact other forms of land use if there are financial incentives for such actions. Firewise, a program run by the National Fire Protection Association, may be one such example. When communities join they assess their wildfire risk and develop an action plan and engage in some outreach and education. The insurance company USAA found that Firewise communities in different states all had lower losses than those not in Firewise communities and is thus providing discounts to residents of these localities (OMB, 2016). Although property values clearly capitalize disaster risk and/or insurance costs, there is little support for the claim that the availability of insurance has altered land-use patterns substantially.

The economic attractiveness of disaster mitigation measures is enhanced by considering the co-benefits that they provide (Benson and Clay, 2004, Hallegatte and Przyluski, 2010, Meyer et al, 2013). For example, natural wetlands that are restored in locations where they will reduce the harmful effects of storm surge will also provide a wide range of ecosystem services. Instances where the co-benefits exceed the cost are sometimes called "no-regrets" measures. Similarly, planned capital improvements can be made hazard-resilient for a low marginal (extra) cost. These measures are sometimes called "low-regrets" measures. As shown in this chapter, critical to the success of linking disaster risk reduction in the context of a changing climate requires (Muir-Wood, 2016):

- High-quality data on the risks to be insured;
- Risk landscapes' information by which to apply technical pricing and diversification strategies;
- Active government engagement in risk management and regulation;
- Customers' appreciation for how insurance works.

Kousky (2019) lays out the risk landscape that needs to be quantified for insurability and presents five idealized conditions for insuring risk:

1. A degree of randomness to loss occurrences and their magnitude;
2. Independent, thin-tailed, and quantifiable risks;
3. Determinable losses;
4. Limited adverse selection or moral hazard; and
5. Demand meets supply (the market clears).

As climate alters extreme event risks around the globe, a deeper appreciation of the role insurance can play in climate adaptation will be required (Kousky, 2019). Much more research is needed on the links between risk transfer and risk reduction:

- Providing a suitable enabling environment for risk management, including insurance.
- Investing in systematic and reliable risk exposure data, historic and forward-looking, that is both accessible and usable.
- Acting on lessons drawn about the role of government in convening and seeding regional public-private partnerships.

Realizing these goals in a changing environment requires anticipatory and active governance. Such agility should include standards, accountability, and alignment across governments, communities, the private sector, NGOs, and academia necessary for financial services and disaster mitigation to function across timescales and at different levels of society as new risks and opportunities emerge.

References

ABI (2005) Financial risks of climate change. Association of British Insurers, London, UK

Adams-Schoen S, Thomas E (2015) A three-legged stool on two legs: recent federal law related to local climate resilience planning and zoning. The Urban Lawyer 47(3):525–542

American Farm Bureau Federation (2019) Farm bankruptcies rise again. URL www.fb.org/market-intel

American Insurance Association (2000) Potential Areas of Focus for the OECD with Regard to Global Catastrophe Mitigation. Unpublished mimeograph, Washington, DC

Benson C, Clay E (2004) Understanding the economic and financial impacts of natural disasters, Disaster Risk Management Series, vol 4. The World Bank, Washington, DC

Booz Allen Hamilton (2013) Reimagining the next generation of homeland security. Tech. Rep. BA12-269, Booz Allen Hamilton

Bretz L (2017) Climate change and homes: Who would lose the most to a rising tide? Zillow Research. URL https://www.zillow.com/research/climate-change-underwater-homes-2-16928/

Brody SD, Highfield WE (2013) Open space protection and flood mitigation: a national study. Land Use Policy 32:89–95

Changnon SA, Pielke Jr RA, Changnon D, Sylves RT, Pulwarty R (2000) Human factors explain the increased losses from weather and climate extremes. Bulletin of the American Meteorological Society 81(3):437–442

Clark KM (1997) Current and potential impact of hurricane variability on the insurance industry. In: Diaz H, Pulwarty R (eds) Hurricanes: Climate and Socioeconomic Impacts, Springer, New York, NY, 273–283

Cook CL, Dowlatabadi H (2011) Learning adaptation: climate-related risk management in the insurance industry. In: Ford JD, Berrang-Ford L (eds) Climate Change Adaptation in Developed Nations: From Theory to Practice, Springer, New York, NY, 255–265

Cooke RM, Nieboer D, Misiewicz J (2014) Fat-tailed Distributions: Data, Diagnostics and Dependence, vol 1. John Wiley & Sons, Hoboken, NJ, USA

Cutler DM, Zeckhauser R (2004) Extending the theory to meet the practice of insurance. Brookings-Wharton Papers on Financial Services 2004(1):1–53

Dixon L, Clancy N, Seabury AS, Overton A (2006) The National Flood Insurance Program's Market Penetration Rate: Estimates and Policy Implications. RAND Corporation, Santa Monica, CA

Easterling DR, Meehl GA, Parmesan C, Changnon SA, Karl TR, Mearns LO (2000) Climate extremes: observations, modeling, and impacts. Science 289(5487):2068–2074

FEMA (2019) National Mitigation Investment Strategy. Federal Emergency Management Agency, Department of Homeland Security, Washington, DC

Freeman PK, Keen M, Mani M (2003) Dealing with Increased Risk of Natural Disasters: Challenge And Options. Working Paper WP 03/197. International Monetary Fund, Washington, DC, USA

GAO (2017) Climate change: Information on potential economic effects could help guide federal efforts to reduce fiscal exposure. Tech. Rep. GAO-17-720, Government Accountability Office, Washington, DC

GAO (2018) Army corps of engineers budget requests. Tech. Rep. GAO 19-99, Government Accountability Office, Washington, DC

GCA (2019) Adapt Now: A Global Call for Leadership on Climate Resilience. Global Center for Adaptation and World Resources Institute, Washington, DC

Ghesquiere F, Mahul O (2010) Financial Protection of the State against Natural Disasters. Working Paper WPS 5429. The World Bank, Washington, DC

Hallegatte S, Przyluski V (2010) The Economics of Natural Disasters: Concepts and Methods. The World Bank, Washington, DC

Healy A, Malhotra N (2009) Myopic voters and natural disaster policy. American Political Science Review 103(3):387–406

Heinz Center (2000) The Hidden Costs of Coastal Hazards: Implications for Risk Assessment and Mitigation. Island Press, Covelo, CA

Howe CW, Cochrane HC (1993) Guidelines for the uniform definition, identification, and measurement of economic damages from natural hazard events: With comments on historical assets, human capital, and natural capital. FMHI Publications. Paper 64

Insurance Information Institute (2000) Catastrophes. Washington, DC

Kahn ME, Casey B, Jones N (2017) How the insurance industry can push us to prepare for climate change. Harvard Business Review, August 28

Knowles SG, Kunreuther HC (2014) Troubled waters: the national flood insurance program in historical perspective. Journal of Policy History 26(3):327–353

Knutson T, Camargo SJ, Chan JCL, Emanuel K, Ho CH, Kossin J, Mohapatra M, Satoh M, Sugi M, Walsh K, Wu L (2020) Tropical cyclones and climate change assessment: Part II. Projected response to anthropogenic warming. Bulletin of the American Meteorological Society 101:E303–E322

Kousky C (2014) Informing climate adaptation: a review of the economic costs of natural disasters. Energy Economics 46:576–592

Kousky C (2019) The role of natural disaster insurance in recovery and risk reduction. Annual Review of Resource Economics 11:399–418

Kousky C, Kunreuther H (2017) Defining the roles of the public and private sector in risk communication, risk reduction, and risk transfer. Resources for the Future Discussion Paper 17–09

Kousky C, Shabman L (2017) Federal funding for flood risk reduction in the US: pre-or post-disaster? Water Economics and Policy 3(01):1771001

Kunreuther H (2006) Disaster mitigation and insurance: learning from Katrina. The Annals of the American Academy of Political and Social Science 604(1):208–227

Kunreuther H, Novemsky N, Kahneman D (2001) Making low probabilities useful. Journal of Risk and Uncertainty 23(2):103–120

Kunreuther HC, Michel-Kerjan EO (2009) At War with the Weather: Managing Large-Scale Risks in a New Era of Catastrophes. MIT Press, Cambridge, MA

Kunreuther HC, Pauly MV, McMorrow S (2013) Insurance and Behavioral Economics: Improving Decisions in the Most Misunderstood Industry. Cambridge University Press, Cambridge, UK

Lindell MK, Prater CS (2003) Assessing community impacts of natural disasters. Natural Hazards Review 4:176–185

Linnerooth-Bayer J, Vari A (2006) Extreme Weather and Burden Sharing in Hungary. MIT Press, Cambridge, MA

Meyer V, Becker N, Markantonis V, Schwarze R, Van Den Bergh J, Bouwer L, Bubeck P, Ciavola P, Genovese E, Green CH, Hallegatte S, Kreibich H, Lequeux Q, Logar I, Papyrakis E, Pfurtscheller C, Poussin J, Przyluski V, Thieken AH, Viavattene C (2013) Assessing the costs of natural hazards-state of the art and knowledge gaps. Natural Hazards and Earth System Sciences 13(5):1351–1373

Michel-Kerjan E (2012) How resilient is your country? Nature 491(7425):497–497

Michel-Kerjan E, Lemoyne de Forges S, Kunreuther H (2012) Policy tenure under the US national flood insurance program (NFIP). Risk Analysis 32(4):644–658

Milken Institute (2008) Financial innovations for catastrophic risk: Cat bonds and beyond

Millennium Ecosystem Assessment (2005) Millennium Ecosystem Assessment: Current Status and Trends. URL www.millenniumassessment.org

Mills E, Roth RJ, Lecomte E (2005) Availability and affordability of insurance under climate change: a growing challenge for the US. Ceres, Boston, MA

MMC (2017) Natural Hazard Mitigation Saves 2017 Interim Report: An Independent Study. Multihazard Mitigation Council, National Institute of Building Sciences, Washington, DC

Muir-Wood R (2016) The Cure for Catastrophe: How We Can Stop Manufacturing Disasters. OneWorld Publications, London

NAS (1999) The Impacts of Natural Disasters: A Framework for Loss Estimation. National Academies of Science, National Academies Press, Washington, DC

Niehörster F, Aichinger M, Murnane R, Ranger N, Surminski S (2013) Warming of the oceans and implications for the (re)insurance industry, A Geneva Association Report

NOAA (2013a) Economics: National Ocean Watch. URL https://coast.noaa.gov/digitalcoast/data/enow.html

NOAA (2013b) Spatial Trends in Coastal Socioeconomics: Total Economy of Coastal Areas. URL https://www.coast.noaa.gov/htdata/SocioEconomic/CoastalEconomy/CoastalEconomy_DataDescription.pdf

NRC (1999) The Impacts of Natural Disasters: A Framework for Loss Estimation. National Research Council, National Academies Press, Washington, DC

OECD (2015) Disaster risk financing: a global survey of practices and challenges. OECD Publishing, Paris, France

OMB (2016) Standards and Finance to Support Community Resilience. Office of the President of the United States, Washington, DC

Prevost L (2013) On floods and rising insurance premiums. New York Times July 14

Pulwarty R, Verdin JP (2013) Crafting early warning systems: the case of drought. In: Birkmann J (ed) Measuring Vulnerability to Natural Hazards: Towards Disaster Resilient Societies, 124–147

Rose A (2004) Defining and measuring economic resilience to disasters. Disaster Prevention and Management 13(4):307–314

SBA (2013) FY 2013 Congressional Budget Justification and FY 2011 Annual Performance Report. Small Business Administration, Washington, DC

Schnitkey G (2019) Historical prevent planting payments: Implications for 2019. Farmdoc Daily 9:126

Scolari B, Pfister M (2018) Strengthening Financial Resilience to Climate Change: The Role of Insurance. Washington, DC, USA, URL www.eesi.org, environmental and Energy Study Institute EESI Factsheet

Seneviratne SI, Nicholls N, Easterling D, Goodess CM, Kanae S, Kossin J, Luo Y, Marengo J, McInnes K, Rahimi M, Reichstein M, Sorteberg A, Vera C, Zhang X (2017) Changes in climate extremes and their impacts on the natural physical environment. In: IPCC Special Report on Managing the Risks of Extreme Events and Disasters to Advance Climate Change Adaptation Field, Cambridge University Press, Cambridge, UK

Smith AB (2020) U.S. billion-dollar weather and climate disasters (1980–2019). URL https://www.ncdc.noaa.gov/billions/

Smith AB, Katz RW (2013) US billion-dollar weather and climate disasters: data sources, trends, accuracy and biases. Natural Hazards 67(2):387–410

Smith AB, Matthews JL (2015) Quantifying uncertainty and variable sensitivity within the US billion-dollar weather and climate disaster cost estimates. Natural Hazards 77(3):1829–1851

Todey D (2019) USDA Climate Hub Director quoted in "A Wet Year Causes Farm Woes Far Beyond the Floodplains". New York Times, 21 November

Tversky A, Kahneman D (1973) Availability: a heuristic for judging frequency and probability. Cognitive Psychology 5(2):207–232

UNDRR (2011) Global Assessment Report on Disaster Risk Reduction: Revealing Risks, Redefining Development. United Nations Office for Disaster Risk Reduction, Washington, DC, USA

USACE (2013) Civil Works Budget of the US Army Corps of Engineers for 2014. Coastal Hydraulics Laboratory, Washington, DC, USA

Vermeiren J (2000) Risk transfer and finance experience in the Caribbean. In: Kreimer A, Arnold M (eds) Managing Disaster Risk in Emerging Economies, World Bank, Washington, DC

Wuebbles DJ, Fahey DW, Hibbard KA, DeAngelo B, Doherty S, Hayhoe K, Horton R, Kossin JP, Taylor PC, Waple AM, Weaver C (2017) Executive summary. In: Wuebbles DJ, Fahey DW, Hibbard KA, Dokken DJ, Stewart BC, Maycock T (eds) Climate Science Special Report: Fourth National Climate Assessment, Volume I, U.S. Global Change Research Program, Washington, DC, pp 12–34

11

Extreme Events, Population, and Risk: An Integrated Modeling Approach

Lelys Bravo de Guenni
University of Illinois at Urbana-Champaign, Champaign, IL, USA

Desireé Villalta
Universidad Simón Bolívar, Caracas, Venezuela

Andrés Sajo-Castelli
The Numerical Algorithms Group Ltd, Oxford, UK

CONTENTS

11.1	Introduction	235
11.2	Conceptual framework for risk modeling	236
	11.2.1 Hazard, exposure, vulnerability, and risk	236
11.3	Applications of the conceptual framework	238
	11.3.1 An example considering hazard counts	238
	11.3.2 An example considering hazard space-time fields	245
11.4	Discussion, conclusions, and future work	252
References		255

11.1 Introduction

According to Munich RE (2017), the number of people worldwide who lost their lives in a natural disaster during year 2017 was about 10,000. Flood events including river flooding and flash floods accounted for 47% of events. The major events were devastating floods in India, Nepal, and Bangladesh. In North America, about 170 events were registered, with the highest losses caused by the three big hurricanes: Harvey, Irma, and Maria. A striking fact is that a higher number of deaths occurred in emerging and developing countries than in industrialized/developed countries.

There is an increasing gap between economic and insured natural disaster losses, with up to 100% of losses being uninsured in developing and emerging countries (Bollman and Wang, 2019), which causes severe disruption on the national development strategies. Aon (2018) reported an amount of $215 billion in economic losses for weather related disasters in 2018 (4th costliest year on record), while only $89 billion (40%) were insured. However, the $215 billion of economic losses were a notable reduction from the $438 billion losses in 2017 (Aon, 2018).

The geography of risk to weather-related events results from the conjunction of human development and population growth and their inherent susceptibility to suffer damage; jointly with magnitude and occurrence of potentially damaging events. The frequency and magnitude of these events are in nature nonstationary spatiotemporal processes, and the potential to suffer damage is also a dynamic process driven by complex social and geophysical changing factors.

Attempts to develop a conceptual framework to estimate risk, considering its main components: hazard, vulnerability, and exposure, have been discussed by many authors (Forzieri et al, 2017, Lin and Shullman, 1997, Liu et al, 2017, Vörösmarty et al, 2013). The vulnerability concept has been used in different ways within the social sciences and the physical sciences. Brooks (2003) discussed the difference between social vulnerability and biophysical vulnerability, concluding that social vulnerability is not a function of the frequency and severity of a given type of hazard, while biophysical vulnerability is concerned with the final impacts of a potentially damaging event. In the social vulnerability case, there are inherent factors as poverty, inequality, marginalization, housing quality, that determine the final outcome experienced by a community impacted by a hazardous event. Hence social vulnerability can be included as one of the determinants of biophysical vulnerability. A more detailed list of definitions of vulnerability as it is used in different disciplines is provided in Nunes (2003). In our approach, we will refer to biophysical vulnerability as vulnerability in plain language.

On the hazard side, we will be referring to natural hazards of hydrometeorological origin and would exclude from our approach the technological hazards. According to Downing et al (1999), a *hazard* is defined as a threatening event or the probability of occurrences of a potentially damaging phenomenon within a given time and area. However, the probabilistic description has also been used by some authors to define risk itself (Stenschion, 1997).

11.2 Conceptual framework for risk modeling

11.2.1 Hazard, exposure, vulnerability, and risk

A hazard is a natural physical event that might potentially cause damage, and it is external to the community or subject of study. It can be normally classified as climatological, hydrological, meteorological, or geophysical hazard. It can cause life losses, injuries, material damage, and social and economic disruptions including environmental degradation. The hazard is essentially a spatiotemporal phenomenon, which can be quantified by its magnitude, intensity, and duration that has a probability associated to it. We will focus on natural hazards, although technological hazards or a combination of them (natech hazards) could be also considered under this framework. Another risk component is the exposure (denoted as E), which is quantified in terms of population, infrastructure, or physical assets potentially subjected to damage due to a hazard occurrence at a particular location and time. In terms of the population, (Vörösmarty et al, 2013) express the exposure as $E = Pop|H$, which represents the population exposed to a hazard level H or conditioned to the occurrence of hazard level H.

From the whole population exposed, the population affected (A) is defined as the number of individuals from a population actually experiencing some damage in absolute terms: the total number of people affected by hydrometeorological phenomena, such as floods, landslides, mass movements, caused by extreme rainfall events. In general, $0 \leqslant A \leqslant E \leqslant Pop$. Following similar arguments, the number of people affected is a spatiotemporal variable conditioned on the hazard magnitude H. We can write $A|H \leqslant E|H$.

Vulnerability is a multidimensional concept, which is dynamic in nature and difficult to quantify. Within this framework, vulnerability (V) is defined as the degree of losses (from 0% to 100%) resulting from a potentially damaging phenomenon. This random process can be quantified in economic terms associated with material or infrastructure damage, or it can be quantified in terms of the proportion of people affected (Downing et al, 1999). If the focus is on human vulnerability, we can quantify the proportion of people affected conditioned on a given hazard level H (Vörösmarty et al, 2013), such that $V = (A/E) \mid H$, where $A \leqslant E \leqslant Pop$.

Risk is defined as the expected losses (number of people affected, material damage, and disrupted economic activity) due to a particular hazard affecting a geographic domain at a particular time. Therefore, the losses are incurred as a result of the hazard level and the vulnerability of the population or assets exposed to the particular hazard (Plate, 1996).

We will consider the hazard and vulnerability as space-time processes written as $H(t, s)$ and $V(t, s)$, where $t \in T$ and $s \in S$ are elements of the spatial and temporal domains S and T, respectively. We consider $E(t, s)$ as the population or assets exposed to a given hazard level $H(t, s)$. The degree of loss $\mathcal{L}$ given $H(t, s)$ can be written as $(\mathcal{L}_{t,s}|H_{t,s}) = (V_{t,s} \mid H_{t,s})E_{t,s}$, which is the degree of vulnerability conditioned to a hazard level multiplied by the exposed subject. Using the previous definitions, the risk for a given location s and time

t ($R_{t,s}$) can be expressed as

$$\begin{aligned} R_{t,s} &= \mathrm{E}_H[\mathrm{E}_{V\mid H}[V_{t,s}\mid H_{t,s}]E_{t,s}] \\ &= \int_{\Omega_H} \mathrm{E}_{V\mid H}[V_{t,s}\mid H_{t,s}]E_{t,s}\mathsf{P}(H_{t,s})\mathrm{d}H_{t,s} \\ &= \int_{\Omega_H}\int_{\Omega_V} V_{t,s}\mathsf{P}(V_{t,s}\mid H_{t,s})E_{t,s}\mathsf{P}(H_{t,s})\,\mathrm{d}V_{t,s}\,\mathrm{d}H_{t,s}, \end{aligned} \quad (11.1)$$

where Ω_H and Ω_V are the hazard and vulnerability domains, and $\mathrm{E}_{V\mid H}[.]$ is the conditional expectation of the vulnerability given the hazard level, and $\mathrm{E}_H[.]$ is the marginal expectation with respect to the hazard. As the exposure ($E_{t,s}$) is not a function of the hazard or the vulnerability, this can be taken out of the integral in the form:

$$R_{t,s} = E_{t,s}\int_{\Omega_H}\int_{\Omega_V} V_{t,s}\mathsf{P}(V_{t,s}\mid H_{t,s})\mathsf{P}(H_{t,s})\,\mathrm{d}V_{t,s}\,\mathrm{d}H_{t,s}. \quad (11.2)$$

Here $\mathsf{P}(H_{t,s})$ is the hazard probability distribution while $\mathsf{P}(V_{t,s}\mid H_{t,s})$ is the vulnerability conditional probability distribution, for a given location s and time t. Big part of the modeling effort is spent in modeling the probability distributions $\mathsf{P}(H_{t,s})$, $\mathsf{P}(V_{t,s}\mid H_{t,s})$ and the exposure quantification. In case the hazard variable $H_{t,s}$ is a counting process with occurrence rate λ_H (for example, number of events per year), (11.2) can be expressed as:

$$R_{t,s} = E_{t,s}\sum_{h=1}^{N_H} \mathrm{E}[V_{t,s}\mid H_{t,s}]\mathsf{P}(H_{t,s}=h\mid\lambda_H),$$

where $\mathsf{P}(H_{t,s}=h\mid\lambda_H)$ is the probability of the hazard counts being equal to h, conditioned on λ_H.

11.3 Applications of the conceptual framework

11.3.1 An example considering hazard counts

In this analysis we used the Spatial Hazard Events and Losses Database for the United States (SHELDUS; CEMHS, 2018) data set to implement this framework in the state of South Carolina. SHELDUS is a county-level hazard data set for the United States and covers natural hazards such as thunderstorms, hurricanes, floods, wildfires, and tornados, as well as perils such as flash floods, heavy rainfall, etc.[1]

---

[1] A metadata description is given on the website `https://cemhs.asu.edu/sheldus`.

Applications of the conceptual framework

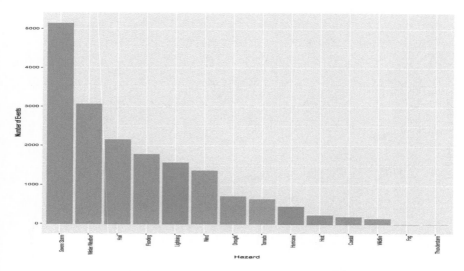

FIGURE 11.1: Number of events during 1960–2016.

Figure 11.1 shows a summary of the number of events that occurred during the period 1960–2016. The total number of fatalities and total injured are presented in Figures 11.2 and 11.3.

To explore the impacts in economic terms, Figure 11.4 presents the property damage per capita in thousands of US dollars (USD). Hurricanes, droughts and coastal hazards are the three hazard types causing major damage in South Carolina.

The highest loss-producing hazards in terms of fatalities are winter weather, lightning, and heat; while the highest injured counts are produced by tornadoes, hurricanes, and lightning. In terms of property damage per capita, the highest losses are produced by hurricanes, droughts, and coastal hazards.

Following our suggested approach, we need to develop a vulnerability function that relates losses as a function of the hazard magnitude, and assess its probability. In this case the focus is not on the hazard magnitude itself, but on its rate of occurrence. In statistical terms, we will refer to the process intensity as the mean number of damaging events per year that a particular county might experience during the study period.

In this example, the rate of occurrence of an event of a given type is used as our predictor variable, and the cumulative consequence of this intensity process on producing damages in a particular location is recognized as the response variable. This relationship defines our vulnerability or loss function. Other predictors shaping the social-demographic information could also be included in the analysis.

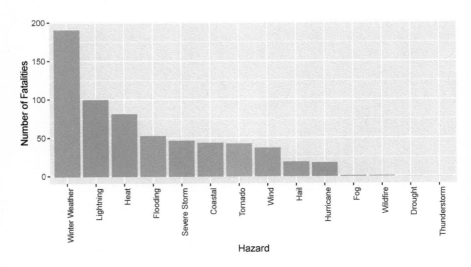

FIGURE 11.2: Total number of fatalities during 1960–2016.

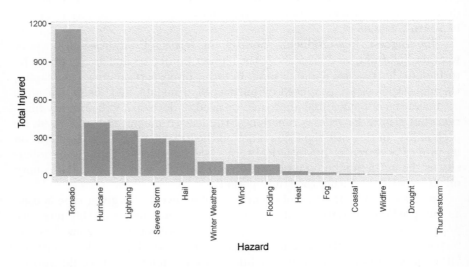

FIGURE 11.3: Total number of people injured during 1960–2016.

Applications of the conceptual framework

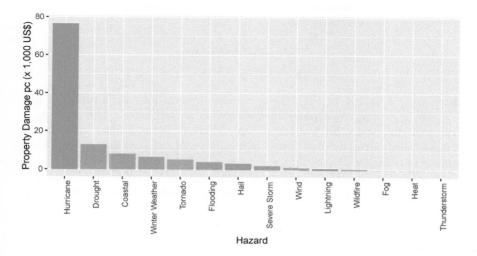

FIGURE 11.4: Property damage per capita during 1960–2016.

Risk is estimated as the expected losses for a particular hazard type i and county j defined as:

$$E[\mathcal{L}_{ij}] = \sum_{k=1}^{M} E[\mathcal{L}_{ij}|Nh_{ij}]P(Nh_{ij} = k) \qquad (11.3)$$

for large M. In this equation $E[\mathcal{L}_{ij}|Nh_{ij}]$ are the expected losses conditioned on the occurrence of the number of events Nh_{ij} of a certain type at county j; and $P(Nh_{ij} = k)$ is the probability that the number of events is equal to a fixed value k. The expectation is taken over a potential large number of events occurring during the study period. The two components, vulnerability and hazard probabilities, need to be modeled before completing the risk estimation.

Hazard model

Our interest is in modeling the number of hazard events Nh of type i on county j for the whole study period. We will call this the spatial random process Nh_{ij}. Since we have count data with potential spatial dependence, we can use a conditional autoregressive (CAR) model to account for spatial dependence. At this point, single hazard types are modeled, but an extension of this approach to model multiple hazard types, as proposed by Wang and Kockelman (2013), could be implemented.

Since the rate of occurrence for each hazard type is modeled individually, we can drop the subscript i in the following paragraphs.

Let Nh_j be the number of events that occurred during the study period at county j. We assumed a model of the form:

$$Nh_j|\lambda_j \sim Poisson(\lambda_j),$$
$$\log(\lambda_j) = \mathbf{x}_j^\top \beta + \phi_j, \qquad (11.4)$$

where $\mathbf{x}_j^\top = (1, x_{1j}, \ldots, x_{jp})$ is a vector of covariates at location j and $\beta = (\beta_0, \beta_1, \ldots, \beta_p)$ is a parameter vector to be estimated. The term ϕ_j is a random effect term for $j = 1, 2, \ldots, N$, where N is the number of counties. ϕ_j is assumed normally distributed with mean and variance depending on the number of neighbors for county j.

Observed values of the number of hurricanes and number of coastal hazards that affected the South Carolina counties during the study period are presented in Figure 11.5(b).

Moran's test for spatial dependence suggests a significant spatial correlation for the number hurricane events (p-value = 0.0195) and number of coastal hazard events (p-value = 0.037). Since the p-values are below 0.05, we reject the spatial independence hypothesis. The Leroux's model (Leroux et al, 1999) was used to account for the spatial correlation effect:

$$\phi_j|\phi_{-k} \sim N\left(\frac{\rho \sum_{i=1}^{N} w_{ji}\phi_i}{\rho \sum_{i=1}^{N} w_{ji} + \rho - 1}, \frac{\tau^2}{\rho \sum_{i=1}^{N} w_{ji} + \rho - 1}\right), \qquad (11.5)$$

where ρ is a spatial autocorrelation parameter; τ^2 is a scale parameter, and w_{ij} are the elements of the proximity matrix W, which depends on the number of neighbors to a particular county, and has values $w_{ij} = 1$ if county j and county i are neighboring counties, while $w_{ij} = 0$ otherwise. Note that the spatial correlation defined in (11.5) plays a similar role to the autocorrelation function in time series analysis.

The model described by (11.4) and (11.5) was fitted using the R library *CARBayes* (Lee, 2019). The estimated parameters for hurricanes and coastal hazards are shown in Table 11.1. No covariates were included into the model, however the model is able to reproduce the spatial occurrence of the two different hazard types.

Vulnerability model

The vulnerability functions can be developed using selected response variables, for example:

- Fatalities and injured (total number of people affected);
- Property damage (damage per capita, USD).

These two variables are measures of the degree of loss, $\mathcal{L}_{ij}$, due to a particular type of hazard i for a given county j. Usually the relationship between losses

Applications of the conceptual framework 243

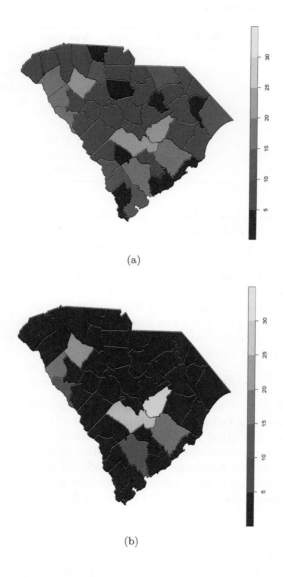

FIGURE 11.5: Observed number of hurricanes (a) and coastal hazards (b) that affected South Carolina counties during the period 1960–2016.

and the hazard intensity is nonlinear, and an appropriate model to quantify this relationship should be investigated.

Vörösmarty et al (2013) proposed a nonlinear model to represent the relationship between the proportion of people affected by a rainfall event and the

TABLE 11.1: Hazard model parameter estimates for South Carolina

Parameter	2.5%	Median	97.5%
	Hurricanes		
β_0	2.1460	2.2503	2.3510
τ^2	0.0682	0.1856	0.4862
ρ	0.0053	0.1418	0.6253
	Coastal hazards		
β_0	0.0258	0.4175	0.7744
τ^2	1.0110	1.9296	4.5514
ρ	0.0021	0.0664	0.4144

rainfall anomalies associated with a particular event. The loss function was developed for rural and urban populations, since the particular events were aggregated by country or states, and population data were available at a higher spatial resolution. In this example, we fitted a loss model to the variables $\mathcal{L}_{ij}$, as a function of the rate of occurrence of hazard type i at county j, γ_{ij}. γ_{ij} is estimated as the mean number of events per year. The most damaging hazard types were used for the analysis. To illustrate the methodology, the amount of property damage per capita was used as our loss variable.

Let $\mathcal{L}_{ij} = Z_{ij}$ be the amount of property damage per capita (in USD). The following model was fitted to the variable $\log(Z_{ij})$:

$$\log(Z_{ij}) = \beta_{0i} + \beta_{1i}\log(\gamma_{ij}) + \varepsilon_{ij},$$

where β_{0i} and β_{1i} are model parameters to be estimated, and ε_{ij} is assumed to be a random error term with distribution $N(0, \sigma^2)$.

This model was fitted separately for hurricane events and coastal hazard events. The regression models explained 41% of the variation of property damage per capita for hurricane events and 85% of the variation of property damage per capita for coastal hazard events. The fitted vulnerability models after log-transformation are shown in Figure 11.6.

Risk model

After modeling the degree of loss conditioned on a given hazard rate and number of damaging events, the expected losses are calculated using (11.3). Samples from the posterior predictive probability distribution are used to estimate the probabilities of occurrence $P(Nh_{ij} = k)$ for a given hazard type i and county j, and the expected losses conditioned on the hazard rate of occurrence are estimated from the vulnerability model. The risk estimate calculated as the expected losses in property damage per capita is presented in Figure 11.7. The three highest risk counties are Claredon, Orangeburg, and Laurens. These counties have over 20% of poverty rate; and the interaction between social and geophysical factors might be triggering the higher risk

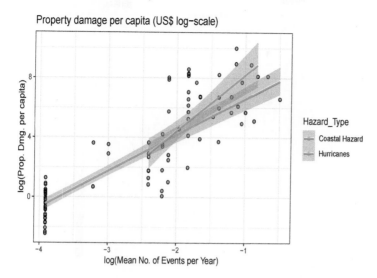

FIGURE 11.6: Property damage per capita (USD) versus mean number of events per year (after log-transformation) for all South Carolina counties affected by hurricanes and coastal hazards.

effects. A more detail analysis with additional information on the vulnerable population locations, might be necessary to better explain the geography of risk. This implies building vulnerability functions that might be able to produce loss estimates in time and space, and consider exposure variability accounting for the mobility of the population.

11.3.2 An example considering hazard space-time fields

In this example the study region is the Vargas state located in the north-central coast of Venezuela, between West 66° 19′ 00″ and West 67° 25′ 00″, and between North 10° 23′ 00″ and North 10° 38′ 00″. The northern limit is the Caribbean Sea while the southern limit is the Avila mountain with highest peak reaching above 2700 MASL. The state has an area of 1,496 km², which corresponds to 0.16% of the country's territory (Carrano and Montenegro, 2006). The state is located along the central mountain chain, covering a thin land strip of about 25 km in length, located between the Caribbean Sea and the Coastal Mountain Chain. This study spans the period 1970–2006.

Rainfall data from 26 climatological stations were obtained from the Argus/CEsMA repository (Bravo et al, 2014, Centro de Estadística y Matemáticas Aplicadas, 2015), which includes meteorological data from several official sources (Figure 11.8). Monthly data on the total number of casualties were obtained from CRED (2013), Desinventar (2014), FUNVISIS (2013). Population census data for years 2001 and 2010 were obtained from the

HURRICANES

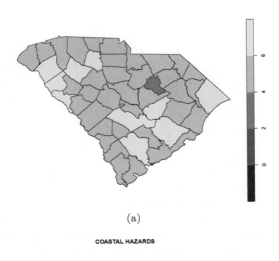

(a)

COASTAL HAZARDS

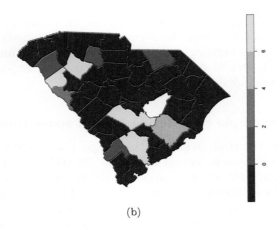

(b)

FIGURE 11.7: Observed number of hurricanes (a) and coastal hazards (b) that affected South Carolina counties during the period 1960–2016.

National Institute of Statistics (INE). An exponential growth model was used to interpolate and extrapolate population values for the remaining years to generate population maps for the whole study domain.

Potential covariates to explain the inter-annual variability of casualties due to extreme rainfall events were introduced in the analysis. These covariates

Applications of the conceptual framework

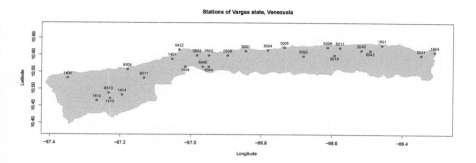

FIGURE 11.8: Locations of hydro-meteorological stations. Numbers represent the station code.

are large-scale climatic indices obtained from the US National Oceanic and Atmospheric Administration (NOAA). The multivariate ENSO index (MEI) and the sea surface temperature anomalies in the Pacific region Niño 3+4 (Niño 3.4) were used as potential covariates.

A categorical variable was also introduced to classify El Niño/La Niña events according to the strength of the phenomenon, measured by the sea surface temperature anomaly at Pacific region 3.4. The values of 1, 2, and 3 were assigned for weak, moderate, and strong El Niño events, respectively; and 4, 5, and 6 for weak, moderate, and strong La Niña events, respectively.

The seasonal variability and extremeness of the data are presented in Figure 11.9 for four locations. The boxplots show that extreme values occur mostly from October to May for most of the locations.

Hazard model

In this framework, the hazard model component was treated as a spatiotemporal prediction problem from rainfall point measurements $y(s_1), y(s_2), \ldots, y(s_g)$ observed in locations $s_1, s_2, \ldots, s_g$. These measurements are considered realizations from a set of random variables $Y(s_1), Y(s_2), \ldots, Y(s_g)$. We wish to estimate a spatial random field $Y(\mathbf{s})$ in a new set of ungauged locations $\mathbf{s} = (\tilde{s}_1, \ldots, \tilde{s}_u)^\top$. This problem is traditionally known as *kriging* or spatial prediction. Following Le and Zidek (2006), the spatiotemporal prediction problem can be written as follows. Assume Y_t a p-dimensional vector of the random field at time t. Assume data at the first u coordinates are not available, while the next g observations are known. Vector Y_t can be partitioned as

$$Y_t = \left(Y_t^{[u]}, Y_t^{[g]} \right)^\top,$$

where $Y_t^{[u]}$ corresponds to the u ungauged locations while, $Y_t^{[g]}$ corresponds to the gauged g locations. We can assume that random variables $\{Y_t\}$ are time

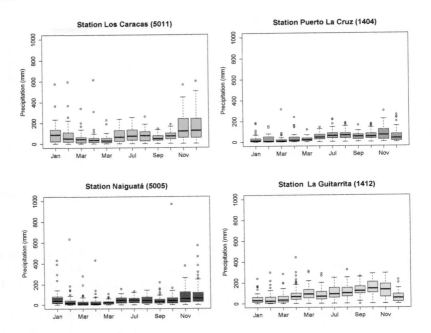

FIGURE 11.9: Boxplots of monthly rainfall at four stations in Vargas state, Venezuela.

independent, and the data vector follows a Gaussian distribution of the form

$$Y_t \mid z_t, B, \Sigma \sim N_p(z_t B, \Sigma),$$

where $N_p(z_t B, \Sigma)$ denotes a normal p-variate distribution with mean $\mu = z_t B$ and variance-covariance matrix Σ; $z_t = (z_{t_1}, \ldots, z_{t_k})$ is a k-dimensional row vector of covariates, and B is a $k \times p$ dimension matrix of regression coefficients, with $p = u + g$. Matrix B can be written as

$$B = \begin{bmatrix} \beta_{1,1} & \cdots & \beta_{p,1} \\ \vdots & \ddots & \vdots \\ \beta_{1,k} & \cdots & \beta_{p,k} \end{bmatrix} = \begin{bmatrix} B^{[u]}, & B^{[g]} \end{bmatrix}.$$

The partitions of matrix B and vector Y_t are in agreement in the sense that covariates can change with time, but should be constant for all locations. On the other hand, regression coefficients β's can vary for the different locations.

The variance-covariance matrix can be decomposed in the following way

$$\Sigma = \begin{bmatrix} \Sigma_{uu} & \Sigma_{ug} \\ \Sigma_{gu} & \Sigma_{gg} \end{bmatrix}.$$

Applications of the conceptual framework

Matrices Σ_{uu} and Σ_{gg} are the covariance matrices of $Y_t^{[u]}$ and $Y_t^{[g]}$, respectively; Σ_{ug} is the cross-covariance matrix between $Y_t^{[u]}$ and $Y_t^{[g]}$.

Following Le and Zidek (2006), conjugate prior distributions for the unknown parameters B and Σ are given by

$$B \mid B_0, \Sigma, F \sim N_{kp}(B_o, F^{-1} \otimes \Sigma)$$
$$\Sigma \mid \psi, \delta \sim W_p^{-1}(\psi, \delta), \qquad (11.6)$$

where $W_p^{-1}(\psi, \delta)$ is the p-dimensional inverse Wishart distribution with scale matrix ψ, and δ degrees of freedom. This is a proper distribution when $p < \delta$. Matrices B_0, F, and ψ are hyperparameter matrices with dimensions $k \times k$, $k \times 1$, and $p \times p$, respectively.

The observed data (D) of the random variable Y_t can be written as

$$D = \left\{ \left(y_1^{[g]}, z_1\right), \ldots, \left(y_T^{[g]}, z_T\right) \right\},$$

where it is assumed that the observations for times $t = 1, \ldots, T$ are independent and that z_t is the vector of covariates for each time t.

Le and Zidek (1992) estimated the posterior predictive distribution for $Y_f = \left(Y_f^{[u]}, Y_f^{[g]}\right)$ conditioned on the covariates vector z_f and the hyperparameters $\{B_0, F, \psi, \delta\}$. This distribution is the product of two Student's t-distributions characterized completely by their hyperparameters and can be factorized as

$$P\left(Y_f^{[u]}, Y_f^{[g]} \mid D\right) = P\left(Y_f^{[u]} \mid Y_f^{[g]}, D\right) P\left(Y_f^{[g]} \mid D\right), \qquad (11.7)$$

where $P\left(Y_f^{[u]}, Y_f^{[g]} \mid D\right)$ is the joint posterior predictive distribution of Y_f at ungauged and gauged locations, $Y_f^{[u]}$ and $Y_f^{[g]}$, respectively.

Once the posterior predictive distribution is calculated, it is possible to obtain samples for future realizations of Y_f, which represent plausible future values of the precipitation variable at future time $f > T$.

Figure 11.10 shows a comparison of the observed values with the 95% posterior probability intervals obtained from simulations of the posterior probability distribution given in (11.7). From these results we conclude that the spatiotemporal hierarchical model is able to represent the complex dynamic of rainfall in this region.

Vulnerability model

The loss variable (number of people affected or number of casualties) is a counting variable and an appropriate discrete probability distribution as a Poisson or a negative binomial should be used for modeling. Since there is a considerable amount of zeroes in the data set, a zero-inflated Poisson or negative binomial model is proposed (Velasco and Cerrillo, 2010). Let

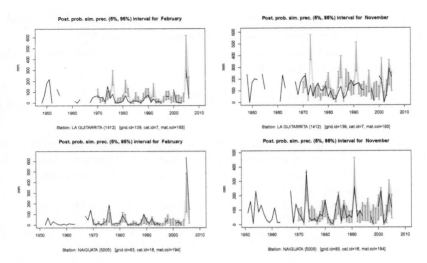

FIGURE 11.10: Observed monthly rainfall (black lines) and 95% posterior probability intervals (blue bands and red tick-marks) for February and November in La Guitarrita (top) and Naiguata (bottom).

$A_1, A_2, \ldots, A_T$ be an observed sample representing the number of people affected or casualties associated with a precipitation event occurred at time $t \in \{1, 2, \ldots, T\}$.

A zero-inflated negative binomial model (ZINB; Lambert, 1992) with parameters λ_t and θ_t was used to model the number of casualties:

$$P(A_t = a_t | \pi_t, \lambda_t, \theta_t) =$$
$$\begin{cases} (1 - \pi_t) + \pi_t \left(\dfrac{\theta_t}{\lambda_t + \theta_t}\right)^{\theta_t} & \text{if } A_t = 0, \\ \pi_t \dfrac{\Gamma(a_t + \theta_t)}{\Gamma(\theta_t)\, a_t!} \left(\dfrac{\theta_t}{\lambda_t + \theta_t}\right)^{\theta_t} \left(\dfrac{\lambda_t}{\lambda_t + \theta_t}\right)^{a_t} & \text{if } A_t > 0, \end{cases} \quad (11.8)$$

where $0 \leqslant \pi_t \leqslant 1$ represents the occurrence probability. Note that $(1 - \pi_t)$ is the probability of 0 occurrences not coming from the f distribution and represents the zero-inflation probability.

In practice, parameters π_t and λ_t can be dependent on additional explanatory variables $\vec{x}_t \in \mathbb{R}^q$ and $\vec{g}_t \in \mathbb{R}^m$:

$$\log(\lambda_t) = \boldsymbol{x}_t^\top \boldsymbol{\beta} \quad \text{and} \quad \log\left(\dfrac{\pi_t}{1 - \pi_t}\right) = \boldsymbol{g}_t^\top \boldsymbol{\gamma}; \quad (11.9)$$

where $\boldsymbol{\beta} = (\beta_1, \ldots, \beta_q)^\top$ and $\boldsymbol{\gamma} = (\gamma_1, \ldots, \gamma_m)^\top$ are unknown parameter vectors of dimensions q and m, respectively. A Bayesian approach was used to fit

Applications of the conceptual framework

model (11.8) to the observed casualties time series for the period 1970–2006. Gibbs sampling and the Metropolis-Hastings (Gamerman and Lopes, 2006) algorithms were used to simulate from the posterior probability distributions to get samples for model parameters $\boldsymbol{\zeta} = (\boldsymbol{\lambda}, \boldsymbol{\pi}, \boldsymbol{\theta}, \boldsymbol{\beta}, \boldsymbol{\gamma}, \sigma_\beta^2, \sigma_\gamma^2)^\top$. Details on the posterior conditional distributions for the parameter vector $\boldsymbol{\zeta}$ and implementation of the Gibbs sampling and Metropolis-Hastings algorithm can be found in Villalta et al (2020).

Risk model

Modeling risk implies the application of (11.1) for location s and time t. A discrete representation of (11.1) was used to get risk estimates to produce risk maps. Since the vulnerability model simulates aggregated values of casualties over the whole region, an *ad hoc* procedure was implemented to disaggregate the simulated casualties, by assuming a degree of loss proportional to the amount of rainfall fallen at each grid cell.

For each grid cell s and time t we estimate disaggregation factors $\nu_{t,s}$, using the Bayesian kriging spatiotemporal average rainfall predictions $\hat{h}_{t,s}$. The total rainfall at time t, H_t, is estimated by aggregating spatially,

$$H_t \approx \widehat{H}_t = \sum_{s \in S} \hat{h}_{t,s},$$

where S is the total number of grid cells covering the spatial domain. With an estimate for the total rainfall $\widehat{H}_t$ and the grid spatial average $\hat{h}_{t,s}$, we can set weights $\nu_{t,s}$ as:

$$\nu_{t,s} \equiv \frac{\hat{h}_{t,s}}{\widehat{H}_t}.$$

The weight $\nu_{t,s}$ is the proportion of precipitation for each grid cell $s \in S$ and time $t \in T$. By assuming that this same relationship holds for the vulnerability model, it is possible to spatially disaggregate $\widehat{V}_t$ as follows:

$$\widehat{V}_{t,s} = \nu_{t,s} \widehat{V}_t \quad \text{for} \quad t \in T, s \in S,$$

After multiplying by the exposure $E_{t,s}$, the expected losses can be calculated as:

$$\mathrm{E}_V\left[[V_{t,s} \mid H_{t,s}]\, E_{t,s}\right] = \mathrm{E}_V[A_{t,s} \mid H_{t,s}], \quad (11.10)$$

where $A_{t,s}$ represents the total number of casualties at time $t \in T$ and grid cell $s \in S$. This identity summarizes the key concept used in this research regarding risk estimation.

By further discretizing the hazard domain, Ω_H, into rainfall sub-intervals (mm/month)

$$H = \{[0, 10), [10, 20), \ldots, [300, 600), \geq 600\},$$

we obtain an approximation of (11.1), that can be numerically evaluated:

$$R_{t,s} = E_{t,s} \sum_{\Delta h \in H} \mathrm{E}_V[V_{t,s} \mid H_{t,s} = h] \mathsf{P}(H_{t,s} \in \Delta h) \Delta h, \qquad (11.11)$$

where Δh is the discrete sub-interval length, and h is Δh interval midpoint. By using the vulnerability spatial disaggregation factors, risk can be expressed as:

$$R_{t,s} = \sum_{\Delta h \in H} \mathrm{E}_V[A_{t,s} \mid H_{t,s} = h] \mathsf{P}(H_{t,s} \in \Delta h) \Delta h. \qquad (11.12)$$

For each precipitation class Δh, the proportion of casualties is estimated from the vulnerability model (using weights $\nu_{t,s}$), and (11.12) provides an estimation of the expected number of casualties after multiplying by the exposure $E_{t,s}$. Using samples from the posterior distribution of the vulnerability model and the hazard model, we can produce risk estimate samples for time t and grid cell s using (11.12). From these samples, it is possible to get relative risk estimates for different percentiles, in particular, 5%, 50%, and 95%.

The main results from the implementation of the presented approach are maps corresponding to the hazard, vulnerability (losses), and risk (relative or absolute figures) for the domain and time span considered. Maps are based on the 50th percentile statistic, and when required, maps for 5th and 95th percentiles can be used as uncertainty measures. Each map for the elements involved in the risk estimation is color-coded. Hazard (rainfall) maps are coded with hues from sand color (0 mm/month) to dark blue (600 mm/month). Loss is represented with a purple color hue (0% to 100%), with more intense colors indicating a higher vulnerability to the corresponding hazard level. Finally, the relative risk (percentage casualties) maps are represented with a red color hue, with more intense tones pointing to areas with higher relative risk. The yellow circles in the map represent the populated centers in the state. Figures 11.11 and 11.12 show example hazard maps (top), vulnerability maps (center), and relative risk maps (bottom) for August and November of 1995.

11.4 Discussion, conclusions, and future work

Risk quantification to weather-related extreme events imposes an important challenge due to the integration of three factors that change in space and time: exposure, hazard, and vulnerability. Sources of data to evaluate each of these components can have disparate spatial and temporal supports, and some assumptions might be needed to proceed with the adequate articulation of these factors.

Extreme events are part of the natural climate variability; however, climate change might increase the frequency and intensity of those events. If the vul-

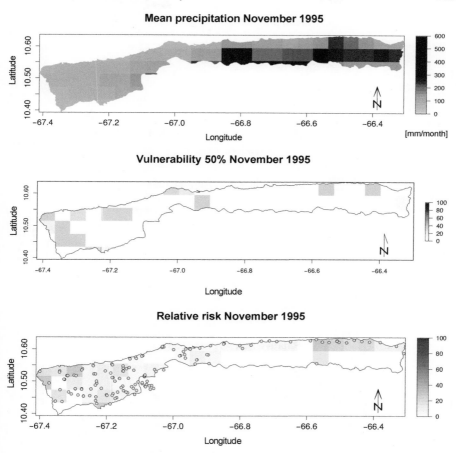

FIGURE 11.11: Hazard map (top), 50th percentile vulnerability map (center) and relative risk map (bottom) in Vargas state, during November 1995 (a wet month).

nerability or degree of loss associated with those events remains unchanged, but the hazard probability increases, the relative risk would increase, and the exposure would determine the expected losses in absolute terms.

In lower-income countries, where population settles in river banks or step slopes prone to landslides, the expected number of people affected or number of casualties will increase due to an adverse exposure condition, even if changes in hazard probabilities and degree of preparedness to disasters remain constant. In wealthier economies where exposed assets increase in value, expected losses also increase. These two increasing risk examples show the complexities involved in risk estimation.

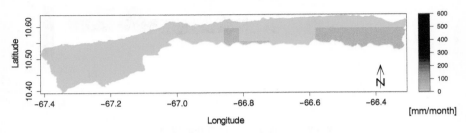
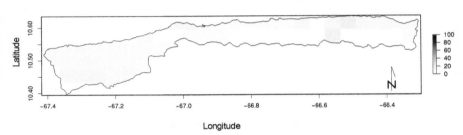
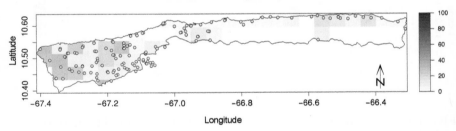

FIGURE 11.12: Hazard map (top), 50th percentile vulnerability map (center) and relative risk map (bottom) in Vargas state, during August 1995 (a dry month).

Adaptation and protection measures are required to lower vulnerability. Bollman and Wang (2019) discuss the protection gap between insured and uninsured losses during 1970–2016, and conclude that the economic losses have outpaced the insured losses. In terms of gross domestic product (GDP), total economic losses have increased from 0.09% to 0.27% of GDP, while the uninsured losses have increased from 0.07% to 0.19% of GDP. This condition has been aggravated by the exposure increases due to urbanization.

As proposed by Downing and Patwardhan (2016), an adaptation process to climate extremes is expected to reduce vulnerability and risk, and its quantification can be assessed directly, by subtracting the term $Ad_{t,s}$ from the vulnerability term. That is, use $(V_{t,s} - Ad_{t,s})$ instead of $V_{t,s}$ in (11.1).

In economic terms, $Ad_{t,s}$ could be understood as the insured losses, while in social terms, $Ad_{t,s}$ can be estimated as the degree of preparedness and response of the exposed population under a potentially damaging event. By including adaptation in the proposed analysis, we would be able to close the risk cycle.

To evaluate each component of this risk cycle, we might need to deal with disparate sources of data, as we discussed in the examples. We have selected a given spatial and temporal scale for the analysis, but we would normally expect complex interactions among different scales. To evaluate vulnerability we might require other techniques that allow us to evaluate cross-scale vulnerability conditions based on multiple socioeconomic indicators. The use of machine learning methods might be a good alternative methodology to evaluate potential losses on exposed population or infrastructure, as a vulnerability estimate. More analysis along this approach will be presented in the near future.

Risk assessment to extreme hydro-meteorological events is a complex and challenging problem requiring the expertise of several specialists working within an interdisciplinary framework. The harmonization of social science related information with biophysical factors is key to developing realistic vulnerability models to quantify damage over several exposed elements. In a multi-hazard context, for example, extreme weather events combined with national security threats, we might need new modeling and risk assessment approaches to account for a complex exposure structure. This and other extensions of the proposed methodology will be explored elsewhere.

Acknowledgments

We are grateful to the SAMSI program on Mathematical and Statistical Methods for Climate and Earth Systems (CLIM), Group XII: Risk and Coastal Hazards lead by Brian Blanton (RENCI), for suggesting and providing the South Carolina Data set from the SHELDUS database, and for useful and stimulating discussions about the methodology.

References

Aon (2018) Weather, climate and catatrophe insight. URL http://thoughtleadership.aonbenfield.com/Documents/20190122-ab-if-annual-weather-climate-report-2018.pdf

Bollman A, Wang SS (2019) International catastrophe pooling for extreme weather. URL https://www.soa.org/globalassets/assets/files/re

sources/research-report/2019/international-catastrophe-pooling.pdf

Bravo L, et al (2014) Repositorio de Datos Hidroclimáticos para la Gestión de Riesgos Epidemiológicos y Ambientales, 1st edn. USB-UCV-FONACIT, Caracas, Venezuela

Brooks N (2003) Working Paper 38. In: Vulnerability, risk and adaptation: A conceptual framework, Tyndall Center for Climate Research, pp 1–16

Carrano AM, Montenegro M (2006) Venezuela en Datos 2007. Editarte, Caracas, Venezuela

CEMHS (2018) Spatial hazard events and losses database for the United States, version 17.0. URL https://cemhs.asu.edu/sheldus

Centro de Estadística y Matemáticas Aplicadas (2015) Repositorio de Datos Hidroclimáticos para la Gestión de Riesgos Epidemiológicos y Ambientales. http://argus.cesma.usb.ve/

CRED (2013) Center for Research on the Epidemiology of Disasters. URL https://www.cred.be, accessed 2013

Desinventar (2014) Sistema de inventario de efectos de desastres. URL https://www.desinventar.org/es/, accessed 2014

Downing TE, Patwardhan A (2016) Assessing Vulnerability for Climate Adaptation. Tech. rep., UNFCCC-NAP, URL https://www4.unfccc.int/sites/NAPC/Country%20Documents/General/apf%20technical%20paper03.pdf

Downing TE, Olsthoorn A, Tol RSJ (eds) (1999) Climate, Change and Risk. Routledge, London, UK

Forzieri G, Cescatti A, Batista e Silva F, Feyen L (2017) Increasing risk over time of weather-related hazards due to the European population: a data-driven prognostic study. Lancet Planet Health 1:e200–e208

FUNVISIS (2013) Estudios y Desastres, Fundación Venezolana de Investigaciones Sismológicas. URL http://www.estudiosydesastres.gob.ve/, accessed 2013

Gamerman D, Lopes H (2006) Markov Chain Monte Carlo: Stochastic Simulation for Bayesian Inference, 2nd edn. Chapman & Hall / CRC

Lambert D (1992) Zero-inflated Poisson regression, with an application to defects in manufacturing. Technometrics 34(1):1–14

Le ND, Zidek JV (1992) Interpolation with uncertain spatial covariances: a Bayesian alternative to kriging. Journal of Multivariate Analysis 43(2):351–374

Le ND, Zidek JV (2006) Statistical Analysis of Environmental Space-Time Processes. Springer, New York

Lee D (2019) CARBayes: Spatial Generalised Linear Mixed Models for Areal Unit Data. URL https://CRAN.R-project.org/package=CARBayes, R package version 5.1.3

Leroux B, Lei X, Breslow N (1999) Estimation of disease rates in small areas: a new mixed model for spatial dependence. In: Halloran M, Berry D (eds)

Statistical Models in Epidemiology, the Environment, and Clinical Trials, 1st edn, Springer-Verlag, 135–178

Lin N, Shullman E (1997) Dealing with hurricane surge flooding in a changing environment: Part I. risk assessment considering storm climatology change, sea level rise, and coastal development. Stochastic Environmental Research and Risk Assessment (31):2379–2400

Liu B, Siu Y, Mitchell G (2017) A quantitative model for estimating risk from multiple interacting natural hazards: an application to northeast Zhejiang, China. Stochastic Environmental Research and Risk Assessment 31:1319–1340

Munich Re (2017) Topics geo: Natural catastrophes 2017. Munich, Germany

Nunes AR (2003) Working Paper 163. In: Assests for Health: Linking Vulnerability, Resilience and Adaptation to Climate Change, Tyndall Center for Climate Research, pp 1–29

Plate E (1996) Risk management for hydraulic systems under hydrologic loads. In: Third Kovacs Colloquium on Risk Reliability,Uncertainty and Robustness of Resources Systems, UNESCO, Paris

Stenschion P (1997) Development and disaster management. Australian Journal of Emergency Management 3(12):40–44

Velasco MLV, Cerrillo SFJ (2010) Un Modelo de Regresión Poisson Inflado con Ceros para Analizar datos de un Experimento de Fungicidas en Jitomate. Memoria del 2 Encuentro Iberoamericano de Biometría y la V Reunión de la Región Centroamericana y del Caribe de la Sociedad Internacional de Biometría, 16

Villalta D, Bravo de Guenni L, Sajo-Castelli A (2020) Spatio-temporal modelling of hydro-meteorological derived risk using a Bayesian approach: A case study in Venezuela. Stochastic Environmental Research and Risk Assessment, 34:513–529

Vörösmarty CJ, Bravo de Guenni L, Wollheim W, Pellerin B, Bjerklie D, Cardoso M, D'Almeida C, Green P, Colón L (2013) Extreme rainfall, vulnerability and risk: a continental-scale assessment for South America. Philosophical Transactions of the Royal Society of London A: Mathematical, Physical and Engineering Sciences 371(2002):20120408

Wang Y, Kockelman KM (2013) A Poisson-lognormal conditional-autoregressive model for multivariate spatial analysis of pedestrian crash counts across neighborhoods. Accident Analysis and Prevention 60:71–84

12

Aspects of Climate-Induced Risk in Property Insurance

Ola Haug

Norwegian Computing Center, Oslo, Norway

CONTENTS

12.1	Introduction	259
12.2	The role of statistics in assessing insurance climate risk	260
12.3	Water damage to properties in Norway	263
12.4	The Gjensidige case study	264
	12.4.1 Data	265
	12.4.2 Modeling	266
	12.4.3 Claim predictions	267
	12.4.4 Extensions	269
12.5	Climate change and property insurance interactions	271
12.6	Conclusions	274
References		275

12.1 Introduction

Climate change is bringing radical consequences for safety and welfare in society. Businesses ranging from health to energy production, from agriculture and food supply to infrastructure and tourism, will all be affected. Among the risk-prone industries is also the financial sector including insurance companies with their public and private clients.

The Intergovernmental Panel on Climate Change (IPCC) warns that a changing climate leads to changes in the frequency, intensity, spatial extent, duration, and timing of weather and climate extremes, and can result in unprecedented extremes (Seneviratne et al, 2012). These changes influence directly the core business operations for the insurance industry, potentially changing the portfolio risk profile substantially. As a consequence, claims of the past may no longer be indicative of future risk exposure.

Additional to weather, in a report from 2014, the Canadian Institute of Actuaries points to aging of infrastructure and human lifestyle changes as other examples of drivers contributing to a new risk landscape (Friedland et al, 2014). For an insurance company, correct apprehension of its risks is imperative for flawless pricing and profitable and sustainable operation. In recent reports (e.g., IPCC, 2018), the IPCC states that climate change is already happening, and impacts on natural and human systems from global warming have already been observed. This makes the situation urgent for the insurance sector, and appropriate measures must be taken to incorporate climate change into insurance risk evaluation.

In this chapter, we discuss the role of statistical analysis as a tool for assessing climate-induced risk within property insurance. In particular, we refer to a case study from Norway on predicting future losses. We also consider interactions and implied consequences of climate change in home insurance beyond the immediate generation of claims.

12.2 The role of statistics in assessing insurance climate risk

Until not too many years ago insurance had the reputation of being a conservative industry advocating old-fashioned perspectives and stuck in traditional business processes. This was in spite of companies relying on data collection and quantitative analyses as cornerstones for their business operation. However, in the era of big data and data science, a silent revolution has hit the sector, and the potential of computational statistics has been explored as a natural extension of traditional actuarial methods.

Also following the new paradigm of computational power is the goal of decision support via artificial intelligence (AI). Human decision making relies on judging multifaceted, often conflicting, knowledge about a system or environment. AI strives to mimic this reasoning and aims at solving problems that involve complex, multi-source interactions for which specific rules are not easily formulated in a traditional framework. Highly skilled algorithms permit capturing subtle patterns in the data not evident from conventional techniques primarily inferring first-order effects. Machine learning (ML) comes as part of AI and has revitalized the first rule-based expert systems by specifying algorithms that learn from data in a dynamic fashion. E.g., see Chapter 14 demonstrating application of random forests for predicting traffic accidents based on weather and other characteristics.

Data science brings insurance one step closer to personalised solutions, and its potential spans a wide range of applications. For instance, AI can assist underwriting by establishing more precise and dynamic customer risk profiles. In home insurance, sensor technologies and the Internet of Things offer supplementary data sources that add information to traditional risk classification. The same holds true for social media activity leaving behavioral patterns for each individual customer, indicative of his background and current risk profile. Considering weather risk, one can think to the following example: before a forecasted rainstorm, real-time smart home sensor recordings identify an open roof window. Along with knowledge of the homeowner's habitual or recent social media activity putting a prior on his likely presence over the next couple of days, an alert service is informed about the property's present risk of being damaged. Of course, missing consent to exploit such data or regulatory restrictions as imposed by the authorities will restrain the use of such systems, but those legal issues are not the topic of this chapter.

Various aspects of claims estimation naturally lend themselves to AI systems. As an example, in the case of a natural perils event, early stage estimates of the loss burden can be obtained from computer vision systems analysing aerial images taken by aircraft or drones over the damaged area or individual property. Pursuing this idea one step further, one can think of simulating impacts of climate change from feeding future climate projections into some kind of weather-claims model and thereby dynamically assessing portfolio risk at various time horizons.

On the administrative side, customer support centers offer chatbots for clients who request help or information. The field of natural language processing (NLP) is making big leaps forward with its focus on un- or semi-supervised learning and envisions significant progress for chatbot technologies over the years to come. In marketing, personalized web page services tailored to each customer follow along the same lines.

A cautionary remark should be issued on blind trust in black box decision-making systems like AI. Results are not transparent, and there is often limited or occasional judgment as to whether the outcome of an algorithm seems reasonable. If operational staff are not sufficiently skilled or trained this might lead to uncritical trust in or interpretation of black box outputs. There is also the *right to explanation* regulation emphasizing the responsibility to illuminate the outcome of algorithmic decisions made, with particular relevance to legal or financial affairs.

Bombarded with the new concepts and terminology of data science it is important to bear in mind that the workhorse underlying the algorithms is most often nothing but well-known concepts from statistical methodology. Building models for assessing impacts of climate change on property water damages, the aim of the modeling should be clarified. Is predicting future claims the overarching goal, or is quantifying the relationship between damages and certain explanatory variables what one is after? From a postulated model, the latter approach provides insight into the mechanisms that influence the losses. Prediction models are concerned with forecasting losses from possibly new combinations of model variables. Well-performing prediction models seek to minimize the deviation or distance of the forecast from real outcomes.

In the era of machine learning and data science, predictive rather than statistical inference modeling seems to gain the most interest. The famous Kaggle competitions[1] have contributed to an escalated focus on models that can demonstrate high predictive power. And in an article in Towards Data Science, July 25th, 2019, Phoebe Wong points out that *"Data science curriculums today largely ignore causal inference methodologies, and the data science industry mostly expects practitioners to focus on predictive models"* (Wong, 2019). However, there is little doubt that parsimonious parametric models are often preferable to black box models as they can also be used for interpretation of associations present in the data. In a home insurance claims setting, this means shifting focus towards causal effects, trying to identify factors that impact a property's disposition towards, e.g., water damage.

Regardless of the methods and techniques used, uncertainty quantification stands out as an extremely valuable piece of information in assessing impacts of climate change. For stakeholders and regulators it is crucial to know how much trust they can put in the basis for their decisions. For relevant quantities, providing confidence bands along with point estimates significantly increases the value of the latter.

Sources of uncertainty in model predictions of future losses include model error, parameter uncertainty and climate projection uncertainty. As any model is just an approximation of reality, the model error is intrinsic. And since the truth is unknown, the model error is not quantifiable. When fitting a claims model to data, the model parameters are estimated with a precision that depends on the data at hand. Finally comes the incertitude about future climate exposure.

Climate projections lean upon two pillars, both of which come with indefiniteness. First, assumptions about the evolvement of society (demographic evolution, energy consumption, technological development, etc.) expressed via future CO_2 emission scenarios are at best qualified guessworks. Second, and imperative for the successful modeling of impacts of climate change in nature and society, is the quality and richness of the earth system models (ESM) and downscaling techniques used for describing the physics that govern the climate.

Ensemble runs produced from combining emission scenarios, earth system models, downscalings, and initial conditions demonstrate the variability present in climate projections. Though not claiming to produce statistical confidence bands, these ensembles somehow span the outcomes of future climate. Often, however, only one single realization exists for each combination of CO_2 emission scenario, ESM, and downscaling. In such situations, for temperature and precipitation the Schaake shuffle (Clark et al, 2004) can be used to synthesize a set of equally likely climate projections over a certain period. Briefly, keeping the marginal distributions for the meteorological variables as told by the climate projection, the method imposes temporal and spatial correlations

---

[1]https://www.kaggle.com/competitions

from observed data of a past control period. Forming the synthetic ensemble is at the cost of reduced temporal extent. For instance, going from one realization with daily values over a ten-year period, leads to ten monthly ensembles each representative of that month's pattern in any of the ten years.

Finally, predictions of future claims with confidence bands can be attained from a large simulation experiment. Stochastically perturbed model parameters are combined with climate projection ensemble values and propagated through the claims model.

12.3 Water damage to properties in Norway

In Norway, there is a twofold system underlying the classification of externally inflicted water damages to insured buildings. Depending on their origin, these claims are categorized as natural perils or ordinary, severe weather water damages.

The first category includes claims that are strictly linked to a defined set of hazards. For water-related damage, riverine flooding, storm surge, and partially landslide are the most relevant. The natural perils arrangement applies to all contracts that have fire insurance as part of their coverage. More specifically, all buildings insured against fire are, by obligation, also insured against natural perils. This regulation is stated in the Act on Natural Perils Insurance dating back to 1989 and administered by the Norwegian Natural Perils Pool[2]. All insurers writing fire cover in Norway have compulsory membership in the Pool. Incurred peril costs are equalized among the members according to their share of the market for fire insurance. Additional to the water related hazards mentioned above, the Pool compensation scheme covers losses due to avalanche, storm, earthquake or volcanic eruption.

The second category comprises damages that are not caused by high sea water level incidents or lakes or watercourses growing beyond their normal size. Rather, these claims typically result from extreme rainfall events leading to pluvial flooding and sewer backflow. Heavy rainstorms are capable of forming local streams away from existing watercourses. From an insurance perspective, such streams are potentially harmful if they develop in the vicinity of buildings. In urban environments where impervious surfaces cover large areas due to asphalt coating, surface runoff has traditionally been transported via the storm water sewer system. In such infrastructures pipeline capacity limitations manifest themselves via increased loss burden.

A substantial change in flood patterns is seen in Norway over the past 20–30 years. Traditionally spring floods due to snowmelt in the mountains were

---

[2] https://www.finanstilsynet.no/en/laws-and-regulations/insurance-and-pensions/activity-of-eea-insurance-companies-in-norway/

the main flood claims driver. More recently, floods due to local cloudbursts or medium- to high-intensity precipitation lasting for several days tend to happen in all seasons. This generates new situations and challenges. For instance, massive amounts of rain falling onto frozen ground with no snow cover typically seen during late fall conceptually resemble the surface runoff problem in urban environments. Combinations of heavy, local precipitation with riverine water transport are also observed. Such a regime can result in simultaneous ordinary bad weather claims (forming of streams in new places, drainage failures, stormwater damage, and backflow) and natural perils (flooding and landslide).

Thinking to the physical phenomena underlying water damages, the splitting into the two categories discussed above may seem somewhat arbitrary or even inconsistent. For instance, extreme precipitation events might well give rise to claims in both categories. A house located close to an existing watercourse will be hit if the massive rainfall causes the river to overrun its edges, thus leading to a Natural Perils Pool claim. In an urban environment the typical extreme rainfall damage event is backflow due to surface water overloading the sewer system. Such pluvial flooding losses do not fall under the definition of flooding adopted by the Perils Pool and thus will be compensated directly by the homeowner's primary property insurance.

Despite claims due to natural hazards getting more attention in media, in Norway damages caused by heavy rainfall generate larger costs. Over the period 2009–2018 weather-related claims on insured properties summed up to more than 24 billion NOK. Out of this, damage due to precipitation constituted 44%, whereas natural perils flooding and storm events were 15% and 21%, respectively (Finans Norge, 2019).

12.4 The Gjensidige case study

Based on data from a 10-year period around the millennium, researchers at Norwegian Computing Center joined forces with Gjensidige ASA, a major Norwegian insurance company operating in Scandinavia and The Baltics, and studied future building loss projections due to climate change. A detailed description of the modeling approach along with some results were published in Scandinavian Actuarial Journal in 2011 (Haug et al, 2011). In brief, the idea was to establish statistical claims models that link daily claim aggregates along with their severities to meteorological and hydrological variables on a municipal level via generalized linear models (GLM). Feeding these models with downscaled and calibrated future climate predictions produces estimates of future losses. The components leading up to these estimates are summarized in Figure 12.1 along with the various data sources involved.

The Gjensidige case study

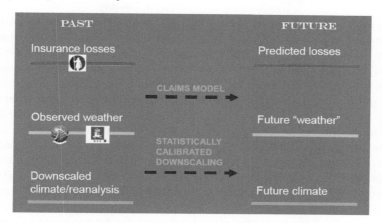

FIGURE 12.1: Flowchart depicting the modeling steps and data sources involved in producing future loss estimates.

Gaining quantitative insight into envisaged threats, insurance companies may update their risk assessment and announce dedicated preventive measures to their clients, regulators, and the construction industry. In the following we present an excerpt of the data and methodology utilized in the case study. In Section 12.4.3, we include unpublished material from the analyses, and we conclude by suggesting some possible extensions identified from an ongoing follow-up study on a richer data set.

12.4.1 Data

Insurance data, weather data, and climate model data are collected from 19 counties across the nation and organised into 431 sets of multivariate time series, each representing one of Norway's municipalities (as of 2006). The study investigates externally inflicted water damages caused by local weather phenomena such as heavy precipitation and melting of snow. The losses typically generated from such events are due to surface water running into basements, undermined drainage and sewer backflow rather than any of the natural hazards mentioned in Section 12.3.

Insurance claims and population data are from Gjensidige's own portfolio confined to a certain subset of buildings for the period 1997–2006. These include privately-owned homes comprised of detached, semi-detached, and townhouse entities. For each municipality, recordings of the number of claims and their index-linked aggregate payment exist on a daily resolution. Population data is monthly and holds the number of coverages.

Weather data includes meteorological and hydrological variables aligned in time and space with the insurance data. First, precipitation and temperature data are obtained on a 1×1 km^2 grid by applying advanced kriging techniques to observations collected by the Norwegian Meteorological Institute (https://www.met.no) on a network of measurement stations across the country. Even for individual municipalities, weather variables may vary considerably due either to a wide range of altitudes or simply large spatial extent. Alleviating this heterogeneity, representative time series for each municipality are produced by averaging temperature and precipitation across the most densely populated grid squares only. Since these are the areas where losses will primarily occur, a desirable basis for increased coherence between claims and weather data is established. The area series of precipitation and temperature are further processed by the Norwegian Water Resources and Energy Directorate (NVE). Daily values of the hydrological variables runoff and snow water equivalent are calculated from a gridded water balance (GWB) model using precipitation and temperature as input data.

Analogously, climate model area series exist for future scenario periods. Comparing climate model control runs of the past to historical observations, local climate data is found to deviate from measured weather records even at aggregate scales in time and space (Palutikof et al, 1997). Hence, raw climate data as provided by met.no has been adjusted by calibrating their annual and monthly means and standard deviations against those of observations over the control period 1961–1990 (Engen-Skaugen, 2007, Engen-Skaugen et al, 2007). The same calibration was applied to future climate scenarios. As for the weather data, population-based municipality series of meteorological and hydrological variables are produced from these gridded, post-processed climate records of temperature and precipitation via spatial averaging in the NVE GWB model.

12.4.2 Modeling

Following the classical approach to modeling aggregate losses (Lundberg, 1903), we assume independence between claim frequency and severity. In our setting, separate frequency and severity models are established, both linking losses to meteorological and hydrological variables. The number of claims is modeled via a binomial model with overdispersion, also named a quasibinomial model. Accounting for what is often observed in claims data, this model allows for more variability in the number of claims than what follows from the binomial model. Letting N_t be the number of claims on day t, its mean and variance are given by

$$\begin{aligned} \mathrm{E}(N_t) &= A_t p_t; \\ \mathrm{Var}(N_t) &= \phi A_t p_t (1 - p_t), \end{aligned} \quad (12.1)$$

where A_t is the number of coverages, p_t is the claim probability on day t, and ϕ is the dispersion parameter. Now, under the framework of generalized linear models, daily claims are modeled using logistic regression

$$\mathrm{logit}(p_t) = \beta_0 + \sum_{i=1}^{m} \beta_i x_{it}, \qquad (12.2)$$

where $\mathrm{logit}(p) = \log(p/(1-p))$ is the log odds ratio. Furthermore, $\beta_0, \ldots, \beta_m$ are model coefficients and $x_{1t}, \ldots, x_{mt}$ are exogenous variables including the weather elements. Alternatively, a Poisson model could have been specified for N_t. However, in a prediction setting the binomial formulation imposes the crucial property that the predicted number of claims will never exceed the number of coverages.

For claim severities, let S_{tj} denote the size of the j'th claim on day t, $j = 1, \ldots, N_t$. Assuming a gamma distribution for S_{tj} with $\mathrm{E}(S_{tj}) = \xi_t$ and $\mathrm{Var}(S_{tj}) = \xi_t^2/\nu$ following the parametrisation in McCullagh and Nelder (1989), and, furthermore, postulating independence between the sizes of individual claims, the average claim size on day t obeys

$$\overline{S}_t | N_t \sim \mathrm{Gamma}(\xi_t, \nu N_t);$$
$$\mathrm{E}(\overline{S}_t | N_t) = \mathrm{E}(\overline{S}_t) = \xi_t; \qquad (12.3)$$
$$\mathrm{Var}(\overline{S}_t | N_t) = \xi_t^2/(\nu N_t).$$

The expectation ξ_t is tied to a set of regressors x_{it}, $i = 1, \ldots, n$, via model coefficients $\alpha_0, \ldots, \alpha_n$ and a logarithmic link function:

$$\log \xi_t = \alpha_0 + \sum_{i=1}^{n} \alpha_i x_{it}. \qquad (12.4)$$

The aggregate payment on day t, U_t, is obtained from summing the individual losses over all claims, $U_t = \sum_{j=1}^{N_t} S_{tj}$. From the expressions derived for the claim frequency and mean claim size, it follows that

$$\mathrm{E}(U_t) = A_t \, p_t \, \xi_t. \qquad (12.5)$$

The weather variables included as covariates in the models (12.2) and (12.4) are summarized in Table 12.1. In addition, to account for effects not explicitly expressed via the weather variables, a trend term and a few seasonal components are included as regressors.

The number of claims and mean claim size models are both fitted via GLM. Final models are selected from a set of candidate models using the Bayesian information criterion (BIC) thus favouring parsimonious models.

12.4.3 Claim predictions

Haug et al (2011) utilize data from the UK Met Office HadAM3H model under two different CO_2 emission scenarios A2 and B2. The scenarios represent

TABLE 12.1: Meteorological and hydrological variables used for modeling claims on day t

Variable	Unit
Precipitation registered day t	mm/day
Mean precipitation over the 5 days prior to day t	mm/day
Mean temperature day t	°C
Runoff day t	mm/day
Snow water equivalent day t	mm

somewhat different future worlds with A2 being the more CO_2-intensive of the two, thus leaving a higher projected global average surface temperature towards the end of the twenty-first century (Nakićenović and Swart, 2000). Presented here are results from the Max Planck Institute's ECHAM4 model under the B2 emission scenario.

Faced with the challenges of climate change, one question that concerns the insurance sector is how bad will it get—and when? That is, insurers want to quantify changes in their risk exposure from the current situation to some time in the future. One way to do this goes via ratios of certain risk measures. Dividing the risk measure value for a future scenario period to that of a past control period, ratios larger than one indicate an increased risk level in the future. For property insurance, relevant risk measures include the number of claims, their severity, and the aggregate payment. Let "scn" and "ctr" denote the scenario and control period, respectively, and assume for simplicity that they are of equal length. For a fixed number of coverages the above risk measure ratios at municipality level (k) then amount to

$$r_k^{freq}(scn, ctr) = \frac{\sum_{t \in scn} \hat{p}_{kt}^{scn}}{\sum_{t \in ctr} \hat{p}_{kt}^{ctr}}, \quad (12.6)$$

$$r_k^{size}(scn, ctr) = \frac{(\sum_{t \in scn} \hat{\xi}_t^{scn} \cdot \hat{p}_t^{scn})/(\sum_{t \in scn} \hat{p}_t^{scn})}{(\sum_{t \in ctr} \hat{\xi}_t^{ctr} \cdot \hat{p}_t^{ctr})/(\sum_{t \in ctr} \hat{p}_t^{ctr})}, \quad (12.7)$$

$$r_k^{payment}(scn, ctr) = \frac{\sum_{t \in scn} \hat{p}_t^{scn} \cdot \hat{\xi}_t^{scn}}{\sum_{t \in ctr} \hat{p}_t^{ctr} \cdot \hat{\xi}_t^{ctr}}, \quad (12.8)$$

where the hats indicate quantities calculated from the fitted models. Maps displaying ratios for calibrated ECHAM4 model B2 runs with control period 1961–1990 and scenario period 2071–2100 are shown in Figure 12.2. Ratios for the number of claims are from −30% to 71%, for mean claim size from −1% to 33% and for aggregate payment between −24% and 102% on a municipal scale.

In another experiment, we switch historical weather records between the two major cities Oslo and Bergen and consider the implied loss ratios. More precisely, Oslo numbers are formed from feeding Bergen control period weather

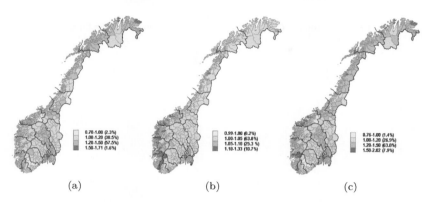

FIGURE 12.2: Ratios of ECHAM4 B2 scenario to control period risk measures at municipality level. (a) Number of claims, (b) mean claim size and (c) aggregate payment. The parenthesized values in the legends define the share of municipalities in each category.

and Oslo control period weather through the Oslo claims models, and then taking their ratio (and vice versa for Bergen). Bergen is situated on the rainy west coast of Norway and experiences on average 2250 mm precipitation annually. Normal precipitation for Oslo located in a more sheltered area in the southeastern part of the country is 763 mm. Figure 12.3 displays the effect of swapping climates to the number of claims, their severities and the aggregate payment. A dramatic increase in Oslo losses is clearly evident from Figure 12.3a, whereas the reduction seen for Bergen when exposed to Oslo weather is more modest (Figure 12.3b).

12.4.4 Extensions

In an ongoing follow-up study, more detailed insurance data is available. Specifically, claims data exists for each individual coverage in the portfolio. Also, information on various building attributes like basement or not, year of construction, quality and roof construction is provided. Combining this with high-resolution weather data allows for comprehensive modeling of the number of claims and their severities.

For claims frequency, every day represents a claim/no claim incident, and the probability of a claim for a specific building depends on its attributes along with current and possibly past weather. Let y_{it} be a Bernoulli distributed 0/1 claim indicator variable for coverage i on day t. In a generalized linear model framework, this can be formalised as

$$y_{it} \sim \text{Bernoulli}(p_{it});$$
$$\text{logit}(p_{it}) = \beta_0 + \sum_k \beta_k x_{kit}, \qquad (12.9)$$

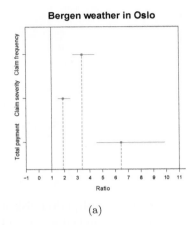
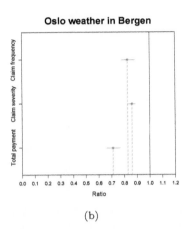

FIGURE 12.3: Effects of swapping Oslo and Bergen control period weather (1961–1990) presented as ratios of losses generated from swapped weather to actual weather, including 95% confidence intervals. (a) Bergen climate in Oslo, (b) Oslo climate in Bergen.

where now p_{it} is the coverage-specific probability of a claim on day t and x_{kit} are regressors describing building attributes and weather variables. To account for unobserved heterogeneity in the data, adding a time-specific random effect $v_t \sim N(0, \sigma_v^2)$ to (12.9) might turn out useful in a prediction setting.

Claim severities may still be modeled according to a gamma distribution, but now we consider the size of each individual claim and introduce property specific mean values ξ_{tj},

$$\log \xi_{tj} = \alpha_0 + \sum_{i=1}^{n} \alpha_i x_{itj}. \qquad (12.10)$$

Exploiting more details in the data substantially increases the computational burden of the analysis. For any coverage, all days, also those without a claim, contribute information to the model in (12.9) and thus should be included. For a portfolio consisting of 100,000 coverages over a ten-year period, the data expands into roughly 3 GB per variable. In models with many regressors, the size of the data object might challenge standard statistical software packages or even computer facilities with respect to memory and speed. In the wake of the big data revolution and in particular the field of machine learning, algorithms have been tailored to specifically handle analyses on big chunks of data. Clever splitting of the data into smaller parts, or even careful sub-sampling, can in certain settings also circumvent these issues without compromising on the outcome of the analyses.

In the original Gjensidige case study, downscaled climate model variables are calibrated by aligning their monthly mean and standard deviations against those of observations as referred in Section 12.4.1. More thorough approaches include a quantile calibration method (Bolin et al, 2016), or via a full distributional correction of the individual weather variables using Doksum's shift function (Bolin et al, 2016, Doksum, 1974). An ultimate procedure performs a coherent calibration of all variables in the full earth model representation simultaneously, pursuing consistency in the covariance and autocorrelation structure among the resulting variables.

Characteristic to Norway is the rugged landscape with large topographic differences over short distances. A key risk driver for stormwater damage and sewer backflow is buildings situated in small, local recesses in the terrain where storm water is likely to accumulate during heavy rainfall. Providing some kind of index expressing the overall concavity (or convexity) of the surrounding topography of every property would possibly contribute valuable risk information. Such data is apparently computable via modern GIS tools.

Extending the Gjensidige case study to other regions around the world would most likely call for some changes and customization. Different mechanisms could turn out relevant in the claims models, also with implications on data resolution and spatial aggregation of results. Norwegian topography undoubtedly is challenging, indicating that conducting a similar study in areas with a smoother topography would most likely turn out simpler.

Furthermore, the Gjensidige case study potentially may act as a template for impact studies in sectors other than insurance as well. The core idea is the fitting of an effects model based on observed data and then propagating future climate scenario runs through that model.

12.5 Climate change and property insurance interactions

It appears as a well-established fact that climate change will affect property insurance risks and thus the generation of future claims. However, thinking about insurance loss data as an invaluable source for climate risk reduction and adaptation priorities is maybe less common. In this section we discuss both aspects.

Insurance data is often considered a scarce resource for those who advertise that they want to publish research on topics involving losses and their risks. This comes as no surprise, as the insurers consider their data a valuable asset, strongly linked to and maintaining their competitive advantages. For that reason, and in combination with confidentiality issues, much of the research and data analysis in this field is undertaken by the companies themselves on proprietary data. This applies to primary insurers, but in particular to the re-insurance companies which hold vast amounts of data on extreme loss events and often employ highly competent staff able to accomplish specific investigations as required by in-house needs.

Over the past decade there has been an increasing awareness from authorities that insurance data can indeed contribute to safeguarding and risk mitigation in society. Often, insurance companies via their loss databases hold more complete data on risk-prone locations than do municipal authorities. Also, there is an emerging acknowledgment among insurance companies that sharing loss data to regulators might prove beneficial to their own business as well. Providing municipalities with knowledge on high-risk locations, municipal staff can spend their often limited resources on initiating targeted efforts locally, often by improving the infrastructure in an area to make it climate resilient. As a result the insurance companies' property risks will diminish, and as a third benefit the homeowner will be exempted from future loss burden. In 2013, a pilot project utilizing high-resolution insurance loss data for understanding municipal risk was initiated by Finance Norway in cooperation with research institutes and a selection of Norwegian municipalities (Brevik et al, 2014). The insight obtained from these loss data served to identify unknown threats, contribute input to risk and vulnerability analyses and expedite priorities in climate adaptation work. The project earned positive mention also outside Norway, and was referred by the World Bank Group[3].

The key idea of loss data sharing as explored in the pilot project was further followed up in a recent study (Hauge et al, 2018) by KLIMA2050[4], a research-based innovation centre directed by SINTEF. The eight largest insurance companies in Norway were asked about their attitudes to sharing such data, what it would take for them to do so and what technical challenges they foresee. It turned out that, in general, companies are willing and even positive towards sharing their data at property level to public organizations working with risk prevention and climate adaptation as long as, by no means, data is made available among the insurance companies. Furthermore, users of the data will be given access to aggregate data only, for example at postcode level. Ideally, the insurance companies prefer that data sharing is collectively imposed on the sector by regulatory authorities. The Norwegian Directorate for Civil Protection (DSB) is assigned responsibility for synthesizing a 'knowledge bank' that holds information on certain weather and climate-related events, including natural perils. The idea is to establish a system that collects such claims data from all the insurance companies on a regular basis, and thereby facilitates 'continuous' climate adaptation.

Internationally, there are a few examples of countries thinking along the same lines of sharing insurance loss data for risk prevention purposes. Maybe inspired by the July 2011 extreme precipitation event in Copenhagen causing massive damage totaling 6 billion DKK, the Danish Insurance Association in 2016 provided municipalities with free access to cloudburst claims data from

---

[3] https://indexinsuranceforum.org/resilience-document/insurance-loss-data-sharing-projects-climate-resilient-municipalities-0

[4] http://www.klima2050.no/

Danish insurers. Also in France there have been initiatives employing insurance data in damage prevention. A thorough review on the use of insurance data in the analysis of surface water flood is available from Gradeci et al (2019).

The impacts of climate change are complex and interwoven with cross-sectoral ramifications. This means that effects seen for the insurance industry will likely propagate through to other sectors. Those cascading effects are often difficult to anticipate. And even if one were able to identify them, linking the chain of impacts quantitatively together would imply a large, holistic model of high complexity.

Nevertheless, it is still possible to envision qualitatively a few examples of plausible inter-connectivities with property insurance. First, using local claim history for producing municipal risk maps would form an extremely useful basis for infrastructure adaptation along the lines mentioned earlier in this section. Maintenance and improvement of public infrastructures like the sewer system has a relatively high cost, especially in urban areas. And like public costs in general, the expenses ultimately reach the taxpayers. However, the alternative cost of not doing anything will most likely prove even higher to society in the long run.

Another immediate consequence of increased claims burden is professionals devising new building codes and design guidelines. Additional to the man-hours needed from architects and engineers to establish the new standards, new materials and products can also be requested. Such inventions may call for new expertise or reorganizing existing industries and thereby affect both education and the labor market as part of the emerging green economy. An example is the blooming of so-called blue-green roofs on buildings for attenuation of stormwater damage in cities.

A major concern for those involved deals with areas or properties that are hit repeatedly by loss-generating weather events. Ultimately, the insurance company refuses to repair or re-build the property and implicitly forces the homeowner to move. On the way there, however, the homeowner might experience that his property is untradable in the market due to a history of multiple losses or soaring insurance premiums, and hence will influence economic mobility.

Eventually, the insurance industry itself can influence climate adaptation and mitigation through their investment policy. Managing large values on behalf of their customers and shareholders, insurance companies can decide to invest in the evolving green economy rather than CO_2-intensive industries, for instance. Care should be exercised, however, so that investing in climate friendly industries does not supersede dismantling environment hostile sectors. For instance, in resource settings, often too much effort is focused on developing new, clean technologies, and too little on reducing existing, dirty activities. The total footprint increases and nothing has been gained. To really mitigate climate change, holistic thinking rather than one-dimensional, technical innovations must be made.

12.6 Conclusions

A harsher climate will leave insurance companies with substantial alterations in their current portfolio risk. New regimes of underwriting will have to incorporate anticipated future weather patterns in the evaluation. Highly skilled algorithms will combine data from multiple sources and aid decision support by capturing patterns and correlations not evident from conventional techniques. The Internet of Things and social media represent new platforms for information, whereas specific knowledge about existing but less accessible risk drivers like sewer system capacity would probably also prove useful.

Statistical methodology remains at the core of many modern techniques like machine learning. Some tasks are best solved via parsimonious modeling providing insight into the risk mechanisms of a portfolio. Black box prediction might be the right option if the focus is on the implications of specific scenarios. Statistics offer an invaluable tool for quantifying and propagating uncertainties along a chain of effects.

In Norway, ordinary bad-weather losses represent a higher cost than natural perils losses over the past decade. A case study established models for the number of claims and their severities from a selection of meteorological and hydrological exogenous variables. Forcing the models with a climate model scenario run from 2071–2100 revealed a municipal change in number of claims in the range from −30% to 71%, and in claim severity in the range from −1% to 33% as compared to a control run from 1961–1990.

Though historical claims alone are not viable for assessing future risks in general, they are still useful for risk reduction and climate adaptation locally. Sharing loss data with municipal authorities, their staff can take action to improve infrastructure and thereby resilience in certain high-risk areas. Increased loss burden may also penetrate through to inventing revised building codes demanding new products and materials, and even new expertise. The reputation of repeatedly damaged properties can eventually influence the economic mobility of the homeowner.

Acknowledgments

I want to thank Magne Aldrin, Xeni K. Dimakos, Elisabeth Orskaug, and Jofrid F. Vårdal for important contributions to the Gjensidige case study summarized in Sections 12.4.1–12.4.3. I would also like to express gratitude to Gjensidige ASA for their kind permission to share results from the project. Claudio Heinrich and Jens C. Wahl have fostered inspiring discussions during the follow-up study referred in Section 12.4.4.

References

Bolin D, Frigessi A, Guttorp P, Haug O, Orskaug E, Scheel I, Wallin J (2016) Calibrating regionally downscaled precipitation over Norway through quantile-based approaches. Adv Stat Clim Meteorol Oceanogr 2:39–47

Brevik R, Aall C, Rød JK (2014) Pilotprosjekt om testing av skadedata fra forsikringsbransjen for vurdering av klimasårbarhet og forebygging av klimarelatert naturskade i utvalgte kommuner. Tech. rep., Vestlandsforskning (in Norwegian)

Clark MR, Gangopadhyay S, Hay L, Rajagopalan B, Wilby R (2004) The Schaake shuffle: a method for reconstructing space-time variability in forecasted precipitation and temperature fields. Journal of Hydrometeorology 5(1):243–262

Doksum K (1974) Empirical probability plots and statistical inference fornonlinear models in the two-sample case. The Annals of Statistics 2(2):267–277

Engen-Skaugen T (2007) Refinement of dynamically downscaled precipitation and temperature scenarios. Climatic Change 84(3–4):365–382

Engen-Skaugen T, Haugen JE, Tveito OE (2007) Temperature scenarios for Norway: from regional to local scale. Climate Dynamics 29(5):441–453

Finans Norge (2019) Klimarapport Finans Norge 2019. Tech. rep., Finans Norge (in Norwegian)

Friedland J, Cheng H, Peleshok A (2014) Water Damage Risk and Canadian Property Insurance Pricing. Tech. rep., KPMG

Gradeci K, Labonnote N, Sivertsen E, Time B (2019) The use of insurance data in the analysis of surface water flood events – a systematic review. Journal of Hydrology 568:194–206

Haug O, Dimakos X, Vårdal J, Aldrin M, Meze-Hausken E (2011) Future building water loss projections posed by climate change. Scandinavian Actuarial Journal 1:1–20

Hauge Å, Flyen C, Venås C, Aall C, Kokkonen A, Ebeltoft M (2018) Attitudes in Norwegian insurance companies towards sharing loss data—public-private cooperation for improved climate adaptation. Tech. rep., KLIMA2050, SINTEF

IPCC (2018) Summary for policymakers. In: Masson-Delmotte V, Zhai P, Pörtner HO, Roberts D, Skea J, Shukla PR, Pirani A, Moufouma-Okia W, Péan C, Pidcock R, Connors S, Matthews JBR, Chen Y, Zhou X, Gomis MI, Lonnoy E, Maycock T, Tignor M, Waterfield T (eds) Global Warming of 1.5°C. An IPCC Special Report on the impacts of global warming of 1.5°C above pre-industrial levels and related global greenhouse gas emission pathways, in the context of strengthening the global response to the threat of climate change, sustainable development, and efforts to eradicate poverty, World Meteorological Organization, Geneva, Switzerland

Lundberg F (1903) Approximerad framställning av sannolikhetsfunktionen. återförsäkring av kollektivrisker. Akademisk afhandling, Almqvist och Wicksell, Uppsala, Sweden (in Swedish)

McCullagh P, Nelder J (1989) Generalized Linear Models, 2nd edn. Chapman & Hall, Boca Raton, FL

Nakićenović N, Swart Re (2000) Special Report on Emissions Scenarios: A special report of Working Group III of the Intergovernmental Panel on Climate Change. Cambridge University Press

Palutikof JP, Winkler JA, Goodess CM, Andresen JA (1997) The simulation of daily temperature time series from GCM output. Part I: Comparison of model data with observations. Journal of Climate 10:2497–2513

Seneviratne SI, Nicholls N, Easterling D, Goodess CM, Kanae S, Kossin J, Luo Y, Marengo J, McInnes K, Rahimi M, Reichstein M, Sorteberg A, Vera C, Zha X (2012) Changes in climate extremes and their impacts on the natural physical environment. In: Field CB, Barros V, Stocker TF, Qin D, Dokken DJ, Ebi KL, Mastrandrea MD, Mach KJ, Plattner GK, Allen SK, Tignor M, Midgle PM (eds) A Special Report of Working Groups I and II of the Intergovernmental Panel on Climate Change (IPCC), Cambridge University Press, Cambridge, United Kingdom and New York, chapter 3, 109–230

Wong P (2019) Predicting vs. Explaining. URL https://towardsdatascience.com/predicting-vs-explaining-69b516f90796

13
Climate Change Impacts on the Nation's Electricity Sector

Craig D. Zamuda
U.S. Department of Energy, Washington, D.C., USA

CONTENTS

13.1	Introduction	277
13.2	Climate impacts and implications for the electricity sector	280
	13.2.1 Specific extreme weather hazards and impacts to the electricity sector	282
13.3	Resilience approaches and options	288
13.4	Analytical approaches for assessing costs and benefits of resilience investments	290
	13.4.1 Consolidated Edison of New York (Con Edison) case study: risk prioritization model	291
	13.4.2 Public Service Electric & Gas (PSE&G) case study: break-even analysis	292
	13.4.3 Entergy's case study: building a resilient Gulf Coast	294
13.5	Gaps and opportunities for improvement in resilience planning	296
References		301

13.1 Introduction

Extreme weather is having a significant impact on the nation's electricity system. Increases in extreme precipitation events, hurricane intensity, and flooding, as well as extreme heat events, drought, and wildfires are adversely affecting electricity assets and operations in many regions (AAAS, 2019, DOE, 2013, 2015a,b, 2017a, Zamuda et al, 2018). These hazards, along with sea level rise and storm surge, are damaging electricity infrastructure and impacting utility operations, further burdening utility customers through disruption of services, and impacting society and the economy. The cost of weather-related outages has also increased, with estimates at $25 to $70 billion annually (Campbell, 2012, COA, 2013, LaCommare et al, 2018, Larsen, 2016a,b). Since 1980, the

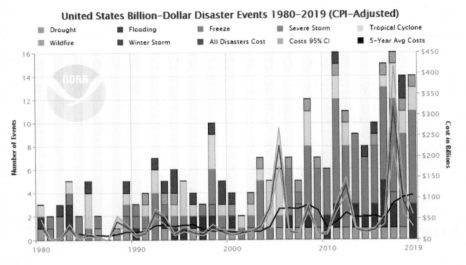

FIGURE 13.1: Billion-dollar climate- and weather-related disaster event types, by year (CPI-adjusted). Source: NOAA (2020).

United States has sustained 258 weather disasters where the overall damage costs reached or exceeded $1 billion (Figure 13.1; NOAA, 2020). The cumulative costs for these events exceed $1.75 trillion in total, direct costs. During 2017, the United States experienced a historic year of weather disasters with 16 separate billion-dollar disaster events, with total damage costs exceeding $300 billion (NOAA, 2018). In 2019, 14 separate US billion-dollar disasters represent the fourth-highest total number of events (tied with 2018). The year 2019 experienced a slightly above average year of costs ($45.0 billion NOAA, 2018). In total, the United States was impacted by 14 separate billion-dollar disasters including: 3 major inland floods, 8 severe storms, 2 tropical cyclones (Dorian and Imelda), and 1 wildfire event. 2019 also marks the fifth consecutive year (2015–2019) in which 10 or more separate billion-dollar disaster events have impacted the United States. Many extreme weather hazards are expected to continue growing in frequency and severity over the century, with accompanying increases in damages and restoration costs, affecting all elements of society and economic security, including the nation's complex electricity system (USGCRP, 2017).

Climate change will act as a stress multiplier, forcing the electricity system, as depicted in Figure 13.2, to operate outside of the normal ranges of the twentieth century for which the majority of existing infrastructure was designed. In addition, the nation's energy infrastructure supplying base load generation is aging with many coal and nuclear plants approaching 40–50 years old, and some of the transmission system over 100 years old (GAO, 2014). Electricity systems have always been shaped by the mix of available energy resources and the end-use demand patterns, as well as the environments in which electric

Introduction

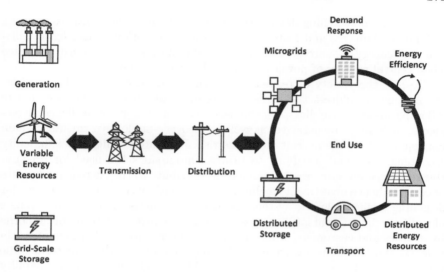

FIGURE 13.2: The electricity system includes four physical components (generation, transmission, distribution, and end-use consumption). The emerging twenty-first-century power grid will incorporate responsive resources, storage, microgrids, and other technologies that enable increased resilience, flexibility, higher system efficiency, reduced energy consumption, and increased consumer options and value. Source: DOE (2017a).

utilities operate. Climate change is one of the most important environmental factors affecting the electricity sector today and in the decades ahead.

The impacts of climate change will affect electricity infrastructure assets and systems in different ways (DOE, 2013, 2015a,b, 2017a, Zamuda, 2018). These climate impacts may affect sector assets fairly directly or more indirectly—as a result of the close interdependencies that have developed with the electricity system and other sectors of the economy. Every sector of the economy depends on electricity from manufacturing to agriculture, banking, healthcare, water treatment and supply, telecommunications, and transportation.

While the nation's electricity system is increasingly vulnerable to extreme weather events, the nation's dependency on electricity is projected to increase in the decades ahead, and will require improved planning and investment to ensure a reliable and resilient supply of electricity is available to power the nation's economy and ensure its security. Actions being taken to enhance the resilience of the electric grid span a wide range of technologies and approaches, including hardening measures (e.g., installing stronger utility poles, undergrounding lines, etc.) and elevating or moving assets to less risk prone areas to avoid damage during extreme events. Adoption of innovative technologies also are providing resilience options including the adoption of smart meters and automated switching devices that can detect and isolate outages to assist in limiting damages and faster recovery times. Adoption of microgrids, distributed energy resources, and storage technologies can enhance resilience when central sources of power are affected during storms.

Despite the variety of resilience strategies and investments that utilities are making to address the threats of extreme weather and climate change following major storm disasters, the pace, scale, and scope of resilience investments, including preventative, as well as recovery-mode investments, remain inadequate given the magnitude of the risk. Regulated utilities face difficulty recouping costs and justifying to utility commissions the need for preemptive resilience investments. Many factors contribute to the current inadequate pace of resilience investments including: (1) the lack of consensus standards for designing resilient electric systems or metrics for measuring the effectiveness of resilience investments; (2) the costs of resilience investments are often borne by utilities and customers, while the benefits accrue to a wide range of stakeholders; and (3) the resilience upgrades may be costly in the near term while the timeframe for associated benefits to address high impact-low probability events may be several years or decades. However, investments in resilience can pay for themselves. For example, studies have demonstrated that programs such as FEMA's (U.S. Federal Emergency Management Agency's) mitigation programs show that every pre-event dollar spent on resilience yields a $4 savings in future losses (Multihazard Mitigation Council, 2005, 2017, Weiss and Weidman, 2013). Thus, an improved understanding of the costs and benefits of resilience solutions is necessary to effectively make the business case to regulators, utility customers, and society that resilience investment are prudent and cost-effective in ensuring the safe and reliable provision of electricity, and establishing a climate-ready electric grid to address present and future risks.

This chapter will highlight the direct and indirect impacts of extreme weather and climate change to the electricity sector, as well as the costs of these vulnerabilities, both current and projected. In addition, the chapter will discuss how utilities or developing strategies and solutions to improve resilience to extreme weather, and employing methodologies to demonstrate the costs and benefits of these investments.

13.2 Climate impacts and implications for the electricity sector

Extreme weather events and damages to critical infrastructure including electricity assets are occurring more frequently and the costs are increasing (Figure 13.1; GAO, 2014, NOAA, 2018). For the last several decades, there has been a steady increase in the number of extreme weather-related grid disruptions, resulting in high costs for utilities and customers, including repair costs for damaged assets, and economic costs related to work disruptions, and lost productivity. The energy sector often bears a significant portion of these costs (USGCRP, 2014, 2017, 2018).

A range of extreme weather events can impact electricity infrastructure and operations. Table 13.1 provides examples of extreme weather trends and potential impacts to the U.S. electricity systems. All regions of the nation can be impacted, and all components of electricity supply and demand are vulnerable (AAAS, 2019, DOE, 2013, 2015a,b). A number of extreme weather hazards are expected to increase in frequency, intensity, and duration due to climate change, including: increasing surface, atmospheric, and oceanic temperatures; melting glaciers; disappearing snow cover; shrinking sea ice; rising sea level; increasing atmospheric water vapor; and changing rainfall patterns and droughts (USGCRP, 2017, 2018). Other trends in severe weather, including the intensity and frequency of tornadoes, hail, and damaging winds, are uncertain and understudied.

TABLE 13.1: Projected climate change hazards and implications relevant to the US electricity systems (DOE, 2013)

Energy sector	Climate projection	Potential implication
Thermoelectric power generation (coal, natural gas, nuclear, geothermal, and concentrating solar power)	Increasing air temperatures	Reduction in power plant efficiencies and available generation capacity
	Increasing water temperatures	Reduction in power plant efficiencies and available generation capacity; increased risk of exceeding thermal discharge limits
	Decreasing water availability	Reduction in available generation capacity; impacts on coal, natural gas, and nuclear fuel supply chains
	Increasing intensity of storm events, sea level rise, and storm surge	Increased risk of physical damage and disruption to coastal facilities
	Increasing intensity and frequency of flooding	Increased risk of physical damage and disruption to inland facilities
Hydropower	Increasing temperatures and evaporative losses	Reduction in available generation capacity and changes in operations
	Changes in precipitation and decreasing snowpack	Reduction in available generation capacity and changes in operations
	Increasing intensity and frequency of flooding	Increased risk of physical damage and changes in operations

Continued on next page

TABLE 13.1 – continued from previous page

Energy sector	Climate projection	Potential implication
Bioenergy and biofuel production	Increasing air temperatures	Increased irrigation demand and risk of crop damage from extreme heat events
	Extended growing season	Increased production
	Decreasing water availability	Decreased production
	Sea level rise and increasing intensity and frequency of flooding	Increased risk of crop damage
Wind energy	Variations in wind patterns	Uncertain impacts on resource potential
Solar energy	Increasing air temperatures	Reduction in potential capacity
	Decreasing water availability	Reduction in concentrating solar potential capacity
Electric grid	Increasing air temperatures	Reduction in transmission efficiency and available transmission capacity
	More frequent and severe wildfires	Increased risk of physical damage and decreased transmission capacity
	Increasing intensity of storm events	Increased risk of physical damage
Energy demand	Increasing air temperatures	Increased electricity demand for cooling
	Increasing magnitude and frequency of extreme heat events	Increased peak electricity demand

13.2.1 Specific extreme weather hazards and impacts to the electricity sector

Hurricanes and extreme winds

Experience with hurricanes over the past decade has revealed the vulnerability of the electric grid to their effects including high winds and flooding (DOE, 2013, 2015a,b). As wind speeds increase, damage to the electrical systems become more common particular to the distribution system, with degradations in system performance, and greater number of customers across wider areas experiencing power outages. High winds can also damage components of the transmission system with similar impacts.

Hurricanes Sandy and Maria illustrate severe impacts of hurricanes upon the electric grid. Hurricane Sandy (2013) caused more than 100 northeast electric substations in four states being inundated, with almost 9 million customers losing power. Substation flooding contributed to outages and severe disruptions to electric power service in the region. The damage to the electric grid affected other sectors as well, including transportation, communications, wastewater treatment, and health care. For example, loss of power to pipelines in the region temporarily disabled pipeline transport of critical fuels to the region, and power outages prevented gas stations from being able to pump available gasoline, resulting in widespread fuel shortages. Power outages at wastewater treatment plants resulted in billions of gallons of raw and partially treated sewage being discharged into the region's waterways, affecting public health and aquatic ecosystems (Kenward et al, 2013).

More recently, Hurricane Maria struck Puerto Rico in 2017 with winds exceeding 150 miles per hour (about 241 km/h) and dumped more than 2 feet (about 610 mm) of rain resulting in a complete failure of the power grid, with power outages to over a million residents, and unprecedented damage to a significant portion of the electricity system, including generation, transmission, and distribution assets. Estimated costs for rebuilding the grid are approximately $18 billion (New York Power Authority et al, 2017). These cost estimates do not include the billions of dollars in lost revenue to the economy of Puerto Rico resulting from the loss of power.

Climate change is expected to increase the intensity of hurricanes, increasing the risk of power outages and damaged infrastructure (USGCRP, 2017, 2018). In addition, coastal flooding caused by hurricane storm surge may be more severe due to rising sea levels.

Sea-level rise

Climate change and the associated warming of the oceans and melting of glaciers and ice sheets is contributing to sea level rise. Globally, sea levels have increased by approximately 7–8 inches since 1900 (USGCRP, 2017, 2018). Global sea level is projected to continue to rise in this century along with the number of routine "nuisance" tidal floods. These flood have increased 5- to 10-fold since the 1960s in several gulf and east coast cities and the rates of tidal flooding will continue increasing in depth, frequency, and extent this century (USGCRP, 2017, 2018).

Sea-level rise can threaten energy infrastructure in coastal zones. The steady increasing sea levels as well as the compounding effects of storm surge from hurricane events can result in inundation and damage to electricity assets. Sea-level rise is projected to increase the depth of inundation associated with storm surges as well as the extent of inland penetration. These compounding factors may increase the frequency with which electricity assets are exposed to inundation as well as the severity of inundation during storm events. A DOE (U.S. Department of Energy) analysis of projected exposure to climate impacts in metropolitan areas indicates that power plants and substations are both potentially vulnerable to future sea-level rise (DOE, 2014a). While some energy assets at potential risk may be retired by the time they would be affected by ongoing sea level rise, replacement assets may face the threat posed by chronic increases in sea level rise and storm surge over the longer term, and in the shorter term, the risks posed by increases in nuisance flooding in coastal communities.

In the Southeast (Atlantic and Gulf Coasts), power plants and oil refineries are especially vulnerable to flooding. The number of electricity generation facilities in the Southeast potentially exposed to hurricane storm surge is estimated at between 69 to 291 for Category 1 and Category 5 storms, respectively (Maloney and Preston, 2014). Nationally, a sea level rise of 3.3 feet (about 1 m) could expose dozens of power plants that are currently out of reach to the risks of a 100-year flood. This would represent an additional cumulative total of 25 gigawatts (GW) of operating or proposed power capacities at risk (Bierkandt et al, 2015). In Florida and Delaware, sea level rise of 3.3 feet would double the number of vulnerable plants (putting an additional 11 GW and 0.8 GW at risk in the two states, respectively); in Texas, vulnerable capacity would more than triple (with an additional 2.8 GW at risk, Bierkandt et al, 2015).

Climate change is expected to continue to contribute to sea level rise in this century. Relative to the year 2000, global sea level is very likely to rise by 0.3–0.6 feet by 2030, and 1–4.3 feet by 2100 (USGCRP, 2017, 2018). Relative sea level rise will vary along the US coastlines and will likely be greater than global averages in the Northeast and western Gulf of Mexico, increasing the frequency and extent of flooding and impacts on electricity infrastructure associated with hurricanes.

Temperatures and extreme heat

Increasing temperatures and extreme heat events will drive increases in demand for cooling energy, while simultaneously threatening power plants and the electric grid with reduced capacity and increased disruptions of power plants and the grid, and potentially increasing electricity prices to consumers. Most utilities experience peak demand during extended heat waves, stressing the existing electric power infrastructure.

On the supply side, high ambient temperatures adversely affect combustion turbines, because warmer air is lower in density causing the efficiency of converting fuel to power to decrease. Increased ambient air and water temperatures across the United States reduce the efficiency of electricity generation in thermoelectric power plants [whether they use nuclear energy, coal, natural gas, concentrating solar power (CSP), bioenergy, or geothermal power], reducing available capacity or increasing fuel consumption at those plants (DOE, 2013). Over time, increasing temperatures will raise the costs of electricity, and more frequent, longer-lasting, and more severe extreme heat events will make blackouts and power disruptions more common (DOE, 2015a, EPA, 2017). Because almost 90% of the electricity generated in the United States comes from thermoelectric power, decreases in power supply and increases in fuel consumption may impair system flexibility and reliability and increase costs of electricity.

Within the past decade alone, over 36 power plants have been forced to shut down or curtail generation due to high temperatures or inadequate water supplies (DOE, 2013). In addition to elevated water temperatures reducing power plant efficiency, in some cases, a plant may have to shut down to comply with discharge temperature regulations designed to avoid damaging aquatic ecosystems (DOE, 2013, 2015a). Such curtailments impact reliability through greater reductions in generation and imposing higher costs due to the dispatch of higher-cost generation technologies. These impacts are expected to increase with climate change. For example, in North America, the output potential of power plants cooled by river water could fall by 7.3%–13.1% by 2050 under the Representative Concentration Pathway (RCP) 2.6 and RCP 8.5 scenarios, respectively[1] (van Vliet et al, 2016).

While higher temperatures increase the electricity demand for cooling, they also reduce the current-carrying capacity and transmission efficiency of electricity lines. Increasing temperatures are therefore expected to increase transmission losses, increase stresses on the distribution system, and decrease substation efficiency and lifespan (DOE, 2013).

At the current pattern of increased greenhouse gas emissions, rising temperatures are projected to increase electricity costs and demand. Costs may increase as a result of increasing demand but also reduced supply by decreased efficiency of power generation and delivery, thereby requiring new generation capacity. This could cost residential and commercial ratepayers up to $12 billion per year (DOE, 2015a, Rhodium Group LLC, 2014). By 2040, nationwide residential and commercial electricity expenditures will likely increase by 6%–18% under RCP 8.5, 4%–15% for a lower scenario (RCP 4.5), and 4%–12% for an even lower scenario (RCP 2.6) (Rhodium Group LLC, 2017). Nationwide electricity demand is projected to increase by 3%–9% by 2040 under the higher scenario and 2%–7% under the lower scenario (Rhodium Group LLC, 2017). This projection includes the reduction in electricity used for space heating in states with warming winters. In a lower scenario (RCP 4.5), temperatures remain on an upward trajectory that could increase net electricity demand by 1.7%–2.0% (EPA, 2017). Because the grid must provide enough power to meet the highest peak load on the hottest day, generating capacity must increase more than total demand, the nation could require up to 25% more power plant capacity in 2040, compared to a scenario without a warming climate (Rhodium Group LLC, 2017).

In addition to thermoelectric generation, hydropower generation of electricity can be impacted by warming temperatures. A warmer climate is causing

---

[1] The RCPs adopted by the Intergovernmental Panel on Climate Change (IPCC) for its Fifth Assessment Report in 2014 are consistent with a wide range of possible changes in future anthropogenic greenhouse gas (GHG) emissions, and represent their atmospheric concentrations. RCP 2.6 assumes that global annual GHG emissions (measured in CO_2-equivalents) peak during 2010–2020, with emissions declining substantially thereafter. Emissions in RCP 4.5 peak around 2040, then decline. In RCP 8.5, emissions continue to rise throughout the twenty-first century.

snowpack to melt earlier in the season, and a greater amount of precipitation falling as rain rather than snow (EPA, 2016, USGCRP, 2017). The timing of streamflow can be just as important for hydropower dams in snowmelt-dominated regions (like the western United States), where both water and hydropower can be much more useful in the dry summer months than the winter and spring. Together, these effects reduce the amount of water – and hydropower – available in the summer (DOE, 2015a). Since 1955, the amount of snowpack remaining on April 1st of each year has declined at over 90% of the sites measured across the west; the average decline across all sites is 23% (EPA, 2016). Projections indicate that by 2050, large areas of the western U.S. could switch from snow-dominated to rain-dominated watersheds, and by 2100, mountain snowpack is expected to be completely eliminated from some watersheds (USGCRP, 2017).

Climate change is projected to result in increases in annual average temperatures over the contiguous United States of about 2.5°F (about 1.4°C) for the period 2021–2050, with much larger increases of 2.8–7.3°F (about 1.6–4.1°C) by late century (2071–2100; USGCRP, 2017, 2018). Extreme temperatures are projected to increase even more than average temperatures with the number of days above 90°F (about 32.2°C) increasing by about 20–30 days per year in most areas by mid century under RCP 8.5, with increases of 40–50 days in much of the Southeast (USGCRP, 2017, 2018).

Drought

Direct impacts from drought affect nearly all aspects of energy supply: how electricity is produced; where future capacity may be sited; the cost of producing electricity; the types of generation or cooling technologies that are cost-effective; and the costs and methods for extracting, producing, and delivering fuels. Restricted access to water for cooling thermoelectric facilities can affect the capacity utilization of power plants. In addition, increased evaporation rates or changes in snowpack may affect the volume and timing of water available for hydropower. Similarly, decreased water availability can affect bioenergy production. Most US power plants, regardless of fuel source (e.g., coal, natural gas, nuclear, concentrated solar, and geothermal) rely upon a steady supply of water for cooling, and operations may be threatened when water availability decreases or water temperatures increase (DOE, 2015a).

Total withdrawals for thermoelectric power for 2010 were 161,000 Mgal/day (about 7,053 $m^3 s^{-1}$), 99% of which was withdrawn from surface water sources, predominantly freshwater. Total withdrawals for thermoelectric power accounted for 38% of total freshwater withdrawals, and 51% of fresh surface-water withdrawals for all uses in the United States (Dieter et al, 2018). In regions where water is already scarce, competition for water between energy production and other uses will increase in this century.

Drought can severely limit the cooling water available for thermoelectric power plants and can lead to plant de-rating because of low water levels, low flow rates, or high water temperatures in rivers and reservoirs. The 2011 drought in Texas, for example, reduced the cooling water available to power plants by 30%. A recent simulation of the weather during the US Dust Bowl disaster in the early 1930s found that generation-capacity losses for California, Arizona, and Texas under such drought conditions would be 17%, 25%, and 30%, respectively (Preston et al, 2016).

Hydropower plants are especially sensitive to the effects of climate change on water availability, either by affecting the amount or timing of precipitation, the persistence of snow and ice accumulating in the mountains, or the rate at which water evaporates from streams and reservoirs. When water levels fall, hydropower facilities must reduce output, or even stop production all together. Drought affects hydropower plants by reducing the total amount of water available to produce power. In 2015, California's historic drought caused the state's hydropower output to fall 59% below the average for the prior two decades (US Energy Information Administration, 2017). The Hoover Dam has had to significantly curtail hydropower output and reduce the capacity of its generators due to a lack of water in the Colorado basin; in 2016, production was 26% lower than in 2001 (US Energy Information Administration, 2017).

Overall, more annual precipitation is projected for the northern United States, while less precipitation is projected for southern regions. Substantial reductions in western US winter and spring snowpack are projected as the climate warms (USGCRP, 2017). Seasonal variations in precipitation, however, are most relevant in understanding regional water availability and competing needs. In particular, the largest declines in precipitation are expected during the summer months, along with long duration droughts increasingly possible by the end of the century (USGCRP, 2017, 2018).

Wildfire

Wildfire events pose a threat to the electricity system, particularly due to the exposure of high-voltage transmission lines (DOE, 2015a,b). Wildfires can trigger emergency line de-rating or shut-downs to prevent line damage. Smoke from wildfires can induce a line fault, resulting in a loss of service. Large fires have damaged and disrupted electricity transmission in recent years (DOE, 2013, 2015a). In some situations, power transmission may be cut for the safety of emergency personnel operating in the area. Utilities may also be liable for wildfire damages associated with their operations. For example, in November 2018, the Camp Fire in Northern California consumed over 153,000 acres, destroyed 13,972 residences, 528 commercial structures, and 4293 other buildings, and claimed the lives of 85 people (SEC, 2019). As the magnitude of the damage and the probable cause became linked to electricity equipment owned and operated by Pacific Gas and Electric (PG&E), the utility declared bankruptcy, estimating at the time that it could face liabilities surpassing $30 billion from the 2017 and 2018 Northern California wildfires. Penetration of wildfires into residential and/or commercial areas can also expose electricity distribution systems and substations to damage, and wildfires have also disrupted generation facilities (DOE, 2013, 2015a). For example, a California wildfire in 2015 damaged five facilities associated with Calpine Corporation's The Geysers—the world's largest geothermal infrastructure. While the absolute number of fires across the country has not increased over the past 50 years, the total area burned has increased markedly. This increase is associated with a lengthening of the fire season (USGCRP, 2017, 2018).

Climate change is projected to further increase the likelihood of major fires in the future, due to continued lengthening of the fire season and projected increases in drought conditions. The incidence of large forest fires in the western United States and Alaska is projected to further increase as the climate warms in this century (USGCRP, 2017, 2018).

13.3 Resilience approaches and options

Options for managing the vulnerabilities of the electric grid span a wide range of costs and long-term effectiveness. These projects may include infrastructure hardening, changing operational procedures, incorporating new technologies, or additional measures to reduce demand or increase reserve capacity (Table 13.2; Con Edison, 2013, DOE, 2015a, Entergy, 2010, Exelon, 2015, PG&E, 2016, Seattle City Light, 2015, Zamuda, 2018). Investments have typically been focused on changes in potential exposure of physical infrastructure, such as building physical barriers or moving equipment, building backup systems, building non-wooden or reinforced poles, and burying lines underground. Reliability and resilience projects have also included operations and maintenance activities, such as aggressive vegetation management. Increasingly, options for managing resilience to extreme weather use new innovative technologies such as smart meters and automated switching devices that allow for faster recovery times from disruptions, or energy efficiency measures that can reduce energy demand. Microgrids and distributed generation and storage technologies also provide options for improved resilience during and after storms. For example, these systems can be "islanded" from the main power grid during power outages.

Adoption of resilience options is happening slowly, and generally is focused on post-disaster recovery and rebuild efforts rather than proactive, preventative investments to avoid or minimize damages and outages. In addition, in many cases adoption of new, more resilient technologies is not the major focus for these investments. For example, about 90% of resilience project funds in response to Hurricane Sandy were spent on infrastructure changes and additional operations and maintenance activities rather than on upgrading infrastructure components with advanced smart grid technologies. Some utilities are doing more than infrastructure changes. For example, after Hurricane Sandy took out Con Edison's substation on the lower East Side, helping to throw lower Manhattan into darkness, the utility's plan of action included construction of walls and barriers; installation of pumping equipment and submersible network equipment; and the deployment of smart grid tools to enhance network flexibility in emergencies (Con Edison, 2013, 2015, 2016).

TABLE 13.2: Examples of resilience measures pursued to address a broad mix of climate and extreme weather threats

Categories of infrastructure and actions	Examples of energy system resilience actions underway
Distributed generation, on-site renewables, and combined heat and power (CHP)	– Greater deployment of distributed generation capacity and back-up power supplies to address peak loads and increase system resiliency – Increased understanding of market opportunities and technical barriers to increasing size of balancing areas for system reliability and risk reduction – Lower cost solar, storage, and system islanding capabilities under development and increasingly deployed to protect critical loads – Increased capture and use of waste heat through locally-generated combined heat and power
Energy efficiency and building codes	– Reduce potential for grid failure by decreasing energy demand and decreasing the likelihood of power outages during peak demand (extreme heat or cold events) – Reduce scale and cost of necessary backup generation by reducing heating, cooling and lighting loads using energy efficient equipment – Reduce dependency on limited water availability and drought impacts – Enhance electricity and oil/gas sector resilience
Smart grid and micro-grids	– Adopt smart grid, microgrids and clean energy sources (PV, wind, biomass) into the existing utility systems – Reduce dependency on vulnerable transmission and distribution from distant power sources
Mechanical and electrical systems	– Harden energy infrastructure, including elevating or relocating water-sensitive equipment – Establish back-up power supply, intelligent controls – Insulate equipment for temperature extremes – Implement dry (air cooled) or low-water hybrid cooling systems for power plants
Electric vehicles and energy storage	– Enhance smart grid and storage capabilities with electric vehicles integration into power systems to accommodate storm related power outages
Green infrastructure	– Reduce cooling demand and energy use – Reduce urban heat island effect – Improved building code design and deployment

Continued on next page

TABLE 13.2 – continued from previous page

Categories of infrastructure and actions	Examples of energy system resilience actions underway
Preparedness and planning	– Improve resistance and resiliency (microgrids, building efficiency, island capabilities, etc.) – Establish policies and codes that support sustainability, security, and safety – Provide protected emergency-response coordination centers – Expand mutual assistance programs to provide critical personnel and equipment to restore power – Develop flood and storm management plans including prepositioning of critical backup equipment – Identification and measures to protect critical infrastructure – Improve vegetation management programs to protect overhead lines
Recovery and rebuilding	– Deploy on-site technology demonstrations (e.g., emergency backup power) – Incorporate energy efficiency, sustainability, and renewable energy measures into disaster recovery efforts – Design sustainable, resilient energy infrastructure (e.g., oil/gas exploration and refining, generation, transmission, and distribution, etc.)
Enabling policies to remove market barriers	– Expand incentives (e.g., tax credits, loans, grants) and standards to enhance technological innovation and bring new technologies to market, including demonstration – Remove barriers to the deployment of existing resilient commercial technologies
Technical information, assistance and decision support tools	– Provide downscaled extreme weather and climate science information to characterize current and future risks – Improve methodologies to quantify costs and benefits, and make the business case for resilience investments – Adopt resilience metrics to allow evaluation of progress and performance of resilience investments
Partnerships with agencies and other stakeholders	– Enhance climate resilience planning and implementation, and sharing of lessons learned, best practices, information, tools, and methods for resilience planning

13.4 Analytical approaches for assessing costs and benefits of resilience investments

Evaluating the costs and benefits of potential resilience improvements is an important step in the analytical process for utilities as they are developing climate resilience strategies. To help prioritize investments and enable cost-recovery, most utilities are required to demonstrate that identified resilience projects would yield net benefits for their customers. However, existing risk management frameworks that apply to reliability projects are not always adequate for planning resilience projects to address climate change. It is therefore necessary to enhance current approaches while developing new tools and methodologies. Another challenge is that there are no established methods for calculating the benefits of resilience improvements, particularly given the probabilistic nature of estimating impacts associated with future events. Utilities will need to develop strategies for prioritizing and implementing their resilience solutions (Dumas et al, 2019, Zamuda et al, 2019a).

In the absence of an industry adopted standard cost-benefit method, a wide variety of methods and approaches are being used. A brief review of methods used by utilities is provided to illustrate the variety of approaches used. The case studies include: (1) Con Edison and their use of a risk reduction prioritization method to evaluate their resiliency investments; (2) Public Service Electric and Gas Energy Strong program that employs data from value of lost load studies into a break-even analysis; and (3) Entergy that employs an Incremental Cost Analysis to prioritize and assess the value of possible resilience improvements (Dumas et al, 2019, Zamuda et al, 2019a).

13.4.1 Consolidated Edison of New York (Con Edison) case study: risk prioritization model

Con Edison developed a resilience plan motivated by its recovery from the impacts of Superstorm Sandy in 2012. Hardening efforts were completed between 2014 and 2016 as part of a plan approved by the New York State Public Service Commission (Con Edison, 2013, 2015). These efforts focused on mitigating the risk of flooding for components of the utility's electric, gas, and steam infrastructure. Example hardening measures for electricity assets undertaken by Con Edison included: (1) Installing submersible components at assets within the FEMA + 3-feet flood zones; (2) Modifying the distribution network to reduce the number of outages that would occur in the case of a failure of part of the overhead network (i.e., due to a downed tree); (3) Undergrounding of select segments of the distribution network; and (4) Taking measures to prevent flooding and water intrusion at substations, e.g., installing flood doors, shrink wrapping equipment, caulking and adding seals, and increasing on-site backup power supply.

Con Edison developed a method for evaluating and prioritizing resilience improvement projects in a model that establishes the value of each of their storm hardening initiatives in terms of the magnitude of risk that is reduced per asset (Con Edison, 2013). The following equation describes the risk reduction potential in terms of change in R or risk:

$$\Delta R = pB \cdot PT \cdot DB - pA \cdot PT \cdot DA$$

In this expression, pB and pA are the flooding or wind damage probabilities before or after the resiliency efforts, respectively, PT is the total population, affected by power outages, and DB and DA are the outage durations before or after the storm hardening initiatives, respectively. Con Edison's method of project prioritization involves these risk assessments, where each project is analyzed to determine its potential to reduce risk; and then individual projects are ranked in order of risk-reducing potential. Con Edison developed this risk-reduction prioritization model to show that proposed capital funding was being appropriately allocated to maximize risk reduction to the most critical assets. The model assumes that all proposed hardening projects will be undertaken. It was not intended to be a standalone tool for determining project value or deciding which projects to undertake.

In Phase III of Con Edison's Storm Hardening and Resiliency Collaborative Report, a model was developed to demonstrate the value of each storm-hardening program from an avoided economic-cost perspective (Con Edison, 2015). This method utilizes LBNL's VOLL database from 2009, along with the annual kWh by customer class data for each asset to determine potential outage costs pre- and post-resiliency investments. Then the simple difference is computed on an asset-by-asset basis between the pre-investment and post-investment impact costs to estimate the monetary impact reduction that can be expected from each storm hardening initiative. Con Edison intends to use its economic cost-benefit analysis alongside its risk prioritization method to determine budgets for resiliency improvements.

13.4.2 Public Service Electric & Gas (PSE&G) case study: break-even analysis

PSE&G identified vulnerabilities to its distribution system and resilience measures for these assets as part of its Energy Strong (ES) program. Much of the development of it resilience program occurred after the impacts of Hurricane Irene in 2011 and Superstorm Sandy in 2012. Resilience response measures were approved by the New Jersey Board of Public Utilities. Some of the approved hardening measures included: (1) Elevating switching and substations to the higher of the FEMA + 1 foot level or 1 foot above the observed flood level in 2011–2012; (2) Installing more efficient HVAC systems at large customers, including hospitals; and (3) Deploying distributed solar generation and microgrids. The utility partnered with a university to develop a sea level rise model it can use to evaluate future elevating requirements.

In the development of the PSE&G resilience plan, and engagement with the New Jersey Board of Public Utilities that must approve plans, PSE&G requested that The Brattle Group review the ES program to estimate the potential benefits that may be realized from these investments (Zarakas et al, 2014). A major challenge to assessing the benefits of resilience investments is the difficulty in estimating and applying the probabilities associated with the occurrence of the severe weather and the impact that such events may have on utility infrastructure. The uncertainty makes it difficult to perform cost-benefit analysis when the expected value of investment costs and benefits are largely unknown and probabilistic.

The Brattle Group introduced the break-even approach as an alternative outlook for evaluating resiliency investments. This approach uses the estimated costs and benefits in a method that incorporates the probability of severe weather to help determine the value of each investment. The benefit of ES investments is calculated by estimating the number of customer outages during major weather events that ES investments would mitigate and estimating the value that PSE&G's customers place on avoiding extended outages during extreme weather events. This analysis uses the value of lost load (VOLL) method to determine how PSE&G's customers value interruptions to their electric services. Then VOLL data is used in a break even analysis to determine the benefit to customers for ES Electric investments.

The value of the investment is given in minutes of customer interruption (CMI) that could be mitigated over the lifetime of the investment. The "break-even" point is the interruption time that has value of lost load equivalent to the cost of the investment (Zarakas et al, 2014). The break-even point can be defined as $E(B) - C = 0$, where $E(B)$ are expected benefits and C is the predetermined cost of the investment.

$$E(B) = \text{(Probability of weather event)} \times \text{(Resiliency investment mitigation impact on outage minutes given)} \quad (13.1)$$

If $E(B) - C = 0$ and C is known, then $E(B)$ or VOLL times unserved kWh can be used to back solve for the components of $E(B)$ in (13.1) to give the number hours/days of outage to "pay-back" resiliency investment. Then the value of the investment can then be compared to historical outage data and the probabilities of outages associated with climate risks in the future to the break-even number of outage days to assess the expected benefits of the investment (Zarakas et al, 2014).

Through this analysis, it was determined that the proposed ES program would result in reductions in the number and duration of outages caused by severe weather events, providing value to customers. The Brattle Group analysis found that this value "breaks even" or is equal to the cost of the proposed ES program for cumulative outage durations of three days (Fox-Penner and Zarakas, 2013). They note that "either through a single major future weather event, such as another Hurricane Sandy, or from the combination of lesser weather events taking place over the course of the life of the ES assets customers would realize the value of the investments." In this analysis, benefits are calculated as avoided costs to customers during outages. The Brattle Group recognized that "additional benefits to society from resilience improvements are apparent" and could further justify the benefit of the ES investments, but those additional benefits were not evaluated in their study.

Addressing indirect cost-benefits to the electricity sector

Costs-benefits analysis of resilience investment should consider the range of categories including direct and indirect costs and benefits (Zamuda et al, 2019a). Typically the focus is on direct costs and benefits to utilities and to customers, but generally not the broader category of costs and benefits to society for a reliable and resilience electricity system. For example, spillover effects can result in lost revenue and increased costs to businesses resulting from long duration outages (Sullivan and Schellenberg, 2013). These indirect costs to commercial and industrial customers represent the chain reaction of economic losses stemming from direct costs: interactions between businesses (e.g., changes in quantities of inputs bought or outputs sold, changes in relative prices) and interactions between consumers and businesses (e.g., lost wages and reduced spending). Indirect costs are thus incurred not only by people and firms subject to an outage, but also to people and firms outside of the affected area. Additionally, outage costs associated with public expenditures (e.g., assistance programs, emergency services, loss of taxes), public goods (e.g., water treatment) and injury or loss of life can be considered a part of indirect costs and inversely, investments that reduce the outages can result in both direct and indirect benefits including operation of government and national security, maintaining critical infrastructure (hospitals, police, water treatment, etc.), safety, tax revenue, economy, jobs, avoided increases in insurance premiums.

In addition to electricity system resilience investments, there are a number of investments that while not traditionally pursued to enhance electricity system resilience may cost-effectively do so. For example, studies have demonstrated the cost effectiveness of wetlands preservation to avoid or minimize coastal flooding.

13.4.3 Entergy's case study: building a resilient Gulf Coast

Entergy dates its company resilience planning to Hurricane Betsy of 1965. After the storm severely impacted Entergy's service territory, the company began installing assets with strengths exceeding the National Electric Safety Code (NESC) requirements. Further system hardening was undertaken since the landfall of Hurricane Katrina in 2005, including additional measures to harden the system, incorporate resilience into long-term planning processes, and investments in studies of the resilience of external systems, like the community and the utility's customers. Specific examples include: (1) No longer using wood poles for transmission lines; (2) Elevating at-risk distribution centers; (3) Deploying Advanced Meter Infrastructure; and (4) Considering an internal Resiliency Peer Group to coordinate resilience actions across business divisions and share information. In 2010, Entergy Corporation partnered with America's Energy Coast, America's Wetlands Foundation, McKinsey & Co.,

Analytical approaches for assessing costs and benefits

and Swiss Re to develop a framework for quantifying climate risks to better inform plans to build a resilient Gulf Coast (Entergy, 2010).

In the analysis, a hazard module, a value module, and a vulnerability module were used to determine expected loses under three different climate change scenarios. The value of current assets is assessed spatially across the coast, then project value of those assets in 2030 was determined. In the Entergy study, Gulf Coast assets were estimated to be worth $2 trillion and are projected to be over $3 trillion by 2030. In addition to asset value information, vulnerability assessments also informed their estimations of expected losses. The expected losses are calculated with data from their assessments of hazard (severity and frequency of hazard for different climate change scenarios), value (assets, incomes, and human elements), and vulnerability (functions of vulnerability to hazards given different climate scenarios and values of assets).

The expected loss values are used to create cost-benefit ratios for various resilience solutions which are represented in a numerical value of cost per unit of benefit (Figure 13.3). In their analysis, all solutions with cost-to-benefit ratios less than 2 are considered to be economically viable, taking into account positive externalities (additional co-benefits) not quantified in the cost-to-benefit analysis. Due to data propriety, the exact methods used to determine costs and benefits for this analysis are not public. However, it would be useful for other utilities interested in duplicating this method, if a publicly available framework with more detailed steps could be created, based upon this methodology.

For the purposes of this analysis, Entergy employed an Incremental Cost Analysis to prioritize and assess the value of possible resilience improvements. They developed their analysis based on estimates of societal costs and benefits rather than a focus on an individual firm. It is worth noting that Entergy's

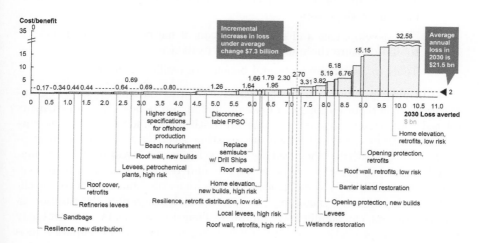

FIGURE 13.3: Cost-benefit ratios for various resilience solutions along the Gulf Coast. Source: Entergy (2010).

society approach to valuing resilience diverges from the norm; most costbenefit studies focus only on the direct costs incurred by the utility or its customers. Different resilience measures are compared on an overall cost curve. The width of each bar in the cost curve represents the total potential of that measure to reduce expected losses up to 2030, for a given scenario. The height of each bar represents the ratio between costs and benefits for that measure.

13.5 Gaps and opportunities for improvement in resilience planning

Significant advances have been made in the methods, tools, and metrics used for evaluating and planning to improve electricity system reliability and resilience. However, there are also still significant gaps and opportunities for improvement in the electricity technologies, tools, and methods in practice (DOE, 2015b, 2017a, NAS, 2017). Several key gaps are discussed in this section and include:

1. The collection, organization, and access to data relevant to climate resiliency planning.
2. Research, development, and deployment of innovative electricity technologies that enhance resilience and are cost effective.
3. The development of resilience codes and standards to foster the design of resilient electricity systems to address current extreme weather threats and projected climate change impacts over the lifespan of the assets.
4. The development and standardization of metrics that are specific to and capture the unique facets of resilience.
5. Tools to determine costs and benefits of resilient solutions.

Multiple gaps exist in accessible extreme weather data at the level of granularity that is required for local decision making on policies and investments related to electricity resilience. Data are critical for understanding the current and future extent to which our existing electricity system is vulnerable and in prioritizing the need for future resilience investments. Informational challenges prevent access to or full understanding of climate projections, vulnerabilities, and resilience solutions. Scientific uncertainty about climate change impacts, including the severity and geographic distribution of certain impacts, can significantly inhibit resilience investments. Planners may lack access to projections of local climate impacts that could support decision making on local resilience solutions, such as facility siting and hardening measures. Informational challenges also arise in translating climate projections into specific actions for energy asset planners, owners, and operators.

Improved informational resources are needed to assess the potential limitations of resilience actions over a range of spatial and temporal scales (including high-impact/low-probability events). Improved approaches could better characterize both the individual and aggregate climate change vulnerabilities of energy systems and lead to a better understanding of the associated probabilities and uncertainties, as well as, the interdependencies among sectors (e.g., manufacturing, transportation, communications, water supply and treatment, and health care) that can lead to cascading impacts.

Efforts are ongoing to increase access to resilience information, tools and methods. For example, DOE has collaborated with NOAA, NASA, and electric utilities to identify useful tools, information, and subject matter expertise to help make the electricity system more resilient. This information has been made available to the public using the US Climate Resilience Toolkit (NOAA, 2020), a federal inter-agency initiative operating under the auspices of the United States Global Change Research Program. The website is managed by NOAA's Climate Program Office and is hosted by NOAA's National Centers for Environmental Information. The Toolkit offers information from all across the US federal government in one easy-to-use location. The goal is to improve people's ability to understand and manage their extreme weather and climate-related risks and opportunities.

Another example of ongoing efforts to enhance information and tools is DOE's development of a comprehensive resilience modeling system for the North American energy sector and its associated infrastructure (DOE, 2019). Initiated in 2019, the North American Energy Resilience Model (NAERM) will advance existing capabilities to model, simulate, and assess the behavior of electric power systems, as well as associated dependencies on natural gas, and other critical energy infrastructures. The NAERM will enable the systematic identification of threats to the nation's energy infrastructure, the development of market approaches for resilience investments to reduce exposure to these threats, and enhanced situational awareness and sophisticated analytics to minimize the impact of threats and increase resiliency as they evolve in real time. The ultimate goal of the project is to provide real-time situational awareness and analysis capabilities for emergency events and optimal operations and recovery, enabling the federal government and industry to quickly and effectively prepare and respond.

Developing innovative electricity technologies that are less vulnerable to extreme weather and climate change is critically important. While many impacts are anticipated, there is no single technology solution, and the resilience of any technology option will ultimately be measured by its ability to remain operational under a broad range of environmental conditions. Opportunities for developing innovative electricity technologies that contribute to enhanced resilience could include: Operational and infrastructure improvements to enhance safety, reliability, and performance of transmission and distribution systems, including measures to create additional system capacity and redundancy; Practical models and tools for integrating renewable resources, demand side management, and alternative energy storage technologies; Improved design standards for specific components of the smart grid and protective measures for lightning, wildfires, wind, flooding, and other extreme events; Optimized storage technologies for varied load profiles, including onsite storage; Improved grid monitoring capabilities and dispatch protocols to manage more varied load scenarios and improve timely restoration of power; Development and use of microgrids, controlled islanding, distributed generation, and technologies to maintain service and minimize system vulnerabilities in response to possible climate disruptions of the power grid; and Placement of substations and other critical local electricity infrastructure in locations that are not anticipated to be affected by flooding and storm surges.

Resilience-based design codes and standards are also critical to ensuring infrastructure is built to withstand current and future extreme weather threats or climate change. The majority of codes and standards applicable to the electricity system are focused on reliability and the design, operation and maintenance of the electricity system. Codes and standards applicable to the electricity system have been developed by several national and international organizations, including: North American Electric Reliability Corporation (NERC); the National Electric Safety Code (NESC) developed by the Institute of Electrical and Electronics Engineers (IEEE); the National Electrical Code (NEC); the American Society of Heating, Refrigerating and Air-Conditioning Engineers (ASHRAE); and the International Code Council (ICC). The ICC codes include the International Building Code, the International Residential Code, the International Fire Code, the International Energy Conservation Code, and the International Woodland and Urban Interface Code.

Generally, the codes and standards developed by these organizations apply to the safety and reliability of the electricity system and typically do not directly address resilience to extreme weather events. In the limited cases where the requirements do address resilience to extreme weather, such as extreme wind, they generally use historic data rather than current or projected data for resilience planning. In many cases, certain components of the electricity system are exempt from compliance. For example, the nation's transmission and distribution infrastructure is designed to meet the NESC standard for extreme weather. NESC 250C is used for higher winds typically found along the coastline and during extreme events. However, the NESC wind maps rely on historic information and do not incorporate current wind profiles or projections of future wind threats to allow resilience over the expected lifespan of the asset. In addition, the extreme wind performance criteria for utility pole structures only apply to poles that are higher than 60 feet above the ground, and poles under 60 feet in height are exempt from compliance with the extreme wind performance criteria. This exemption results in significant reductions in size and strength of utility poles in vulnerable areas. For example, approximately 90% of the utility poles in Puerto Rico, Florida, and other southeastern states subject to extreme wind conditions are exempt from compliance with the extreme wind standard. During hurricanes Irma and Maria over 50,000 and 20,000 utility poles were damaged or destroyed in Puerto Rico and Florida, respectively (APPA, 2017).

Advances are needed in the development and the adoption of resilience-based codes and standards. While many studies have demonstrated the value of resilience investments (Multihazard Mitigation Council, 2005, 2017), many states and communities have not adopted building codes and standards. However, federal legislation is expanding the use of codes and standards for federally funded resilience programs. For example, the Disaster Recovery Reform Act of 2018 (DRRA; FEMA, 2018) directed FEMA to adopt hazard-based codes and standards for building back better after major disasters. As amended by Section 1235(b) of the DRRA, Section 406(e) requires FEMA to fund repair, restoration, reconstruction, or replacement of residential structures and facilities (e.g., electric power, buildings, roads, bridges, potable water supply, wastewater, etc.) in conformity with the latest published editions of relevant consensus-based codes, specifications, and standards that incorporate the latest hazard-resistant design (FEMA, 2019b).

There is a lack of qualitative and quantitative resilience metrics that are widely used today to measure the vulnerability of electricity systems and the effectiveness of resilience investments. Due to lack of resilience metrics some utilities are using reliability metrics to evaluate resilience investments. However, reliability metrics do not adequately characterize the full suite benefits of resilience investments. The reliability metrics and tools primarily only measure "blue-sky" conditions, not extreme weather conditions. They also primarily rely on customer survey data for short-term outages rather than the long-term outages that tend to follow extreme weather.

Development of resilience metrics for the electricity system is ongoing across the public and private sector. For example, the US Department of Energy in collaboration with the National Laboratories are developing metrics for quantifying resilience as part of a multi-year project under the DOE Grid Modernization Consortium (GMLC, 2017). The work has focused on performance-based metrics that provide a quantitative characterization of how resilient is the electricity system, as well as attribute-based metrics that evaluate the presence of key electricity system characteristics in the system that contribute to resilience. In addition, maturity models have been used by utilities to assess an organization's resilience capabilities to a range of threats (i.e., extreme weather, cyber and physical threats). For example, DOE's Electricity Subsector Cybersecurity Capability Maturity Model provides a set of characteristics, attributes, indicators that represent capability and progression for a electric grid resilient to cybersecurity threats (DOE, 2014b). Zamuda et al (2019b) offer one such model for evaluating electric utility resilience capabilities to extreme weather and climate threats. The model focuses on eight domains (i.e., Governance and Accountability, Stakeholder Engagement, Communication, Risk Management, Investments, Supply Chains, Services, and Employees). For each domain, a discussion of management practices is provided along with illustrative examples. In addition, the discussion addresses how these management practices could be structured in a framework progressing through five levels of maturity (i.e., Initiating, Progressing, Optimizing, Leading, and Pioneering). The five levels represent defined stages of an organization's progress toward achieving its resilience vision. By assessing its current maturity level for each attribute and taking steps to increase its levels as appropriate, an organization will move closer to obtaining the desired benefits of an effective resilience strategy.

Limitations have been identified in the current tools and methods that are being used to determine costs and benefits of resilience projects. There are currently many approaches as highlighted in this chapter for guiding resilience planning but having a common framework could be helpful for utilities in their resilience planning.

As the DOE's Quadrennial Energy Review suggests, common analytical frameworks and tools are needed to help set priorities for and justify expenditures in climate resilience (DOE, 2015b). Particularly, there are specific cost-benefit tools, such as the Interruption Cost Estimate (ICE) Calculator (DOE, 2017b), used to estimate the value of lost load. FEMA has developed the Benefit Cost Tool (FEMA, 2019a), used to perform benefit-cost analysis for applications submitted under FEMA's Hazard Mitigation Assistance grant programs (including applications for electricity system mitigation). Both of these tools have limitations and may not be appropriate for evaluating resilience projects because they cannot accurately predict the customer costs for long-term outages.

Work is ongoing at DOE, by other federal agencies and in other venues to address the challenges in quantifying the costs of climate impacts and the benefits of resilience improvements (for example, see Chapter 8 on detection of trends in losses from extreme weather and Chapter 9 on attribution of specific extreme events to climate change impacts).

As described in this chapter, climate change and extreme weather threaten the sustainable, affordable, and reliable supply of electricity across all regions of the United States. The exact character, severity, and timing of impacts will depend not only on changes in extreme weather events and climate, but also on the electricity system's exposure to risks and ability to enhance resilience in a timely manner. Given that electricity infrastructure investments made today will likely be in place for many decades, it is important that decision-makers have enough information, tools, and cost-effective resilient technologies to make sound technical and economic decisions. Continuing to identify potential impacts to the existing and future US electricity infrastructure is essential, as is improving understanding of the technical and economic potential of alternative innovative technologies and possible limits of those options. Innovative research and development efforts involving both private and public stakeholders and supporting policy frameworks could address existing market barriers and enable the development and deployment of the next generation of resilient electricity technologies.

Resilience to extreme weather and climate change requires ongoing improvements in multiple areas, many of which are described in this chapter, as well as an improved understanding and commitment by individuals, businesses, governments, and others. Efforts to improve the capacity to predict, prepare for, and avoid adverse impacts must span multiple economic sectors and levels of government. These efforts include the deployment of electricity technologies that are more resilient, assessment of vulnerabilities in the electricity system, resilience planning efforts, and policies that can facilitate these efforts. A significant number of actions underway described in this chapter may have been undertaken for reasons other than creation of a more resilient energy system and may have co-benefits in addition to increasing preparedness to extreme weather and climate change. These benefits include energy and national security, economic growth and job creation, emergency management and preparedness, public health, agricultural productivity, and ecosystem conservation, among others. The motivation and mechanisms to address electricity system vulnerabilities may vary across the nation and should be recognized in framing effective resilience strategies.

References

AAAS (2019) How We Respond: Community Responses to Climate Change. URL https://howwerespond.aaas.org, American Association for the Advancement of Science

APPA (2017) Puerto Rico needs 50,000 utility poles, 6,500 miles of cable. American Public Power Association. 10 October 2017

Bierkandt R, Auffhammer M, Levermann A (2015) US power plant sites at risk of future sea-level rise. Environmental Research Letters 10(12):124022

Campbell RJ (2012) Weather-related power outages and electric system resiliency. Tech. Rep. R42696, Congressional Research Service, Washington, DC, USA

COA (2013) Economic benefits of increasing electric grid resilience to weather outages. Tech. rep., The President's Council of Economic Advisers, Washington, DC

Con Edison (2013) Storm hardening and resiliency collaborative report. Tech. rep., Consolidated Edison Company of New York Inc., New York

Con Edison (2015) Storm hardening and resiliency collaborative phase three report. Tech. rep., Consolidated Edison Company of New York Inc., New York

Con Edison (2016) Con Edison close to completing $1 billion in post-Sandy storm protections. Tech. rep., Consolidated Edison Company of New York Inc., New York

Dieter CA, Maupin MA, Caldwell RR, Harris MA, Ivahnenko TI, Lovelace JK, Barber NL, Linsey KS (2018) Estimated use of water in the United States in 2015. US Geological Survey Circular 1441

DOE (2013) U.S. energy sector vulnerabilities to climate change and extreme weather. Tech. rep., U.S. Department of Energy, Washington, DC

DOE (2014a) Effects of sea level rise and storm surge on energy assets for select major metropolitan areas. Tech. rep., US Department of Energy, Washington, DC, USA

DOE (2014b) Electricity Subsector Cybersecurity Capability Maturity Model (ES-C2M2). Version 1.1 February 2014. US Department of Energy

DOE (2015a) Climate change and the US energy sector: Regional vulnerabilities and resilience solutions. Tech. rep., US Department of Energy, Washington, DC

DOE (2015b) Transforming US energy infrastructures in a time of rapid change: The first installment of the quadrennial energy review. Tech. rep., US Department of Energy, Washington, DC

DOE (2017a) Transforming the nation's electricity system: The second installment of the QER. Tech. rep., US Department of Energy, Washington, DC

DOE (2017b) Valuation of energy security for the United States. Tech. rep., US Department of Energy, Washington, DC

DOE (2019) North American Energy Resilience Model. Office of Electricity. Tech. rep., US Department of Energy, Washington, DC

Dumas MR, Binita K, Cunliff C (2019) Extreme weather and climate vulnerabilities of the electric grid: A summary of environmental sensitivity of quantification methods. Tech. Rep. ORNL/TM-2019/1252, Oak Ridge National Laboratory, Oak Ridge, TN

Entergy (2010) Building a resilient energy gulf coast: Executive report. Tech. rep., Entergy, Inc., New Orleans, LA

EPA (2016) Climate change indicators in the United States. Tech. rep., US Environmental Protection Agency (EPA), Washington, DC

EPA (2017) Multi-model Framework for Quantitative Sectoral Impacts Analysis: A Technical Report for the Fourth National Climate Assessment. Tech. Rep. EPA 430-R-17-001, US Environmental Protection Agency (EPA), Washington, DC

Exelon (2015) The Exelon Corporation Sustainability Report. Tech. rep., Exelon, Inc., Chicago, IL

FEMA (2018) Disaster Recovery Reform Act of 2018. Washington, DC, US Federal Emergency Management Agency (FEMA)

FEMA (2019a) Benefit Cost Toolkit Version 6.0. US Federal Emergency Management Agency (FEMA)

FEMA (2019b) Consensus-Based Codes, Specifications and Standards for Public Assistance FEMA Recovery Interim Policy FP-104-009-11 Version 2.1. US Federal Emergency Management Agency (FEMA)

Fox-Penner P, Zarakas W (2013) Analysis of benefits: PSE&G's energy strong program. Tech. rep., Public Service Electric and Gas

References

GAO (2014) Climate change: Energy infrastructure risks and adaptation efforts. Tech. rep., Government Accounting Office (GAO), Washington, DC

GMLC (2017) Grid Modernization: Metrics Analysis (GML C1.1). Reference Document. Version 2.1. May 2017

Kenward A, Yawitz D, Raja U (2013) Sewage overflows from Hurricane Sandy. Tech. rep., Climate Central

LaCommare KH, Eto JH, Dunn LN, Sohn MD (2018) Improving the estimated cost of sustained power interruptions to electricity customers. Energy 153:1038–1047

Larsen PH (2016a) A method to estimate the costs and benefits of undergrounding electricity transmission and distribution lines. Energy Economics 60:47–61

Larsen PH (2016b) Severe weather, power outages, and a decision to improve electric utility reliability. PhD thesis, Stanford University

Maloney MC, Preston BL (2014) A geospatial dataset for US hurricane storm surge and sea-level rise vulnerability: development and case study applications. Climate Risk Management 2:26–41

Multihazard Mitigation Council (2005) Natural hazard mitigation saves: An independent study to assess the future savings from mitigation activities. Tech. rep., National Institute of Building Sciences Multihazard Mitigation Council, Washington, DC

Multihazard Mitigation Council (2017) Natural hazard mitigation saves: 2017 interim report – summary of findings. Tech. rep., National Institute of Building Sciences Multihazard Mitigation Council, Washington, DC

NAS (2017) Enhancing the Resilience of the Nation's Electricity System. National Academies of Science, National Academies Press, Washington, DC

New York Power Authority et al (2017) Build back better: Reimagining and strengthening the power grid of Puerto Rico. Tech. rep., New York Power Authority, Puerto Rico Electric Power Authority, Puerto Rico Energy Commission, Consolidated Edison Company of New York, Inc., Edison International, Electric Power Research Institute, Long Island Power Authority, Smart Electric Power Alliance, US Department of Energy, Brookhaven National Laboratory, National Renewable Energy Laboratory, Pacific Northwest National Laboratory, Grid Modernization Lab Consortium, and PSEG Long Island, an agent for and on behalf of the Long Island Lighting Company d/b/a LIPA, and Navigant Consulting, Inc.

NOAA (2018) US Billion-Dollar Weather and Climate Disasters: Summary Stats. NOAA National Centers for Environmental Information (NCEI)

NOAA (2020) 2010–2019: A landmark decade of US billion-dollar weather and climate disasters. URL https://www.climate.gov/news-features/blogs/beyond-data/2010-2019-landmark-decade-us-billion-dollar-weather-and-climate, National Oceanic and Atmospheric Administration (NOAA)

PG&E (2016) Climate change vulnerability assessment and resilience strategies. Tech. rep., Pacific Gas and Electric Company, San Francisco, CA

Preston BL, Backhaus SN, Ewers M, Phillips JA, Silva-Monroy CA, Dagle JE, Tarditi AG, Looney J, King Jr TJ (2016) Resilience of the U.S. electricity system: A multi-hazards perspective. Tech. rep., Argonne National Laboratory, Brookhaven National Laboratory, Los Alamos National Laboratory, Oak Ridge National Laboratory, Pacific Northwest National Laboratory, Sandia National Laboratories

Rhodium Group LLC (2014) American Climate Prospectus: Economic Risks in the United States. Prepared as input to the Risky Business Project. Rhodium Group, New York, NY

Rhodium Group LLC (2017) Assessing the Effect of Rising Temperatures: The Cost of Climate Change to the US Power Sector. Rhodium Group, New York, NY

Seattle City Light (2015) Climate change vulnerability assessment and adaptation plan. Tech. rep., Seattle City Light, Seattle, WA

SEC (2019) Pacific Gas and Electric Annual Report Pursuant to Sections 13 or 15(d) of the Securities Exchange Act of 1934 for the fiscal year ended December 31, 2018. Securities and Exchange Commission (SEC)

Sullivan MJ, Schellenberg J (2013) Downtown San Francisco Long Duration Outage Cost Study. Freeman, Sullivan & Company, San Francisco, CA

US Energy Information Administration (2017) Electricity Data Browser. URL https://www.eia.gov/electricity/data/browser/#/, accessed on 2017-03-21

USGCRP (2014) Third National Climate Assessment. Washington, DC, URL https://nca2014.globalchange.gov/report

USGCRP (2017) Climate science special report. In: Wuebbles DJ, Fahey DW, Hibbard KA, Dokken DJ, Stewart BC, Maycock TK (eds) Fourth National Climate Assessment, vol 1, US Global Change Research Program, Washington, DC

USGCRP (2018) Impacts, risks, and adaptation in the United States. In: Reidmiller DR, Avery CW, Easterling DR, Kunkel KE, Lewis KLM, Maycock TK, C SB (eds) Fourth National Climate Assessment, vol 2, U.S. Global Change Research Program, Washington, DC

van Vliet MTH, Wiberg D, Leduc S, Riahi K (2016) Power-generation system vulnerability and adaptation to changes in climate and water resources. Nature Climate Change 6(4):375–380

Weiss DJ, Weidman J (2013) Pound foolish: Federal community-resilience investments swamped by disaster damages. Tech. rep., Center for American Progress

Zamuda CD (2018) Electricity sector resilience strategies: Current practices and lessons learned. Tech. rep., US Department of Energy, Washington, DC, USA

Zamuda CD, Bilello DE, Conzelmann G, Mecray E, Satsangi A, Tidwell V, Walker BJ (2018) Energy supply, delivery, and demand. In: Reidmiller DR, Avery CW, Easterling DR, Kunkel KE, Lewis KLM, Maycock TK, C SB (eds) Impacts, Risks, and Adaptation in the United States: Fourth National

Climate Assessment, vol 2, U.S. Global Change Research Program, Washington, DC, 174–201

Zamuda CD, Larsen PH, Collins MT, Bieler S, Schellenberg J, Hees S (2019a) Monetization methods for evaluating investments in electricity system resilience to extreme weather and climate change. The Electricity Journal 32(9):106641

Zamuda CD, Wall T, Guzowski L, Bergerson J, Ford J, Lewis LP, Jeffers R, DeRosa S (2019b) Resilience management practices for electric utilities and extreme weather. The Electricity Journal 32(9):106642

Zarakas WP, Sergici S, Bishop H, Zahniser-Word J, Fox-Penner P (2014) Utility investments in resiliency: Balancing benefits with cost in an uncertain environment. The Electricity Journal 27(5):31–41

14

Impacts of Inclement Weather on Traffic Accidents in Mexico City

Sophie Bailey
University of Plymouth, Plymouth, United Kingdom

S. Marcelo Olivera-Villarroel
Metropolitan Autonomous University Cuajimalpa, Mexico City, Mexico

Vyacheslav Lyubchich
Chesapeake Biological Laboratory, University of Maryland Center for Environmental Science, Solomons, MD, USA

CONTENTS

14.1	Introduction	307
14.2	Data description	310
14.3	Methods	313
14.4	Results	316
14.5	Conclusions	320
References		321

14.1 Introduction

Traffic accidents are the leading cause of death amongst young people worldwide (aged 5–29 years; WHO, 2018) and is in the top-ten causes of overall mortality and morbidity. The majority of the victims are economically active people in developing countries—the accidents throw many families into poverty. Economic losses due to traffic accidents (including direct costs of emergency and long-term medical treatment and indirect costs) are high; in developing countries, the losses are twice the amount of international development assistance (Kapp, 2003). This chapter demonstrates analysis and forecasting of traffic accidents (Mexico City is taken as an example) using two well-established multivariate techniques that can be employed in assessing the impacts of inclement weather and forecasting traffic conditions for the intelligent transportation systems.

The main risks of traffic accidents include driving under the influence of alcohol or other psychoactive substances, the use of distractors, and breach of traffic regulations (Rolison et al, 2018, WHO, 2018). These risks are amplified in bad weather conditions, which cause restricted motorists' vision, decreased traction on tires, and increased stopping distance, especially when motorists are traveling at higher speeds (e.g., see Morris et al, 1977, Sun et al, 2011). By assessing the effects of the weather on traffic accidents we can better prepare for climate change, which is expected to make the weather events of a low individual but high cumulative impact more frequent and more severe (such events include severe rainstorms, snowfall, heat waves, etc. that are not classified as catastrophic).

Mexico has experienced a rapid growth of its motor vehicle fleet (from 15.6 million motor vehicles in 2000 to 40.0 million vehicles in 2015; INEGI, 2019), and road injuries have been identified as a public health problem (Aguirre Quezada, 2015, Valencia et al, 2009). In 2016, 7.8 out of 100,000 inhabitants of Mexico City died due to traffic accidents (SEDESA, 2019). In 2017, both in Mexico and its capital, Mexico City, road injuries were the second-most severe cause of death of people aged 15–49 (surpassed by interpersonal violence; IHME, 2019). Despite this, there has been no systematic quantitative analysis on the factors associated with the accidents in Mexico City and the relative place of weather effects within such factors.

Mexico City has subtropical highland climate, hence the main weather impacts are due to rain and heat events, not freezing rain or snow. Rain reduces visibility (increases the risk of collisions), but also makes drivers reduce their speed to avoid collisions with other vehicles and objects (e.g., see Black et al, 2017 and references therein). Once the rain has passed, the drivers are more confident to drive at higher speeds. In cities with flat topographies such as Mexico City, rainwater fills potholes on the road increasing the probability of a vehicle to fall into potholes that become invisible underwater. Potholes have become a common problem causing traffic jams and accidents, because the vehicles have to reduce the speed or do forced maneuvers (Rojas Barreth, 2018, Wambold et al, 1984).

Another risk factor that increases the probability of traffic accidents is excessive temperature. The heat accentuates the feeling of fatigue, which decreases alertness and concentration, and increases the reaction time of the drivers (Gao et al, 2016, Yaacob et al, 2019). Excessive heat also puts a burden on the engine cooling system and air circulation system inside the vehicle, which need to prevent moisture from fogging the glass and causing visibility problems or too dry air causing eye itching and irritation that can disturb driving.

Our literature search identified a number of studies that have researched how the weather impacts road traffic accidents. The studies use such methods as the matched pairs analysis (Black et al, 2017, Jaroszweski and McNamara, 2014, Omranian et al, 2018, Sun et al, 2011, Tamerius et al, 2016), case-crossover (Liu et al, 2017), regression analysis (Yaacob et al, 2019), and

Introduction

machine learning methods (Dong et al, 2018, Sathiaraj et al, 2018, Wahab and Jiang, 2019). For references on analysis of the distribution of accidents along road network, see Section 1.2.2 by Okabe and Sugihara (2012). The most popular method, matched pairs, can be summarized as quantifying the difference or ratio of the average number of accidents in a rainy period (usually, a day) and in a paired dry period of the same length and similar other characteristics. The definitions of dry and rainy periods and characteristics for selecting a pair differ from study to study and may require the paired days to be of the same type (holiday or not), of the same weekday, to be within a certain relatively short period from each other (to assume a similar traffic density for the pairs), etc. As a result, many (sometimes, arguable) choices make the studies hard to replicate or compare across; too restrictive rules for selecting a pair lead to small sample sizes; the results often quantify the effect of presence of rain, without interaction effects with temperature or other weather factors and without assessing how much of the accident variability is explained by weather compared to the other factors, such as traffic volume, season, or time of the day. The power of more advanced techniques, such as nonlinear statistical models and machine learning, for analysis of the factors affecting traffic accidents, remains underemployed.

The highlights of our study are as follows:

1. Our study provides both regression and machine learning perspectives to the problem of assessing the impacts of inclement weather on traffic accidents in Mexico City.

2. We use a larger data set compared to the previous studies (we use hourly data from 2001-01-01 to 2015-11-30).

3. Both of our methods (generalized additive modeling and random forest) are nonlinear and allow us to model interactions of different factors.

4. We model the accident rate based on weather variables and other factors (holidays, weekend effects, etc.) together, which allows us to compare the importance of the factors in predicting the number of accidents, without restricting our analysis just to the weather effects.

5. We normalize the number of accidents only by the annual number of registered cars, which implies we treat reductions of the traffic volume during inclement weather as an integral part of the weather effects and do not remove it from our analysis.

6. We compare the utility of our two methods and two data resolutions (hourly and daily) using out-of-sample forecasts on the testing set not used to train the models.

The workflow of our analysis is shown in Figure 14.1. We repeat it twice, using hourly and daily aggregated data, which yields four different types of

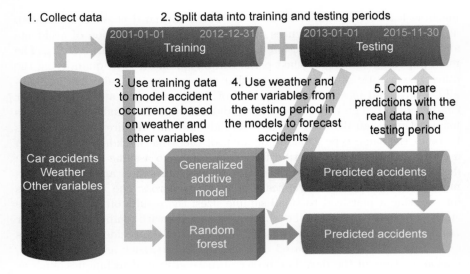

FIGURE 14.1: The implemented analysis workflow.

predictions we further compare to one another. The separate sections in the remainder of the chapter describe the data we used, applied methods, results, and conclusions of this study.

14.2 Data description

Here we present the data we used to study the effect of inclement weather on the number of car accidents in Mexico City, Mexico. The compiled data are available on GitHub.[1]

The accident database containing the date, time, and characteristics of each car accident in 2001–2015 was obtained from INEGI (2017). During this period, the total number of accidents was rising on average by 130 accidents (or 1.6%) per year (Figure 14.2). Collisions with motorcycles increased by 3.5 times (from 378 to 1320 per year), while collisions with pedestrians decreased by almost 3.9 times (from 1455 to 377 per year). Among the twelve types of accidents, the most frequent was a collision with other vehicles (65.6% of all accidents), followed by collisions with fixed objects (8.9%) and with motorcycles (8.0%).

One of the factors of the growing number of car accidents could be the increasing number of cars in the city. The number of vehicles registered in all

---

[1] https://github.com/vlyubchich/trafficMexicoCity (Lyubchich et al, 2020).

Data description

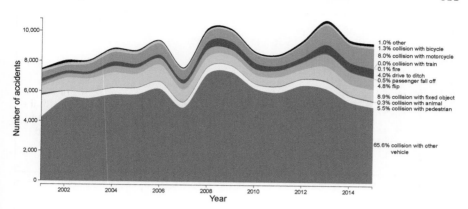

FIGURE 14.2: Number of car accidents per year in Mexico City, with percentages for each type in 2001–2015.

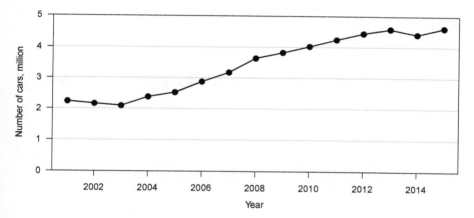

FIGURE 14.3: Number of cars registered in Mexico City, 2001–2015.

the municipalities of Mexico City (including official, public, and private vehicles) increased on average by 5.3% each year during the observed period, from 2.2 million vehicles in 2001 to 4.6 million in 2015 (Figure 14.3, the data were obtained from INEGI, 2019). To remove the effect of such an increase from our analysis, we calculated the *accident rate* as the number of car accidents per 100,000 registered vehicles.

We matched the accident data with hourly observations of *rainfall* and *air temperature* from five weather stations located in the city and its outskirts (PEMBU, 2017). The weather data were averaged across stations, which enabled us to characterize average weather conditions in the city and create consistent hourly time series with almost no missing values (less than 0.1% of missing values) from 2001-01-01 to 2015-11-30.

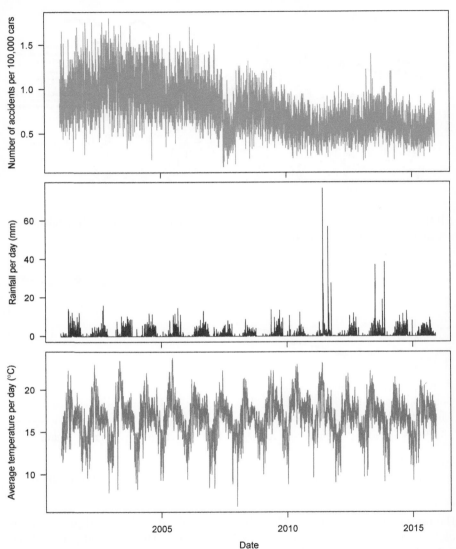

FIGURE 14.4: Time series plots of daily accident rate, total rainfall, and average air temperature in Mexico City, from 2001-01-01 to 2015-11-30.

The accidents and weather data were also aggregated within each day to obtain daily time series (Figure 14.4). One of the data issues we identified is that the hourly rainfall observations underestimate total daily or annual rainfall, which could be due to low sensitivity of the installed monitoring equipment unable to detect and record small amounts of rainfall.

Methods

Among other factors that could affect the number of accidents we considered *weekday* (as a categorical variable), *holiday* (a categorical variable denoting the days when the Mexico statutory holidays were observed[2]), and the implementation of the emissions control program Hoy No Circula. This environmental program restricts the operation of certain vehicles in Mexico City on certain days of the week (based on the last digit of the vehicle license plate number) from 5:00 to 22:00. The program has been operational Monday–Friday since 1990 (started well before our analysis period), but additional Saturday restrictions were implemented from 2008-07-05 (during the period of our analysis). The effects of the traffic restrictions on Monday–Friday can be captured by the weekday variable, but to account for the new restrictions on Saturdays we created a new categorical variable *HNCS* (Hoy No Circula Saturday) that takes on the value of 1 each Saturday starting 2008-07-05 and the value of 0 on all other days. The diurnal cycle in hourly data was captured using the numeric *hour* variable. Seasonal variations were captured with a categorical variable for the *months*, while the combined effect of all other factors influencing the year-to-year variability of the accident rate was represented by numeric *year*.

14.3 Methods

With an expectation of encountering complex relationships in the data (including nonlinear effects and interactions responsible for a combined effect), we chose flexible methods from statistics and machine learning for modeling the accident rate.

Generalized additive modeling

Let Y_t denote the accident rate at time t, and let $m_t \equiv E(Y_t)$ be the respective expected values. Using the framework of generalized additive modeling (GAM; Hastie et al, 2009, Wood, 2006), we estimate a semi-parametric model

$$\begin{aligned}m_t = {} & \alpha_{Month} + \alpha_{Weekday} + \alpha_{HNCS} + \alpha_{Holiday} \\ & + f_1(Year_t) + g_1(Rain_t, Temp_t) \\ & + f_2(Hour_t) + g_2(Rain_{t-1}, Temp_{t-1}),\end{aligned} \quad (14.1)$$

where the parametric part of the model is represented by the effects of categorical variables, α's; the nonparametric part includes smooth functions of the covariates approximated with cubic regression splines (f_1 and f_2) and tensor product smooths (g_1 and g_2). Model (14.1) is the full model for hourly

---

[2]The list of holidays was obtained from https://www.officeholidays.com/countries/mexico.

data. The same model built for daily data omits the hour effect, $f_2(\cdot)$, and the effect of inclement weather in the previous period, $g_2(\cdot)$. We used the R package mgcv (Wood, 2019) to fit these models.

The spline functions in GAM allow us to model a nonlinear interannual trend in m_t and complex shapes of relationships between accident rate and weather conditions. Penalization techniques employed in GAM protect against overfitting the data with excessively wiggly functions. For a not very technical introduction to smoothing methods and GAM, we refer the reader to Berk (2016). Also, see an example of applying GAMs to biodiversity indices in Chapter 5.

Random forest

Random forest (RF; Breiman, 2001) is a completely data-driven technique that is based on averaging predictions from a large number of individual regression trees (regression trees were introduced by Breiman et al, 1984).

Let $X_{i,t}$ ($i = 1, \ldots, p$) represent all independent variables, both categorical and numeric, employed for modeling the accident rate ($p = 10$ variables for hourly data and $p = 7$ variables for daily data). Without assuming any particular shape of relationship between the variables and the variable of interest (also termed the response variable, Y_t), a regression tree starts by selecting among all values of $X_{i,t}$ such a threshold value (let $X_{j,t} = s$ be such a value; $j = 1, \ldots, p$) that splits the response variable into two most distinct subsets:

$$R_1(j,s) = \{X|X_{j,t} \leqslant s\} \text{ and } R_2(j,s) = \{X|X_{j,t} > s\}.$$

If $X_{j,t}$ is a categorical variable, then s represents a specific category of $X_{j,t}$, and the subsets are formed as follows:

$$R_1(j,s) = \{X|X_{j,t} = s\} \text{ and } R_2(j,s) = \{X|X_{j,t} \neq s\}.$$

The subsets R_1 and R_2 can be split further, using another value of the same or another variable from $X_{i,t}$ ($i = 1, \ldots, p$). Let the resulting (terminal) subsets be indexed by k, then the fitted value or regression tree prediction of Y_t for a specific combination of x_i is the observed average value within the corresponding subset:

$$\hat{Y}_t(x_i) = \text{ave}(Y_t|x_i \in R_k).$$

Growing big (saturated) trees with many splits can reduce in-sample errors drastically (perfect goodness-of-fit); however, such trees are unstable (adding or removing a few observations may change the tree dramatically) and hard to interpret or generalize to other data sets.

The algorithm of random forest provides a better performance by aggregating predictions from a large number of trees. To grow many different regression trees from a single data set, two randomization techniques are implemented:

Methods

1. Each tree of a random forest is grown on a sample with replacement (bootstrap sample) of the original data.
2. Each split within a tree is attempted considering not all p variables, but a random subset of those. In the algorithms we implemented, the size of the subset was (rounded down) $\sqrt{p}$ (Wright and Ziegler, 2017).

After growing a random forest, the relative importance of each i-th variable $X_{i,t}$ for predicting Y_t can be assessed by permuting values of $X_{i,t}$ and comparing the prediction errors with the original, not permuted, case (the larger the difference between the errors, the more this i-th variable is important).

The relationships between Y_t and each $X_{j,t}$ learned by a random forest can be visualized using partial dependence plots, where averaged predictions are obtained by replacing all values of $X_{j,t}$ with each unique value of this variable, keeping all other variables $X_{i,t}$ intact $(i, j = 1, \ldots, p;\ i \neq j)$.

We used the R package `ranger` (Wright et al, 2020) to grow random forests and assess relative importance of the variables, and R packages `randomForest` (Breiman et al, 2018) and `plotmo` (Milborrow, 2019) to obtain partial dependence plots. Our random forest for hourly data contained 100 trees, for daily data—500 trees.

Performance evaluation

To assess and compare performance of the two very different modeling techniques (GAM and random forest), we split our data into two periods: training (2001-01-01 to 2012-12-31) and testing (2013-01-01 to 2015-11-30). We use the training period to fit the models, then use these models to forecast the accident rate for each hour or day of the testing period. We assume that forecasting performance reflects the quality of the model, i.e., how well the model represents the relationships in the data.

If Y_t is the observed accident rate in the testing period and $\hat{Y}_t$ is the predicted rate, then the prediction mean absolute error (PMAE) and root mean squared error (PRMSE) for each model and temporal resolution are calculated as follows:

$$PMAE = \frac{\sum_{t=1}^{n} |Y_t - \hat{Y}_t|}{n}; \quad PRMSE = \sqrt{\frac{\sum_{t=1}^{n}(Y_t - \hat{Y}_t)^2}{n}}, \quad (14.2)$$

where n is the size of the testing set ($n = 1064$ days or 25,536 hours).

The PMAE and PRMSE from (14.2) can be compared for models only of the same temporal resolution (for daily or hourly predictions). To compare the predictive accuracy across these resolutions, we calculate totals within each yearly subperiod of the testing set ($\sum_{t \in 2013} \hat{Y}_t$, $\sum_{t \in 2014} \hat{Y}_t$, and $\sum_{t \in 2015} \hat{Y}_t$) and compare with the observed totals ($\sum_{t \in 2013} Y_t$, $\sum_{t \in 2014} Y_t$, and $\sum_{t \in 2015} Y_t$).

14.4 Results

We started analysis of the accidents data in Mexico City by looking for potential combined effects of temperature and rainfall. Table 14.1 gives a coarse picture of such effects by segmenting the data using the temperature and rain quartiles. Within each column, we observe a slight decrease of average accident rates (when moving from low to high temperature). Among the rows, the changes in the first row are the strongest (accident rate increases when moving from light to heavy rain), i.e., the effect of heavy rain is different under different temperature conditions. Thus, Table 14.1 informs us about the existent interaction effects that can be modeled more precisely using the GAM and random forest techniques.

Generalized additive models

All parametric and smooth terms of GAMs applied to the daily and hourly data in the training period were considered statistically significant, based on the p-values for each model term. Model diagnostic checks did not identify serious violations of randomness of the residuals and non-concurvity[3] of the GAM smooth terms.

Based on the estimated coefficients, holidays and Saturdays with driving restrictions (HNCS) corresponded to a reduced accident rate. During the week, more accidents happened on Saturday, followed by Sunday and Friday. The seasonality was not strong, but generally fewer accidents happened during July–October. At the same time, June–September is the season with major precipitation amounts in Mexico City. Hence, the impact of heavy rain is dampened by generally better weather (higher temperatures), which is good for lessening the number of accidents.

TABLE 14.1: Average accident rate (number of accidents per 100,000 cars) under different weather conditions (standard deviations for the sample averages are in parentheses). The temperature thresholds are the quartiles of daily temperature; the rain thresholds are quartiles for days with rain, but the first interval also includes dry days

Temp. \ Rain	0–0.1 mm	0.2–0.7 mm	0.8–2.1 mm	2.2–76.9 mm
6.3–15.3 °C	0.79 (0.01)	0.80 (0.03)	0.85 (0.04)	0.80 (0.03)
15.4–16.8 °C	0.78 (0.01)	0.79 (0.02)	0.80 (0.02)	0.79 (0.02)
16.9–18.1 °C	0.75 (0.01)	0.74 (0.02)	0.74 (0.02)	0.79 (0.02)
18.2–23.9 °C	0.74 (0.01)	0.69 (0.02)	0.72 (0.02)	0.73 (0.03)

---

[3]Concurvity of terms in nonlinear model is analogous to collinearity of regressors in linear models.

Results

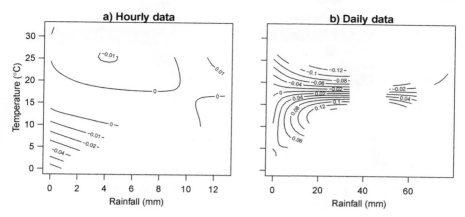

FIGURE 14.5: Contour plots of the tensor smooth terms $g_1(\cdot)$ from GAM (14.1). The numbers show estimated relative effect (the smooths are centered).

The contour plots in Figure 14.5 show the relative impact of rainfall and temperature represented in the tensor smooths. The contour lines connect weather conditions that are estimated to impact the accident rate in the same way. The density of the lines is chosen automatically to ensure readability, while some areas of the graph have no lines because of the data sparsity (there are not enough observations for a reliable estimation of the effects). Figure 14.5a shows an increase of the accident rate with more rain and decrease of the rate when both temperature and precipitation are low. The highest contour values are observed at high hourly temperature and rainfall. (A plot of the term $g_2(\cdot)$ for lagged hourly weather data showed a similar pattern and was omitted for brevity.) Figure 14.5b is a finer representation of Table 14.1, where the daily data cloud is separated by the zero-level line at approximately 17°C with two sets of concentric contours: the upper set shows a decrease of the accident rate at higher temperatures; the other set, below 17°C, shows an increase of the accident rate with lower temperatures and more rain (notice the contour lines in the bottom of Figure 14.5b are more curved, showing the effect of both rain and temperature, while the lines in the top part are less curved, with temperature having the primary effect).

Random forests

The random forests for hourly and daily data showed decreasing, then stabilizing errors with increasing number of trees. The stabilization of error suggested that the used number of trees was sufficient for stability of the results.

The rankings of the variables by their importance in the random forests (Figure 14.6) show that the time variables are the primary predictors of the accident rates: hour and year for the hourly accident rate, year, and weekday

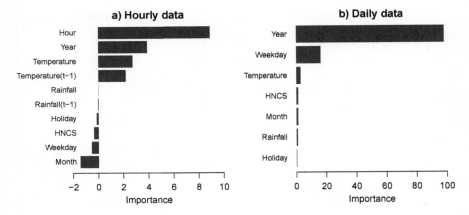

FIGURE 14.6: Relative importance of the variables in random forests.

for the daily rate. The weather variables demonstrate approximately median importance, with temperature being more important than rain in both random forests. Based on Figure 14.6a, the current weather conditions are more important than from the previous hour. The remaining variables representing month, holidays, and HNCS are generally ranked as less important for predicting the accident rate.

By using different variables in consecutive tree splits, random forests are capable of capturing complex interactions of the variables. The visualized interaction effects of temperature and rainfall captured by the random forests (Figure 14.7) are similar to the ones recorded in the GAM smooths (Figure 14.5), while contours by the random forests are more wiggly. Based on Figure 14.7, the random forest models identify high accident rates correspond

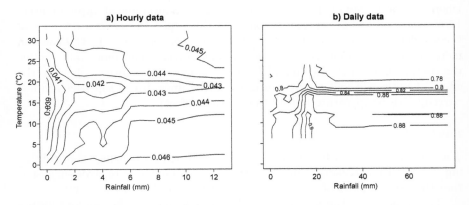

FIGURE 14.7: Partial dependence interaction plots from the random forests. The numbers show average predicted accident rate (noncentered).

Results

to low temperatures and high rainfall. Based on the hourly data, the accident rate is also high when both temperature and rainfall are high (top-right corner of Figure 14.7a), which agrees with the GAM findings.

Performance evaluation

Based on the after-sample evaluation of the models using the testing set (Table 14.2), random forests produce more accurate forecasts (lower PMAE and PRMSE) than GAMs. The differences are obvious when comparing the errors of models for daily data. The errors of GAM and RF using hourly data look more similar, but the hourly data set contains 24 times more observations than the daily data set, and even tiny errors can accumulate over many hours.

We compared all four models by calculating the aggregated predictions within each year (Table 14.3). In the testing period, we observe an overall decline of the accident rate from the training period (the average annual rate in the training period was 296 accidents per 100,000 registered cars). The aggregated predictions of random forests are much closer to the observed rates than GAM predictions are. With the aggregated values, the difference between the two types of models is evident in both hourly and daily data: random forest performs better than GAM, with particularly accurate predictions for 2014.

TABLE 14.2: Prediction mean absolute errors (PMAE) and prediction root mean squared errors (PRMSE) for the four models in the testing set from 2013-01-01 to 2015-11-30

Data	Model	PMAE	PRMSE
Hourly	GAM	0.019	0.026
	RF	0.019	0.025
Daily	GAM	0.189	0.223
	RF	0.113	0.143

TABLE 14.3: Total number of accidents per 100,000 cars registered in Mexico City: observed and predicted by four types of models in each of the annual sub-period of the testing set

Data	Model	2013	2014	2015 Jan–Nov
Observed	—	235	215	179
Predicted hourly	GAM	176	155	121
	RF	218	216	197
Predicted daily	GAM	174	152	116
	RF	216	217	198

Since all the numbers in Table 14.3 are on the same (annual) scale, we can compare models for hourly and daily data. Interestingly, the higher-frequency hourly data give only trivial advantage over daily data (total predictions from the models for hourly data are marginally closer to the observed rates than predictions from the models for daily data). Based on this specific example, the choice of a method for the analysis (GAM vs. random forest) plays a more important role than the data resolution (hourly vs. daily).

The compiled data and R code are available on GitHub[4] and can be used to reproduce the presented results.

14.5 Conclusions

This chapter presented a framework of statistical and machine learning analysis that can be implemented for assessing the impacts of inclement weather on road traffic accidents as well as for scenario analysis and predictions within intelligent transportation systems. The demonstrated methods—generalized additive models and random forests—are flexible and relatively easy to implement. The methods can be used to assess the role of each considered variable in explaining the variability of accident rate and, for example using the random forest, rank importance of the variables. While random forest is largely a "black box," its stellar performance in this study demonstrates a great potential of machine learning techniques in improving our forecasts for proactive adaptation to changing weather. See Chapter 12 for more examples where artificial intelligence and machine learning can step in.

We used a large data set to study the impact of inclement weather on the accident rate in Mexico City, using the two methods and two temporal resolutions, which resulted in four models. Based on the out-of-sample model evaluation, random forests performed considerably better than generalized additive models, high-frequency data (hourly) gave only a trivial advantage over lower-frequency data (daily).

The modeling results demonstrate a high importance of the temporal variables: hour and weekday (these variables mainly represent the relative traffic volumes in the city, hour of the day is also related to visibility conditions) and year (the interannual trend represents all other factors not included specifically into the models, such as the general changes in traffic regulations, road conditions, accumulated drivers' experience, and improving driving culture).

The discovered effects of temperature and rainfall on accidents in Mexico City are consistent with the literature on other locations. Intense heat increases the probability of accidents, which is particularly evident from the hourly data. Unfortunately, the hottest hours in Mexico City coincide with

---

[4]https://github.com/vlyubchich/trafficMexicoCity (Lyubchich et al, 2020).

the busiest hours between 14:30 and 16:30, lunchtime and school departure time.

The effects of the rain tend to be less pronounced in Mexico City compared with other locations studied in the literature because in Mexico City 1) rain mostly falls in summer, when weather is generally better, and 2) most rainy hours are 18:00 to 21:00 when the traffic volume goes down. The significance of lagged hourly data for predicting the accidents can be attributed to the waterlogging effect and the potholes invisible underwater, and the sudden reactions of drivers to these types of obstacles.

The joint analysis of temperature and rainfall in this study allows us to study the interaction effects of these factors, which are often analyzed separately in the literature. The temperature has a lethargic effect decreasing the reaction times of the drivers, while the rain has a multi-fold effect including decreasing traffic speeds, decreasing visibility of the road and, even after the rain stops, hiding the potholes underwater. Temperature and rainfall jointly generate the third effect very little analyzed in the literature—the fogging of the car windows leading to lower visibility. The effect of fogging is higher in older vehicles, which do not have modern defogging systems. Since Mexico City has a warm climate, we did not observe the frost effects that occur at low temperatures (e.g., icy roads, freezing rain, and snowfall). To account for the effect of long dry spells making roads more oily and dangerous if suddenly wet, we would need to consider longer lags of the weather variables in our analysis.

The results of studying interaction effects of multiple variables on the traffic accidents allow us to see beyond traditional analyses and to focus on joint solutions, such as revising the vehicle defogging systems, properties of tires, road surface, and drainage infrastructure in Mexico City.

Acknowledgments

SB and SMOV would like to thank the Chesapeake Biological Laboratory (CBL) of the University of Maryland Center for Environmental Science for support and hospitality during their stays at CBL, which helped to complete the work on this chapter.

References

Aguirre Quezada JP (2015) Accidentes automotrices como problema de salud pública. Tech. Rep. 17, Dirección General de Análisis Legislativo, Mexico City

Berk RA (2016) Statistical Learning from a Regression Perspective, 2nd edn. Springer Texts in Statistics, Springer, Cham, Switzerland

Black AW, Villarini G, Mote TL (2017) Effects of rainfall on vehicle crashes in six US states. Weather, Climate, and Society 9(1):53–70

Breiman L (2001) Random forests. Machine Learning 45(1):5–32

Breiman L, Friedman JH, Olshen RA, Stone CJ (1984) Classification and Regression Trees. Taylor & Francis, New York

Breiman L, Cutler A, Liaw A, Wiener M (2018) randomForest: Breiman and Cutler's Random Forests for Classification and Regression. URL https://CRAN.R-project.org/package=randomForest, R package version 4.6-14

Dong C, Shao C, Li J, Xiong Z (2018) An improved deep learning model for traffic crash prediction. Journal of Advanced Transportation 2018:3869106

Gao J, Chen X, Woodward A, Liu X, Wu H, Lu Y, Li L, Liu Q (2016) The association between meteorological factors and road traffic injuries: a case analysis from Shantou city, China. Scientific Reports 6:37300

Hastie TJ, Tibshirani RJ, Friedman JH (2009) The Elements of Statistical Learning: Data Mining, Inference, and Prediction, 2nd edn. Springer, New York

IHME (2019) Causes of death. Institute for Health Metrics and Evaluation (IHME), University of Washington. URL https://vizhub.healthdata.org/gbd-compare/, accessed 2019-10-17

INEGI (2017) Accidentes de tránsito terrestre en zonas urbanas y suburbanas. Instituto Nacional de Estadistica y Geografia (INEGI). URL https://www.inegi.org.mx/sistemas/olap/proyectos/bd/continuas/transporte/accidentes.asp, accessed 2017-04-04

INEGI (2019) Vehiculos de motor registrados en circulacion. Instituto Nacional de Estadistica y Geografia (INEGI). URL https://www.inegi.org.mx/programas/vehiculosmotor/, accessed 2019-11-26

Jaroszweski D, McNamara T (2014) The influence of rainfall on road accidents in urban areas: A weather radar approach. Travel Behaviour and Society 1(1):15–21

Kapp C (2003) WHO acts on road safety to reverse accident trends. The Lancet 362(9390):1125

Liu A, Soneja SI, Jiang C, Huang C, Kerns T, Beck K, Mitchell C, Sapkota A (2017) Frequency of extreme weather events and increased risk of motor vehicle collision in Maryland. Science of the Total Environment 580:550–555

Lyubchich V, Bailey S, Olivera-Villarroel SM (2020) Analysis of car accidents in Mexico City. URL https://doi.org/10.5281/zenodo.3723688, Zenodo

Milborrow S (2019) plotmo: Plot a Model's Residuals, Response, and Partial Dependence Plots. URL https://CRAN.R-project.org/package=plotmo, R package version 3.5.6

Morris RS, Mounce JM, Button JW, Walton NE (1977) Visual performance of drivers during rainfall. Transportation Research Record 628:19–25

Okabe A, Sugihara K (2012) Spatial Analysis along Networks: Statistical and Computational Methods. John Wiley & Sons, West Sussex, UK

Omranian E, Sharif H, Dessouky S, Weissmann J (2018) Exploring rainfall impacts on the crash risk on Texas roadways: a crash-based matched-pairs analysis approach. Accident Analysis & Prevention 117:10–20

PEMBU (2017) Programa de Estaciones Meteorológicas del Bachillerato Universitario. University Network of Atmospheric Observatories of the National Autonomous University of Mexico. URL https://www.ruoa.unam.mx/pembu/datos_historicos.html, accessed 2017-04-04

Rojas Barreth VH (2018) Diseño de un sistema electrónico de detección de baches para asistencia vehicular. PhD thesis, Universidad de Guayaquil. Facultad de Ingeniería Industrial, Guayaquil, Ecuador

Rolison JJ, Regev S, Moutari S, Feeney A (2018) What are the factors that contribute to road accidents? An assessment of law enforcement views, ordinary drivers' opinions, and road accident records. Accident Analysis & Prevention 115:11–24

Sathiaraj D, Punkasem To, Wang F, Seedah DPK (2018) Data-driven analysis on the effects of extreme weather elements on traffic volume in Atlanta, GA, USA. Computers, Environment and Urban Systems 72:212–220

SEDESA (2019) Mortalidad en Ciudad de México. Secretaría de Salud de la Ciudad de México (SEDESA). URL http://data.salud.cdmx.gob.mx/portal/index.php/informacion-en-salud/103-informacion-salud/354-mortalidad, accessed 2019-10-01

Sun X, Hu H, Habib E, Magri D (2011) Quantifying crash risk under inclement weather with radar rainfall data and matched-pair method. Journal of Transportation Safety & Security 3(1):1–14

Tamerius JD, Zhou X, Mantilla R, Greenfield-Huitt T (2016) Precipitation effects on motor vehicle crashes vary by space, time, and environmental conditions. Weather, Climate, and Society 8(4):399–407

Valencia JAA, Mondragón M, García AH, Aureoles EH (2009) Los accidentes viales, un grave problema de salud en el Distrito Federal. Acta Ortopédica Mexicana 23(4):204–208

Wahab L, Jiang H (2019) A comparative study on machine learning based algorithms for prediction of motorcycle crash severity. PloS One 14(4):e0214966

Wambold JC, Zimmer RA, Ross Jr HE, Ivey DL (1984) Roughness, holes, and bumps. In: The Influence of Roadway Surface Discontinuities on Safety, Transportation Research Board, Washington, D.C., chap 3, 5–10

WHO (2018) Road traffic injuries. World Health Organization (WHO). URL https://www.who.int/news-room/fact-sheets/detail/road-traffic-injuries, accessed 2019-11-26

Wood SN (2006) Generalized Additive Models: An Introduction with R. Chapman & Hall/CRC, New York

Wood SN (2019) mgcv: Mixed GAM Computation Vehicle with Automatic Smoothness Estimation. URL https://CRAN.R-project.org/package=mgcv, R package version 1.8-28

Wright MN, Ziegler A (2017) ranger: A fast implementation of random forests for high dimensional data in C++ and R. Journal of Statistical Software 77(1):1–17

Wright MN, Wager S, Probst P (2020) ranger: A Fast Implementation of Random Forests. URL https://CRAN.R-project.org/package=ranger, R package version 0.12.1

Yaacob NFF, Rusli N, Bohari SN (2019) Relationship of environmental factors toward accident cases using GIS application in Kedah. In: 15th International Colloquium on Signal Processing & Its Applications (CSPA), IEEE, 137–141

15

Statistical Modeling of Dynamic Greenhouse Gas Emissions

Nathaniel K. Newlands

Agriculture and Agri-Food Canada, Summerland, BC, Canada

CONTENTS

15.1	Overview	325
15.2	Background	326
15.3	Introduction	326
15.4	Statistical framework	328
15.5	Ecosystem dynamical optimization	331
15.6	Numerical results	334
15.7	Summary	338
15.8	Appendix: model parameters and variables	339
References		343

15.1 Overview

Farms are intensively managed, complex systems. Finding ways to reduce harmful emissions of greenhouse gases (CO_2, N_2O, and CH_4) relies on an integrated understanding of coupled ecosystem processes and farm operations. Model-based estimates of greenhouse gas (GHG) emissions for farms are quantified under a selected set of crop and livestock production scenarios. Emission equations are adapted to Canadian farm activities and conditions based on the International Panel on Climate Change (IPCC) estimation methodology and are linked to dynamic ecosystem carbon and nitrogen flows under mass-balance constraints. The design and application of a dynamic agroecosystem model, integrated within a statistical framework (i.e., mass-balance optimization, calibration, scaling, and sensitivity analysis) is demonstrated. This approach can provide more robust estimates of GHG reduction potentials for assessing mitigation and adaptation management strategies, especially for dynamic, farm-scale emissions.

15.2 Background

Global warming and its enhancement by increasing amounts of greenhouse gases present in the earth's atmosphere (e.g., carbon dioxide—CO_2, nitrous oxide—N_2O, and methane CH_4) is an international problem that poses enormous challenges for science and society. Under the 2016 Paris Agreement, Canada has committed to reducing its GHG emissions by 30% below the 2005 level of 730 megatonnes of carbon dioxide equivalent (Mt $CO_{2,eq}$) by 2030 to 511 Mt $CO_{2,eq}$.[1] From the starting point in Canada's Second Biennial Report (2016), Canada needed a 304 Mt $CO_{2,eq}$ reduction in projected 2030 emissions that were projected in 2016 to be 815 Mt $CO_{2,eq}$. To reach the 2030 target based on current total emissions of 743 Mt $CO_{2,eq}$ (2019), Canada now needs a 232 Mt $CO_{2,eq}$ reduction (Environment and Climate Change Canada (ECCC), 2019). Emissions from Canadian farms have remained essentially unchanged in the recent decades at 59 Mt $CO_{2,eq}$ or 8.2% of Canada's net GHG emissions. Fuel and fertilizer use and industrial livestock operations contribute significantly to increasing agricultural GHG emissions. Zero and reduced tillage practices, along with other soil management practices, can significantly lower emissions (Agriculture and Agri-Food Canada (AAFC), 2008, Chipanshi et al, 2015), but soil CO_2 emissions can switch between a source and a sink at the regional and national scale (i.e., soil was an emission source in 1991 (8.1 Tg CO_2), switching to a sink in 2002 (-4.4 Tg CO_2) (Desjardins et al, 2005). This points to the need for a multi-scale approach that integrates sensitivity and uncertainty statistical analysis. Overall, total GHG emissions per Gross Domestic Product (GDP) and GHG emissions per capita have declined since the 1990s, despite the fact that Canada's economy and population have grown.[2]

15.3 Introduction

Reliable emission estimates and compliance to standardized accounting, reporting, and review methodologies are critical in attaining targeted national emission reductions. Reliability and international standards also have a leading role in strengthening intergovernmental cooperation, sharing, and broad climate adaptation in science, technology and policy. While international guidelines for estimating GHG emission have been established by the

---

[1] https://www.canada.ca/en/environment-climate-change/services/environmental-indicators/progress-towards-canada-greenhouse-gas-emissions-reduction-target.html

[2] http://prairieclimatecentre.ca/2018/03/where-do-canadas-greenhouse-gas-emissions-come-from/

Introduction

International Panel on Climate Change (IPCC, 1997, 2001) for the agricultural sector, there are many outstanding questions concerning the reliability of estimation equations and their ability to accurately quantify and reflect source-sink dynamics (i.e., changes in the sign or direction of emission). Concerns also highlight how resulting estimates, obtained from different data sources and models, can be effectively integrated within the IPCC or a single methodology. While default (tier 1) IPCC methods are intended for application in any country, based on readily available national statistics, there are many concerns that the methodology is not specific enough to take into account local conditions and as a result lead to over-estimation or under-estimation of emission (Silgram et al, 2001). In many cases, such estimation problems are the result of over simplistic assumptions. More realistic, and likely more complex and cross-sector interaction assumptions are needed. Such reliability issues will likely only be addressed in a comprehensive way if repeated experimentation is conducted in tandem with the application of dynamic emission models within a statistically-based, guiding framework.

Mathematical and statistical models can integrate historical and new knowledge, multiple data-sets, and multiple GHG gases, enabling validation of measured estimates, thereby either preventing or providing an explanation of over- and under-estimation problems (Raupach et al, 2005). Ecosystem-scale models enable the examination of both direct and indirect linkages and can readily test assumptions, offering new interpretations of data. If such models are to help solve the problem of reliably estimating GHG emissions, then several key questions arise; How can models be constructed that utilize IPCC emission equations? What framework might effectively link various model results together? How can models be integrated within the IPCC methodology?

When attempting to deal with the complexity of nature, models that describe chemical, biological and ecological processes can become large (i.e., overparameterized) and involve many interconnected assumptions, making it very difficult to reuse and understand them according to their various functional parts (Lui et al, 2002). Such difficulties are further confounded by a lack of consensus on what spatial and temporal scale various model simulation results can be reliably compared. Ecosystem models can provide invaluable insights of ecological, economic and social indicators. Ecosystem models can also be applied at various spatial and temporal scales; from plot to field, farm, watershed, and up to regional and national scales. Their heterogeneous structure also makes them very flexible and adaptable to different types of ecosystems under both closed and open boundary conditions in both terrestrial and aquatic environments (Belcher et al, 2004, Rastetter et al, 1991, Seppelt, 1999, Vézina et al, 2004). Dynamic ecosystem models under mass-balance constraints may offer the best way to improve the responsiveness, flexibility, robustness, and reliability of model-based GHG emission estimates. While the challenge of describing an entire functional system in sufficient detail is great, an even greater challenge exists for establishing an effective bridge between experimental sampling and validation of system-level models. For this reason, an overarching statistical framework is needed that includes sensitivity and validation (uncertainty) analysis. A statistical framework may enable a more robust, integrated understanding of the impact of farm operations on current and future emission levels (Aggarwal et al, 2006a,b, Beauchemin et al, 2011, Grosso et al, 2002, Kröbel et al, 2016, Li, 2000, Schils et al, 2005, Seppelt, 2000). Such an approach is amenable to integrating Big Data, and incorporating artificial intelligence, machine learning/deep learning algorithms (Newlands, 2016).

A statistical framework is presented here for estimating GHG emissions at the farm-scale linked with carbon and nitrogen flows, mass-balance constraints, scaling factors, and emission losses. The ecosystem model consists of vegetation/shelterbelt, crop, soil, livestock and manure as main components. Equations describing the emission loss from each ecosystem component are based upon default (tier 1), international estimation guidelines established by the International Panel on Climate Change (IPCC, 1997, 2001). These tier 1 equations have been adapted and applied to Canadian farm conditions and context (i.e., tier 2 equations) based on experimental results of measured emission factors under Canadian soil and climatic conditions [Agriculture and Agri-Food Canada (AAFC), 2008, Beauchemin et al, 2011, Janzen et al, 2005, Kröbel et al, 2016, Newlands, 2007, Newlands et al, 2006]. This effort has involved the collaboration of agricultural, atmospheric and environmental scientists, measuring emissions across a range of spatial and temporal scales on different sampling platforms (i.e., aircraft, tower, soil core, and chamber measurements). Emission factors that are scaled by experts to account for changes in farm operations (i.e., management and activities), such as tillage depth, crop rotation frequency, types of fertilizer input and manure handling, as well as quality of feed given to different livestock.

15.4 Statistical framework

The statistical framework for developing the farm-scale dynamic ecosystem model consists of four main steps: estimation, validation, prediction, and verification (Figure 15.1). These steps are standard to good practice in building mathematical models (Jorgensen and Bendoricchio, 2001). The modeled ecosystem components, nutrient, and emission flows are shown in Figure 15.2. The framework links components, parameters, and variables in a special way that reflects the customized technical needs and requirements in predicting GHG emission while maintaining links to IPCC estimation methodology. For example, within the estimation step, emission factors as fixed parameters, activity and climate variables are specified that are linked with the default-IPCC (tier 1) assessment and reporting methodology. Figure 15.6 in the

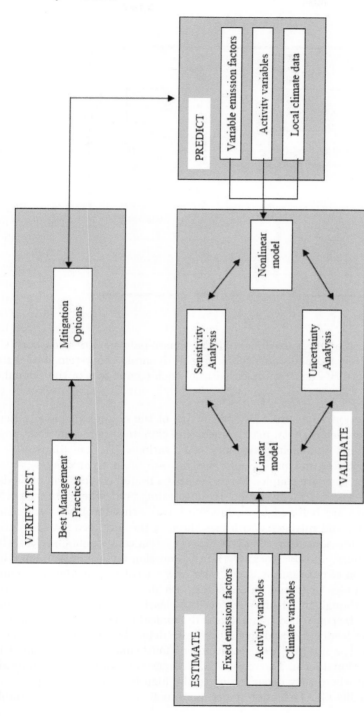

FIGURE 15.1: Statistical framework for developing a dynamic ecosystem model of farms that integrates estimation, validation, prediction, and verification in obtaining reliable estimates of current and future GHG emissions.

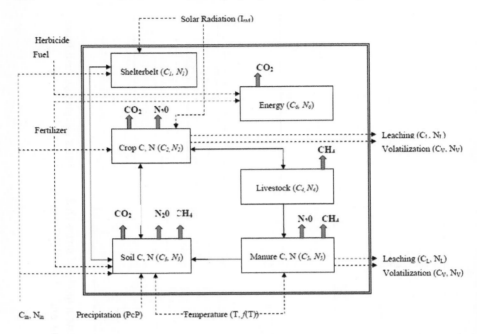

FIGURE 15.2: Main ecosystem components, mass-balance flow of carbon (C) and nitrogen (N) storage and cycling in the dynamic ecosystem model for farms, showing GHG emission released from each component of the system.

Appendix (Section 15.8) provides a summary of the ecosystem model interconnections between activity, management and climate variables for soil, crop, livestock, manure, and shelterbelt linked with various GHG emissions.

While sensitivity and uncertainty analysis are often treated as separate modeling steps, they are coupled here to enable a nested comparison of model estimates, placing special attention to uncertainty and where the greatest knowledge gaps are believed to occur. Specifically, this involves quantifying how carbon (C) and nitrogen (N) fluxes through the farm ecosystem jointly control GHG emissions from the dynamic ecosystem components: shelterbelt, crop, soil, manure, and livestock. Currently, emission factors are obtained by linear regression of data and it is not clear how considering nonlinear cycling and flow dynamics of C and N improves such fits and associated interpretations, even though in nature such cycling clearly does exist. While many emissions may be controlled by nonlinear dynamical behavior, such as thresholds, irregular feedbacks, and cyclic/periodic dependencies, in many cases, such behavior has not yet been quantified or mathematically represented in nonlinear functional form. The reason modelers need to know what nonlinearities exist and where they occur is due to the high level of detail required to accurately predict GHG emission under more realistic assumptions of variable emission factors.

The statistical framework is applied to the simplified case of a linear model and nominal sensitivity analysis for identifying leading parameters/variables that control emission. Results from these estimation and validation steps help to: (1) identify where the largest uncertainties exist, (2) identify where in the ecosystem the highest potential exists for measuring and modeling nonlinearities, and (3) select key parameters and variables in structuring a nonlinear model formulation. The sensitivity of net-emission with respect to nitrogen input into soil from fertilizer, or manure applied in spring and/or fall (Nappl$_{spring}$ and Nappl$_{fall}$, respectively), provides an indication of how important a nonlinear description of N_2O emission from soil is compared to emission from other ecosystem components. In the verification step, "mitigation options" are distinguished as "best management practices" that are strategies that have the highest likelihood of being adopted by farmers. Ultimately, the successful adoption of mitigation practices depends on social and economic factors, not just ecological ones.

15.5 Ecosystem dynamical optimization

We define x as a $n \times 1$ vector of unknown model flows, b is a m vector of measured flow, ϵ is a $m \times 1$ vector of residuals, E is a $m \times 1$ vector of net-emission (i.e., linear summation of contributions of each gas, CO_2, N_2O, CH_4). A is a $m \times n$ matrix comprising elements that are coefficients of the linear mass-balance and data constraints for inflow $i \to j$ and outflow $j \to i$ linking each compartment $j = (1, \ldots, p)$, $i = (1, \ldots, p)$. The ecosystem of differential equations describing carbon and nitrogen storage and flow are given by:

$$Shelterbelt : \frac{dC_1}{dt} = -I_{rad}(C_1), \quad \frac{dN_1}{dt} = -I_{rad}(N_1)$$

$$CropC : \frac{dC_2}{dt} = -I_{rad}(C_1) - C_4 + C_L + E_2^{CO_2}$$

$$CropN : \frac{dN_2}{dt} = -I_{rad}(N_1) - N_4 + N_V + E_2^{N_2O}$$

$$SoilC : \frac{dC_3}{dt} = -(P + T + C_{in}) - C_1 - C_5 + E_3^{CO_2} + E_3^{CH_4}$$

$$SoilN : \frac{dN_3}{dt} = -(P + T + N_{in}) - N_1 - N_5 + E_3^{N_2O}$$

$$LivestockC : \frac{dC_4}{dt} = -C_2 + C_5 + E_4^{CH_4}$$

$$LivestockN : \frac{dN_4}{dt} = -N_2 + N_5 + E_4^{N_2O}$$

$$ManureC : \frac{dC_5}{dt} = -f(C_5, T) - C_4 + C_3 + C_L + E_5^{CH_4}$$

$$ManureN : \frac{dN_5}{dt} = -f(N_5, T) - N_4 + N_3 + N_V + E_5^{N_2O} \quad (15.1)$$

The mathematical programming equations (15.1) and in Figure 15.3 are formulated to attain mass-balance of flows constrained by emission losses. This involves minimizing the squared differences between modeled flow and data (Vézina et al, 2004). The framework integrates constraints for C, N, CO_2, CH_4, and N_2O flows. While achieving mass-balance involves balancing both the C and N flows simultaneously, the mass-balance constraints assume CO_2 and CH_4 emission is independent of N_2O emission, and that C and N flow are independent ecosystem processes. It is in the emission equations themselves that dependencies between emissions of each type are represented. It is assumed that emission losses can be decomposed into three contributions; one that is associated with farm management or activities (perturbed conditions), a second that is associated with C and N flow in the ecosystem (unperturbed conditions), and a third that links the first two. The first of these contributions is termed an activity or scaling factor (γ) and the second, an emission factor or coefficient (K). The third contribution comprises parameters and variables that are not strictly related to farm activity or C and N flow, but instead are related to both, whereby they mediate changes in the "state" (i.e., stored amount of C and N) within each ecosystem component (m_j).

Under the IPCC methodology, the scaling coefficient and emission factors may be constant or non-constant, but the activity or scaling factor is independent of the emission coefficient. We define a set of state-mediator parameter and variables (Tables 15.2–15.8) that enable IPCC-derived emission equations to be expressed in the general form (15.1), whereby the scaling factor is dependent on both management variables, and those that are dependent on C and N flow. Where data is available, modeled flow can be substituted by measured flow data in achieving a mass-balanced solution, i.e., mass-balance constraint becomes a data constraint with known variance and covariance. In the formulation on the next page we also assume that the ecosystem flows are unknown and the emission losses are known. The hydrological cycle and water transport processes are not modeled explicitly, but instead are considered implicitly as they influence various modeled parameters and variables.

Model formulation (C/N flow, mass-balance, emission losses, eco-physiological constraints)

Minimize $(Ax-b)^{-1} S^{-1}(Ax-b)$ (1)

and $Ax = (b+E) + \varepsilon$ (linear system) such that; (2)

$$A = \begin{bmatrix} M \\ D \end{bmatrix}_{m \times n}, \ b = \begin{bmatrix} \Delta Y \\ O \end{bmatrix}_{m \times 1}, \Delta Y \in (\Delta C \text{ or } \Delta N), \ \varepsilon = [\varepsilon]_{m \times 1}, x = [x]_{n \times 1}$$

where m=(p+q) and n total flow, S^{-1} is a data variance-covariance matrix

Subject to:

Mass-balance constraints (j=1,…,p):
carbon (C) flow, with CO_2, CH_4 emission
(contributions denoted with superscript C):

$$M_j^C \equiv \sum_{i=1}^{p} F_{ij}^C - \sum_{i=1}^{p} F_{ji}^C = \Delta C_j + (E_j^{CO_2} + E_j^{CH_4}) + \varepsilon_j^C \quad (3)$$

nitrogen (N) flow with N_2O emission
(contributions denoted with superscript N):

$$M_j^N \equiv \sum_{i=1}^{p} F_{ij}^N - \sum_{i=1}^{p} F_{ji}^N = \Delta N_j + E_j^{N_2O} + \varepsilon_j^N \quad (4)$$

with uncertainty ε_j and k data-constraints (k=1,…,q).

Data-constraints (k=1,…,q):

$$D_k \equiv f(F_{ij}, F_{ji}) = O_k + \varepsilon_k, \quad (5)$$

where a known function, $f(F_{ij}, F_{ji})$, relates inflow and outflow to specify modeled, net-flow, D_k, to measured flow, O_k with uncertainty, ε_k, for compartment k. (i.e., specified from available flow data).

Emission-constraints (j=1,…,p):

$$E_j^{CO_2, CH_4, N_2O} \equiv \sum_{i=1}^{p} f(\gamma_j, m_j, K_j, \Delta Y_j), \quad (6)$$

where f denotes some function relating γ_j as a $m \times 1$ vector termed an "activity/scaling factor", K_j is a $m \times 1$ vector "emission factor" and m_j is a $m \times 1$ vector of "state-mediator" parameters.

Eco-physiological constraints (r=1,…,u; s=1,…,v) for bounds on ecosystem flows

Upper bound: $G_r^U = f(F_{ij}, F_{ji}) \leq h_r^U$ (7)
Lower bound: $G_s^L = f(F_{ij}, F_{ji}) \leq -h_s^L$ (8)

FIGURE 15.3: Ecosystem optimization/programming equations.

TABLE 15.1: Default and imposed ranges in nominal sensitivity analysis of model parameters under the identified six farm mitigation options for reducing GHG emissions: (1) Reduce soil tillage, (2) Apply fertilizer to soil that better matches crop uptake, (3) Increase livestock weight gain, (4) Improve livestock feed quality, (5) Change numbers of livestock, and (6) Change size of areas allocated for crop, fallow, and pasture. Mitigation option is denoted by M, variable by VAR, and step-size by SS. Lower and upper bounds are denoted D-LB, D-UB for default, and I-LB, I-UB for the imposed range, respectively

M	VAR	Units	SS	D-LB	D-UB	I-LB	I-UB
1	$SC_{tillage}$ $\gamma_{3,1}$	Mg C ha^{-1}	0.073	−0.365	0.365	−0.511	0.511
2	N_{rate} $\lambda_{3,1}$	kg N ha^{-1}	10.0	10	110	0.00	120
	$N_{appl_{stubble}}$ $\lambda_{3,3}$	kg N ha^{-1}	11.5	5	120	0.00	143
	$N_{appl_{fallow}}$ $\lambda_{3,4}$	kg N ha^{-1}	11.5	5	120	0.00	143
3	W_{cattle} $m_{4,1}$	kg	60.0	400	1000	400	1000
4	DE_{cattle} $m_{4,6}$	%	3.60	45	81.0	37.8	88.2
	DE_{sheep} $m_{4,7}$	%	3.60	45	81.0	37.8	88.2
	DE_{swine} $m_{4,9}$	Kcal kg^{-1}	60.0	2800	3400	2680	3520
	$Y_{m,cattle}$ $\gamma_{4,1}$	%	0.005	0.03	0.08	0.02	0.09
	$Y_{m,sheep}$ $\gamma_{4,2}$	%	0.0015	0.009	0.024	0.006	0.027
	$C_{a,cattle}$ $\lambda_{4,4}$	—	0.036	0	0.360	−0.072	0.432
	$C_{a,sheep}$ $\lambda_{4,5}$	—	0.0015	0.009	0.024	0.006	0.027
	N_d $\gamma_{4,5}$	day	36.5	1	365	0.00	365
5	$n_{type,age-class}$	—	10.0	0	100	0.00	100
6	A_{crop} $\lambda_{2,1}$	ha	100	0	1000	0.00	1000
	A_{fallow} $\lambda_{2,2}$	ha	100	0	1000	0.00	1000
	$A_{pasture}$ $\lambda_{4,1}$	ha	100	0	1000	0.00	1000
	A_{total} λ'	ha	—	1000	1000	0.00	1000

15.6 Numerical results

Numerical results from nominal sensitivity analysis of the model were obtained assuming closed boundary conditions. The purpose of this sensitivity analysis was to estimate net-GHG under changes in key model variables and to compare estimates between leading variables associated with mitigation options. Static conditions are assumed that avoids the need to couple emission equations to time-dependent ecosystem flow equations. This simplifies the interpretation of sensitivity results, providing a first-order evaluation of net-GHG estimates generated by the model equations, while also making it easier to compare directly between mitigation options. The emission equations (15.1) and Equation 6 in Figure 15.3 were implemented and independent model runs were performed by first selecting a model variable associated with a mitigation

Numerical results

option and then systematically varying its value (i.e., with a given step size) within either the default and imposed range (Table 15.1). The default ranges were specified from observed variation, determined either directly from measurement data or indirectly from expert knowledge from Canadian farms and environmental conditions. The sensitivity of each model variable was tested also by imposing larger ranges in each variable above the default ranges that are based on *a priori* expert knowledge of farm operations and conditions. Simulation runs for six mitigation options were performed:

1. Reduce soil tillage—$SC_{tillage}$ ($\gamma_{(3,1)}$)
2. Apply fertilizer to soil that balances nitrogen crop uptake—Nrate ($\lambda_{(3,1)}$), $Nappl_{fallow}$ ($\lambda_{(3,4)}$), $Nappl_{stubble}$ ($\lambda_{(3,3)}$)
3. Increase livestock weight gain—W_{cattle} ($m_{(4,1)}$)
4. Improve livestock feed quality—DE ($m_{(4,6)}$, $m_{(4,7)}$, $m_{(4,9)}$), Y_m ($\gamma_{(4,1)}$, $\gamma_{(4,2)}$), C_a ($\lambda_{(4,4)}$, $\lambda_{(4,5)}$), N_d ($\gamma_{(4,5)}$)
5. Balance animal numbers by emission level—$n_{type,age}$
6. Balance areas for crop, fallow, pasture areas by emission level—A ($\lambda_{(2,1)}$, $\lambda_{(2,2)}$, $\lambda_{(4,1)}$)

Figures 15.4 and 15.5 show the results of net-GHG farm emission under default and imposed sensitivity analysis ranges. The highest estimated farm emissions are from N_2O from manure and CH_4 from livestock. Manure N_2O emissions are unaffected by all mitigation options, except option 4 where improvements to feed quality have the largest potential to decrease manure N_2O emission and reduce effective methane emission days (N_d), where further decreases would be expected according to storage of various type of manure.

Decreases in N_d may reduce manure N_2O emission levels by up to 50% from 8321 to 4553 kg $CO_{2,eq}ha^{-1}yr^{-1}$. Under such reductions, emission levels are consistent in magnitude with the reported estimate of 4200 Tg $CO_{2,eq}yr^{-1}$ (Matin et al, 2004) for farm area of 1000 ha and 246,934 approximate number of total Canadian farms, while also consistent with the reported range (3237–4597 kg $CO_{2,eq}ha^{-1}yr^{-1}$) of N_2O emission from ruminant livestock farms under contrasting livestock numbers and grassland management (Schils et al, 2005). These results were relatively robust to changes in input range (refer to Figures 15.4 and 15.5). However, for manure CH_4 emission we estimate 27–53 kg $CO_{2,eq}ha^{-1}yr^{-1}$ with highest levels of 403 kg $CO_{2,eq}ha^{-1}yr^{-1}$ attained for option 5 under variation of livestock numbers, a value that appears to overestimate emission when compared to reported ranges of 1–4 Tg $CO_{2,eq}yr^{-1}$ in the literature with a relative difference of a factor of 10 (Matin et al, 2004, Schils et al, 2005).

The modeled estimates of N_2O emissions from soil range between 294–1290 kg $CO_{2,eq}ha^{-1}yr^{-1}$, with farm area having a leading impact (option 6). All other options are better at mitigating increases in this emission because

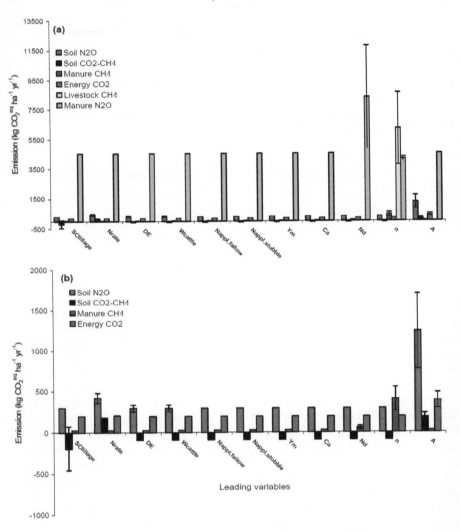

FIGURE 15.4: Sensitivity analysis results yielding net-GHG emission estimates obtained by varying selected model variables within default ranges determined by expert opinion. Comparing estimates across variables associated with six different mitigation options (refer to Table 15.1) yields the relative potential of each individual option; (a) all ecosystem component, (b) same as (a) but with manure and livestock components excluded.

variation in crop, fallow and pasture area do not directly offer reasonable mitigation potential. Also, increases in CO_2 emission from on-farm energy use are accompanied by increases in N_2O emission. The other options do not provide any indirect reduction, thus, we infer that either nitrogen (fertilizer or manure)

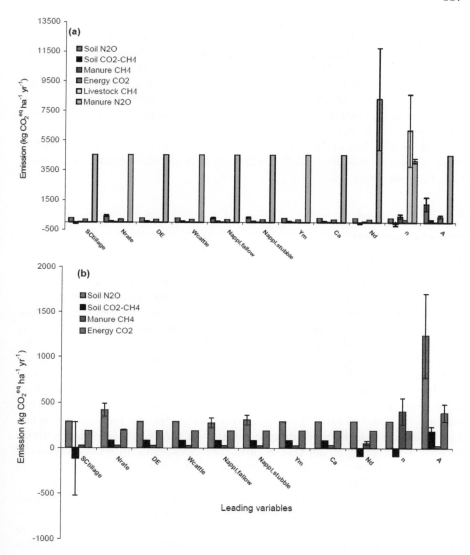

FIGURE 15.5: Same as Figure 15.4, but with imposed ranges for each variable (refer to Table 15.1).

input to soil or the control (i.e., in time) of the emission process of N_2O from soil itself may have a greater potential at reducing emission levels (Gregorich et al, 2005, Janzen et al, 2003, Smith et al, 2004). Our estimates of soil N_2O emission lie within the reported range of 441 kg $CO_{2,eq} ha^{-1} yr^{-1}$ (Schils et al, 2005).

Net emission of CO_2 and CH_4 from the soil exhibits source-sink dynamics where values may decrease or increase. Surprisingly, reducing soil tillage did not exclusively sequester carbon, but the potential for increasing CO_2 emission is shown to exist (Figure 15.4). Increasing variation in soil tillage lead to greater potential for increasing CO_2 emission (option 1), suggesting that other indirect ways of mitigating this emission exist but are limited. This is evident from the switch from decreasing CO_2 emission under default ranges for options 2–5 in Figure 15.4, to increasing emission under imposed ranges for options 2–4. Results for option 6 show that balancing areas dedicated to crop, fallow and pasture is likely ineffective at mitigation against increases in CO_2 emission from soil.

15.7 Summary

The statistical framework showcased here provides a framework for formulating and refining models to estimate and predict GHG emission for farms or regional networks of farms. It includes a direct link to IPCC emission estimation methodology. Modeled emissions lie within previously reported ranges. A high sensitivity of soil CO_2 emission to tillage and source-sink dynamics is evident confirming other published findings (Janzen, 2004, Janzen et al, 1998, Sauerbeck, 2001). Variation in fertilizer input under mitigation option 2 was less than was expected in terms of both direct and indirect impacts on farm emissions. Changes to the mass-balance of C and N within the ecosystem are expected to alter the current results significantly both in magnitude and sign, and lead to more dramatic variation than the nominal sensitivity results. The refined model that is presented exemplifies an ecosystem model capable of describing carbon and nitrogen cycling within, and emissions from farms. By describing the state and changes of state over time for main components of a farm, the model provides a basic structure capable of generating new insights and being tested against emission data. The statistical framework presented here could be further applied to use GHG time-series satellite data (see Hardwick and Graven, 2016). In the future, big data obtained from sensors and unmanned aerial vehicles (UAVs) from Smartfarms could also be integrated into the framework, alongside Earth Observational monitoring data. The core model could also be further extended to estimate and predict fully time-dependent, dynamic changes in net-GHG across spatial and temporal scales.

Acknowledgments

This research was funded by the Canadian Agricultural Innovation (CAP) Program, Agriculture and Agri-Food Canada (AAFC).

15.8 Appendix: model parameters and variables

TABLE 15.2: Farm activity/management parameters and variables

Component	Parameter	IPCC-derived
Crop	λ'	Total area (A_{total})
	$\lambda_{2,1}$	Crop (A_{crop})
	$\lambda_{2,2}, \lambda_{2,3}$	Present, Past fallow area (A_{fallow}, $A_{fallow,20yr}$)
	$\lambda_{2,4}$	Crop residue removal (ReR)
Soil	$\lambda_{3,1}, \lambda_{3,2}, \lambda_{3,3}, \lambda_{3,4}$	Fertilization (N_{rate}, P_2O_5, $Nappl_{stubble}$, $Nappl_{fallow}$)
Livestock	$\lambda_{4,1}$	Pasture area ($A_{pasture}$)
	$\lambda_{4,2}$	Number of animals ($N_{animal,type,age\text{-}class}$)
	$\lambda_{4,3}$	Number of life-cycles per year ($N_{life\text{-}cycles}$)
	$\lambda_{4,4}$	Feed activity coefficient cattle (Ca_{cattle})
	$\lambda_{4,5}$	Feed activity coefficient sheep (Ca_{sheep})
Manure	$\lambda_{5,1}$	Quantity (Q_{manure})
Shelterbelt	$\lambda_{1,1}, \lambda_{1,2}, \lambda_{1,3}, \lambda_{1,4}$	Length, Age, Number of rows, Planting space
	$\lambda_{1,5}$	Permanent cover (A_{perm})

TABLE 15.3: Livestock population matrix ($n_{age\text{-}class,type}$)

Parameter	Type	Age-class
$n_{1,k}$	Cattle	Back-steers, Back-heifers, Finishers, Finishers-steers
		Finishers-heifers, Dairy-milking, Beef milking, Dry cows, Bulls
$n_{2,k}$	Sheep	Rams, Wethers, Ewes
$n_{3,k}$	Swine	Boars, Finishers, Gestating sows, Lactating sows, Weaners
$n_{4,k}$	Other	Chickens-broilers, Chicken-broiler/breeder, Chicken-layers
		Turkey-breeders, Goats, Small ruminants, Horses, Buffalo

TABLE 15.4: Ecosystem state variables – carbon, nitrogen cycling

Variable	Component	C/N Flow—Inputs and Outputs
$C_1 N_1$	Shelterbelt	Soil C
$C_2 N_2$	Crop	Organic soil N, Crop leached N, Crop volatilized N
$C_3 N_3$	Soil	Crop residue N, Shelterbelt C, Permanent cover C
		Fertilizer N (stubble/fallow), Soil tillage C, Soil oxidation C
$C_4 N_4$	Livestock	Cattle/Calves C, Sheep C, Other C
	Manure	Livestock grazing C/N, Other Livestock C/N, Poultry C
$C_5 N_5$		Manure type (liquid, semi-solid, solid, anaerobic digestor)
		Manure land-applied N, Manure imported C/N
		Manure leached C/N, Manure volatilization N
$C_6 N_6$	Energy	Fertilizer C

TABLE 15.5: Environmental (climate) variables

Variable	Description
T	Mean temperature
$f(T)$	temperature sensitivity factor
P	Mean precipitation
I_{rad}	Incident solar radiation

TABLE 15.6: IPCC-derived emission coefficients (EC), $kgCO_{2,eq} ha^{-1}$

Parameter	EC	Component – Emission type
$K_{2,1}, K_{2,2}$	EF_{leach}, EF_{volat}	Crop—CO_2
$K_{2,3}, K_{2,4}$	EF_{fert}, EF_{app}	Crop—N_2O
$K_{3,1}$	EF_{till}	Soil—CO_2
$K_{3,2}, K_{3,3}$	EF_{stored}, EF_{other}	Soil—N_2O
$K_{3,4}$	EF_{oxid}	Soil—CH_4
$K_{4,1}$	EF_{rumin}	Livestock—CH_4
$K_{5,1}, K'_{5,1}$	$EF_{manure,fall}, EF_{manure,spring}$	Manure—N_2O
$K_{5,2}, K_{5,3}$	$EF_{L,manure}, EF_{VD,manure}$	Manure—CH_4

Appendix: model parameters and variables

TABLE 15.7: Ecosystem state-mediator parameters and variables

Type	Parameter	IPCC-derived
Shelterbelt	$m_{1,1}, m_{1,2}$	Growth threshold (L_o), Growth rate (t_o)
Crop	$m_{2,1}$	Grain Yield (GY)
	$m_{2,2}$	Harvest Index (HI)
	$m_{2,3}$	Crop residue concentration (C_R)
Soil	$m_{3,1}$	Nitrogen dry matter input ($C_{nitrogen}$)
Livestock	$m_{4,1}, m_{4,2}$	Average weight (Wt_{cow}, Wt_{sheep})
	$m_{4,3}$	Daily weight gain (ADG)
	$m_{4,4}$	Dry matter intake (DMI)
	$m_{4,5}$	Gross energy (GE)
	$m_{4,6}, m_{4,7}, m_{4,8}, m_{4,9}$	Nutrients ($DE_{cattle}, DE_{sheep}, DE_{swine}, C_d$)
	$m_{4,10}, m_{4,11}, m_{4,12}, m_{4,13}$	Protein intake, retention, excretion (PI, PR, PE)
	$m_{4,14}, m_{4,15}, m_{4,16}$	Milk ($Milk_{prod}, Milk_{fat}, Milk_{yield}$)
	$m_{4,17}$	Wool production
	$m_{4,18}, m_{4,19}$	Probability of birth/twins (%B, %T)
	$m_{4,20}, m_{4,21}$	N excretion ($N_e, N_{e,other}$)
	$m_{4,21}$	Maximum CH_4 excretion (B_o)
	$m_{4,22}, m_{4,23}$	Volatile solids (VS_{prod}, VS_{cons})
	$m_{4,24}$	Animal type coefficient
Manure	$m_{5,1}, m_{5,2}$	Moisture and ash content ($C_{moisture}$, ASH)
Energy	$m_{6,1}, m_{6,2}, m_{6,3}$	Herbicide, Fuel ($E_{herbicide}, E_{fuel}, E_{machinery}$)

TABLE 15.8: IPCC-derived emission scaling factors

Emission type	Parameter	Description
Soil – CO_2	$\gamma_{3,1}$	Tillage ($SC_{tillage}$)
	$\gamma_{3,2}$	Cropping frequency (SC_{freq})
	$\gamma_{3,3}$	Permanent cover (SC_{perm})
Soil – N_2O	$\gamma_{3,4}$	Leaching fraction (R_L)
	$\gamma_{3,5}$	Volatilization fraction (R_{VD})
Livestock – CH_4	$\gamma_{4,1}$	Cattle methane conversion ($Y_{m,cattle}$)
	$\gamma_{4,2}$	Sheep methane conversion ($Y_{m,sheep}$)
	$\gamma_{4,3}$	Feed additive reduction factors ($CH_{4,reduction}$)
	$\gamma_{4,4}$	Activity reduction factor (RF)
	$\gamma_{4,5}$	Emission days (N_d)
Manure – N_2O	$\gamma_{5,1}$	Manure leaching ($R_{L,manure}$)
	$\gamma_{5,2}$	Manure volatilization ($R_{VD,manure}$)

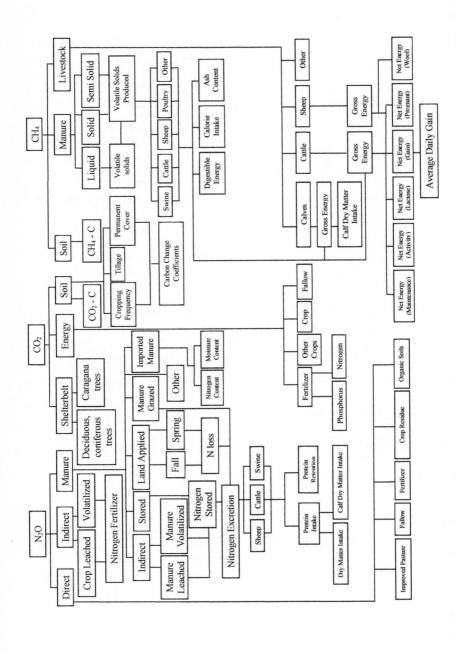

FIGURE 15.6: Main interconnections between activity/management and climate variables for modeling net-GHG emission.

References

Aggarwal P, Kalra N, Chander S, Pathak H (2006a) InfoCrop: a dynamic simulation model for the assessment of crop yields, losses due to pests, and environmental impact of agro-ecosystems in tropical environments, I. Model description. Agricultural Systems 89:1–25

Aggarwal PK, Banerjee B, Daryaei MG, Bhatia A, Bala A, Rani S, Chander S, Pathak H, Kalra N (2006b) InfoCrop: a dynamic simulation model for the assessment of crop yields, losses due to pests, and environmental impact of agro-ecosystems in tropical environments, II. Performance of the model. Agricultural Systems 89:47–67

Agriculture and Agri-Food Canada (AAFC) (2008) In: Janzen HH, Desjardins RL, Rochette P, Boehm M, Worth D (eds) Better Farming, Better Air: A scientific analysis of farming practice and greenhouse gases in Canada, Government of Canada, Ottawa

Beauchemin KA, Janzen HH, Little SM, McAllister TA, McGinn SM (2011) Mitigation of greenhouse gas emissions from beef production in western Canada—Evaluation using farm-based life cycle assessment. Animal Feed Science and Technology 166-167:663–677

Belcher KW, Boehm MM, Fulton ME (2004) Agroecosystem sustainability: a system simulation model approach. Agricultural Systems 79:225–241

Chipanshi A, Newlands NK, Cherneski P, Hill HS, Howard A (2015) Mitigation and adaptation strategies for reducing greenhouse gases in Canada – a review. In: Lac S, McHenry M, Kulshreshtha S (eds) Agriculture Management for Climate Change, Nova Science Publishers Inc., New York, 137–146

Desjardins RL, Vergé X, Hutchinson JJ, Smith W, Grant WN, McConkey B, Worth D (2005) Greenhouse gases. In: Lefebvre A, Eilers W, Chun B (eds) Agri-Environmental Indicators Report, Agriculture and Agri-Food Canada, Ottawa, 142–148

Environment and Climate Change Canada (ECCC) (2019) In: Canadian Environmental Sustainability Indicators: Progress towards Canada's greenhouse gas emissions reduction target, Government of Canada, Ottawa

Gregorich EG, Rochette P, VandenBygaart AJ, Angers DA (2005) Greenhouse gas contributions of agricultural soils and potential mitigation practices in Eastern Canada. Soil and Tillage Research 83(1):53–72

Grosso SD, Ojima D, Parton W, Mosier A, Peterson G, Schimel D (2002) Simulated effects of dryland cropping intensification on soil organic matter and greenhouse gas exchanges using the DAYCENT ecosystem model. Environmental Pollution 116:S75–S83

Hardwick S, Graven H (2016) Satellite observations to support monitoring of greenhouse gas emissions. Grantham Institute Briefing Paper 16:1–16

IPCC (1997) Revised 1996 IPCC Guidelines for National Greenhouse Gas Inventories, Organization for Economic Cooperation and Development and International Energy Agency (IEA), Geneva

IPCC (2001) Good Practice Guidelines and Uncertainty Management in National Greenhouse Gas Inventories, IPCC National Greenhouse Gas Inventories Programme, Japan

Janzen HH (2004) Carbon cycling in earth systems – a soil science perspective. Agriculture, Ecosystems and Environment 104:339–417

Janzen HH, Campbell CA, Izaurralde RC, Ellert BH, Juma N, McGill WB, Zentner RP (1998) Management effects on soil C storage on the Canadian prairies. Soil & Tillage Research 47:181–195

Janzen HH, Beauchemi KA, Bruinsma Y, Campbell CA, Desjardins RL, Ellert BH, Smith EG (2003) The fate of nitrogen in agroecosystems: An illustration using Canadian estimates. Nutrient Cycling in Agroecosystems 67:85–102

Janzen HH, Boehm M, Desjardins RL, Rochette P, Angers DA, Bolinder M, Dyer J, Ellert BH, Gibb D, Gregorich EG, Helgason BL, Lemke R, McGinn SM, McAllister T, Newlands N, Pattey E, Smith W, VandenBygaart AJ, Wang H (2005) Building a virtual farm: an approach for reducing greenhouse gas emissions? Canadian Journal of Soil Science 86:401–418

Jorgensen SE, Bendoricchio G (2001) Fundamentals of Ecological Modelling, vol 21, 3rd edn. Elsevier, London

Kröbel R, Bolinder MA, Janzen HH, Little SM, VandenBygaart AJ, Kätterer T (2016) Canadian farm-level soil carbon change assessment by merging the greenhouse gas model Holos with the Introductory Carbon Balance Model (ICBM). Agricultural Systems 143:76–85

Li CS (2000) Modeling trace gas emissions from agricultural ecosystems. Nutrient Cycling in Agroecosystems 58:259–276

Lui J, Peng C, Dang Q, Apps M, Jiang H (2002) A component object model strategy for reusing ecosystem models. Computers and Electronics in Agriculture 35:17–33

Matin A, Collas P, Blain D, Ha C, Liang C, MacDonald L, McKibbon S, Palmer C, Rhoades K (2004) Canada's greenhouse gas inventory: 1990–2002. Environment Canada, Ottawa

Newlands NK (2007) GHGFarm—a software tool to estimate and reduce net-greenhouse gas emission from farms in Canada. ACTA Press, Calgary, Canada

Newlands NK (2016) Future Sustainable Ecosystems: Complexity, Risk, Uncertainty. Taylor & Francis Group LCC, (Chapman & Hall/CRC Applied Environmental Statistics Series), Boca Raton, Florida

Newlands NK, Foyle J, Yang LL (2006) Potential net reductions in greenhouse gas emissions from farm bioenergy production in Canada. Computers in Agriculture and Natural Resources, 4th World Congress Conference, American Society of Agricultural and Biological Engineers, St. Joseph, Michigan, 5, vol 4, 770–774

References

Rastetter EB, Ryan MG, Shaver GR, Melillo JM, Nadelhoffer KJ, Hobbie JE, Aber JD (1991) A general biogeochemical model describing the responses of C and N cycle in terrestrial ecosystems to changes in CO2, climate and N deposition. Tree Physiology 9:101–126

Raupach MR, Tayner PJ, Barrett DJ, Defriess RS, Heimann M, Ojima DS, Quegan S, Schmullius CC (2005) Model-data synthesis in terrestrial carbon observation: methods, data requirements and data uncertainty specifications. Global Change Biology 11:1–20

Sauerbeck DR (2001) CO_2 emissions and C sequestration by agriculture – perspectives and limitations. Nutrient Cycling in Agroecosystems 60:253–266

Schils RLM, Verhagen A, Aart HFM, Sebek LBJ (2005) A farm level approach to define successful mitigation strategies for GHG emissions from ruminant livestock systems. Nutrient Cycling in Agroecosystems 71:163–175

Seppelt R (1999) Applications of optimum control theory to agroecosystem modeling. Ecosystem Modelling 121:161–163

Seppelt R (2000) Regionalized optimum control problems for agroecosystems management. Ecosystem Modelling 131:121–132

Silgram M, Waring R, Anthony S, Webb J (2001) Intercomparison of national and IPCC methods for estimating N loss from agricultural land. Nutrient Cycling in Agroecosystems 60:189–195

Smith WN, Grant R, Desjardins RL, Lemke R, Li C (2004) Estimates of the interannual variations of N2O emissions from agricultural soils in Canada. Nutrient Cycling in Agroecosystems 68:37–45

Vézina AF, Berrevile F, Loza S (2004) Inverse reconstructions of ecosystem flows in investigation regime shifts: impacts of the choice of objective function. Progress in Oceanography 60:321–341

16

Agricultural Climate Risk Management and Global Food Security: Recent Progress in Southeast Asia

Louis Kouadio
University of Southern Queensland, Toowoomba, Queensland, Australia

Eric Rahn
International Centre for Tropical Agriculture (CIAT), Hanoi, Vietnam

CONTENTS

16.1	Climate risks management in agriculture—use of climate prediction in crop models	348
16.2	Current approaches integrating SCFs and crop simulation models applied in Southeast Asia	349
16.3	Examples of integrated SCF-crop modeling approach for climate risk management in Southeast Asia	350
16.3.1	The climate-agriculture-modeling and decision tool (CAMDT)	350
16.3.2	The integrated seasonal climate-crop yield forecasting system for robusta coffee (ICCFS-Robusta)	352
16.4	Challenges for operationalizing seasonal climate-crop modeling frameworks in Southeast Asia	355
16.4.1	Data scarcity	355
16.4.2	Assessing the skills of seasonal climate forecasts	356
16.4.3	Communicating SCF outputs to farmers	356
16.4.4	Extending the range of applications of integrated SCF-crop modeling systems	356
16.5	Improved climate risk management in Southeast Asia—the way forward	357
References		359

16.1 Climate risks management in agriculture—use of climate prediction in crop models

Agriculture is sensitive to climate variability. The connection between the fluctuations of climate drivers (e.g., El Niño/La Niña Southern Oscillation – ENSO) and crop yields has been well documented (see, for example, Allan, 2000, Cirino et al, 2015, Hansen et al, 1998, Liu et al, 2014, Stone et al, 2000). Dry spells, frosts, changes in precipitation patterns and frequencies of extreme weather events have direct impacts on agro-biophysical processes and crop yields. Given the importance of climate risks and vulnerabilities for the agricultural industry in tropical and sub-tropical regions, a special attention is required in regard to the use of seasonal climate forecasts (SCFs) throughout a given crop value chain at reliable and relevant spatial and temporal coverage and scales. Seasonal climate forecasts are forecasts of the expected climate conditions for the next three to six months (Stone et al, 2000). By providing information early enough to adjust critical agricultural decisions, SCFs can contribute to the efficiency of agricultural management, and to food and livelihood security (Hansen et al, 2006, Meinke and Stone, 2005, Stone et al, 2000).

Risks can be estimated as the probability of occurrence given prior information, while uncertainty refers to situations where probabilities of occurrence cannot be estimated (Shelia et al, 2019). Climate risk management entails integrating adequate climate information services with agricultural advisory systems. This requires investments in climate data sourcing and analysis using meteorological measurements and satellite-derived products to enable risk assessments of sufficient quality. Reliable SCFs benefit from long-term climate monitoring. While there are globally available climate information services (e.g., from the World Meteorological Organization (WMO), International Research Institute for Climate and Society (IRI), etc.), there is a need to verify their local relevance using local data and tailor them to local conditions and decision contexts.

One way of translating SCFs to locally actionable decisions is using crop models, with SCF outputs being converted into relevant data formats beforehand (Stone et al, 2000). Linking SCFs to crop simulation models is generally achieved through four main approaches (Hansen and Indeje, 2004, Hansen et al, 2006): use of daily climate model outputs as inputs in the crop model; use of synthetic daily weather conditioned on climate forecasts; statistical prediction of crop response simulated with historic weather; and classification and analogue methods. Such integration requires i) adequate data availability for evaluating the forecasting skill of seasonal climate forecasts, ii) crop information for crop model calibration, iii) historical crop yield observations for crop model validation, and iv) appropriate ways for temporal downscaling of seasonal climate forecasts to provide daily weather inputs to crop models. Crop models are used often to translate seasonal climate forecasts into actionable decision making for farmers. Many seasonal climate forecasts are provided in tercile probabilities for temperature and rainfall, for example as 30% below normal, 50% near normal, and 20% above normal, requiring temporal downscaling for use in crop models.

16.2 Current approaches integrating SCFs and crop simulation models applied in Southeast Asia

We reviewed published literature on the use of integrated SCF-crop models for crop growth monitoring and climate risk management in Southeast Asia through a systematic research of prominent science databases including Scopus, Web of Science and Science Direct. Peer-reviewed and relevant reports from governmental departments and research institutions spanning the period 2009–2018 were selected and their abstracts were screened to find the most relevant to our review. Additionally, for all relevant papers, we reviewed the reference lists for papers missed in the initial search. We also referred to pioneering studies published before the selected review period. The use of SCF information for agricultural and natural ecosystems applications have been investigated globally (Iizumi et al, 2018) as well as for several different regions of the world (Cantelaube and Terres, 2005, Coelho and Costa, 2010, Crane et al, 2010, Hammer et al, 2000, Hansen et al, 2011, Stephens et al, 2000).

The recent literature contains examples of the use of climate forecasts within crop models to producing relevant information for decision making in agriculture at various spatial scales in Southeast Asian countries. Some were carried out at the global scale for crops such as rice, wheat, maize and soybean, and provided example outputs for Southeast Asian countries (Iizumi et al, 2013, 2015, 2018). For example, Iizumi et al (2015) denoted that reliable in-season yield predictions at the national scale of maize, wheat, rice or soybean based on SCFs can be produced in regions where crop yield is temperature-sensitive and temperature forecasts are reliable. In these studies statistical crop yield models were used. Given the changes in yield responses to temperature and precipitation with time due to technological improvements, operationalizing such approaches requires the statistical crop yield models be recalibrated regularly to account for these changes (Iizumi et al, 2018). Sheinkman (2015) described several national and regional research efforts across Southeast Asia countries including the Food and Agriculture Organization (FAO) Analysis and Mapping of Impacts Under Climate Change for Adaptation and Food Security (AMICAF) project in Asia, the Remote Sensing-based Information and Insurance for Crops in emerging Economies (RIICE; http://www.riice.org/) project, and research activities from the CGIAR Research Program on Climate Change, Agriculture and Food Security (CCAFS) and the International Rice Research Institute.

One of the tools developed through CCAFS research activities is the CCAFS Regional Agricultural Forecasting Toolbox (CRAFT). The CRAFT provides a user-friendly interface to integrate SCF into crop models (Shelia et al, 2019). It has been tested for rice and wheat yield forecasting in Bangladesh and India (Shelia et al, 2019), and it offers a potential application for gridded crop modeling and yield forecasting, as well as impact studies risk assessment in Southeast Asia countries. SCFs in CRAFT are produced using the Climate Predictability Tool (CPT; Mason and Tippett, 2016), which was developed by the IRI and designed as a statistical forecast package for producing SCF using gridded outputs from atmospheric general circulation models (GCMs) and sea surface temperatures (SSTs). The pre-installed crop models or modeling platforms are the Decision Support System for Agrotechnology Transfer (DSSAT; Jones et al, 2003) software application program, the Agricultural Production Systems Simulator (APSIM; Holzworth et al, 2014), and the System for Regional Analysis of Agro-Climatic Risks (SARRA-H; Baron et al, 2003). DSSAT and APSIM have already been evaluated in Southeast Asia countries (see for example Gaydon et al, 2017, Kontgis et al, 2019, Pasuquin et al, 2014), which would facilitate the use of CRAFT for improved agricultural climate risk management in these countries. CRAFT uses the statistical approach proposed by Hansen and Indeje (2004) to integrate SCF with the crop yield forecast. Probabilistic crop yield forecasts are derived from cross-validated hindcast residuals, centered on the expected value of the current forecast (Hansen and Indeje, 2004, Shelia et al, 2019). Hindcast residuals are obtained from a multivariate statistical model in which simulated yields (using observed antecedent weather data for the current year up to the forecast date and then complemented with weather data from available historic years until final harvest) are treated as predictand and the relevant seasonal climate predictor fields (calculated using CPT) are predictors.

Other forecasting systems also used in some Southeast Asian countries for managing climate risks in agricultural production systems include the Climate-Agriculture-Modeling and Decision Tool (CAMDT; Han et al, 2017) and the integrated seasonal climate-crop yield forecasting system for Robusta coffee (ICCFS-Robusta; Kouadio et al, 2015). They are discussed in Section 16.3.

16.3 Examples of integrated SCF-crop modeling approach for climate risk management in Southeast Asia

16.3.1 The climate-agriculture-modeling and decision tool (CAMDT)

The CAMDT is a software framework that links tercile-based SCFs with DSSAT dynamic crop growth simulation models for investigating various crop management scenarios under projected climate patterns (Han et al, 2017). The temporal downscaling of SCFs is achieved through two approaches: i) a parametric method, predictWTD, which is based on a conditional stochastic weather generator; and ii) a non-parametric method, FResampler1, which randomly samples a block of daily time series of weather data for the season of interest from historical observations conditioned on the tercile probabilities (e.g., being below, near and above-normal) (Han and Ines, 2017). Both methods benefit from climate data longer than 30 years. Although CAMDT can be used for yield forecasting, its main purpose is to explore the expected impact of technology options on crop yields and income for different seasonal climate scenarios, which meet agricultural stakeholders' needs, rather than identifying optimal solutions (Han et al, 2017).

An example application of this tool for assessing optimal planting date and fertilizer use in rice farming systems was carried out for the Bicol River Basin, Philippines (Han et al, 2017). In their study, the tercile-based seasonal climate forecasting system was linked to the DSSAT-CSM-Rice crop model within CAMDT. The DSSAT-CSM-Rice crop model was first calibrated and evaluated based on field experiments data, which were made available through the research undertaken by the International Rice Research Institute (IRRI) and the Philippine Rice Research Institute (PhilRice). ENSO influences strongly climate and rice production in the Philippines, making SCFs very skillful for such an analysis, with highest SCFs skill in the October-November-December season (Lyon and Camargo, 2009, Lyon et al, 2006). Different scenarios of fertilizer application and planting date under variable environmental conditions were run and the rice response to climate was analyzed in terms of yield impact and from an economic perspective to increase the value for farmers' decision making. These scenarios include three levels of nitrogen (N) application (i.e., no nitrogen, two- and three-time N application throughout the cropping season) and three different planting dates. Forecasted yields and gross margins of all scenarios were assessed through exceedance probability curves, with the exceedance probability (P) computed as $P = m \times (n+1)^{-1}$, where m is the rank of a forecasted yield or gross margin ($m = 1$ is the largest value) and n is the total number of simulated years. Uncertainties in forecasted yields are reflected by the spread of the probability curves.

For their analysis and because of an El Niño event during the study period 2009-2010, drier SCFs (45% below-normal, 35% near-normal and 20% above-normal) for January-February-March of 2010 were used. The exceedance distribution of yield forecasts, along with the resulting gross margins, indicated that insightful information on the likely impact of fertilizer rates and delays in planting on rice yield based on SCFs. Such tailored information can be used as decision support, and there have been several training workshops conducted in the Bicol region, Philippines for increasing the adoption of this tool as a decision support system. Also, the CAMDT is being used to produce crop yield outlooks for the Seasonal Climate Forecast and Extension Advisory (CLEA) in the same region.

16.3.2 The integrated seasonal climate-crop yield forecasting system for robusta coffee (ICCFS-Robusta)

Coffee is one of the most important commodities in the international agricultural trade, playing a crucial role in the economy of several African, American and Asian countries. In Vietnam, the world's second-largest coffee-producing and exporting country (ICO, 2019), more than 97% of coffee beans are produced in the Central Highlands region; a region listed among the most drought-prone ones in the country (GSOV, 2017, ICO, 2019, Nguyen, 2005). Rainfall over the Central Highlands is mainly governed by monsoon. To help the coffee industry prepare to climate variability and adapt their agricultural planning and operations accordingly, the ICCFS-Robusta was developed (Kouadio et al, 2015). The ICCFS-Robusta is an integrated system consisting of a simplified biophysical model (the USQ-Robusta coffee model) for simulating Robusta coffee growth and seasonal climate forecasting systems (Figure 16.1), through which targeted seasonal climate and coffee potential

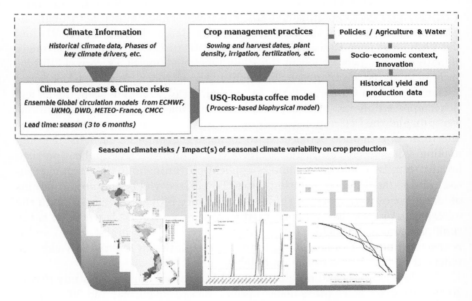

FIGURE 16.1: The integrated seasonal climate-crop yield forecasting system for Robusta coffee (ICCFS-Robusta). The USQ-Robusta coffee model simulates the growth of different organs and the phenology of coffee plants at a daily time step based on information on crop management practices (e.g., harvest date, yield, irrigation, etc.) and daily meteorological data (minimum and maximum temperatures, solar radiation, rainfall). Outputs of the ICCFS-Robusta include simulated coffee yields, probabilistic information (e.g., probability of exceeding median or average) for coffee yields, as well as for climate variables such as rainfall, and maximum and minimum temperatures.

yield forecasts are delivered for nominated key coffee-producing regions, as required. SCFs are derived from the CACS-USQ in-house seasonal climate forecasting systems, as well as latest advanced GCMs. Probabilistic coffee yield forecasts, along with SCFs are pivotal for the success of any agricultural industry that plans or sells ahead of the annual harvest (Meinke and Stone, 2005, Stone et al, 2000). When an impending outlook of likely drier (wetter) than normal is on the horizon, decision-makers can take actions such as forward buying (selling), or made strategic resource mobilization in the most insecure areas.

Historical climate data up to the forecast date (spanning a period of at least 30 years) (see Figure 16.1), along with crop management practices and historical yield data are used as inputs in the biophysical model to simulate the crop response (i.e., potential yield) for each coffee-growing province. Note that prior to the analysis, the USQ-Robusta coffee model was calibrated and tested for three major coffee-producing provinces (Dak Lak, Gia Lai, and Lam Dong), with satisfactory results: the inter-annual yield variability during a 13-year period (2002–2014) was satisfactorily captured, with prediction errors (i.e., root mean square error) ranging from 0.23 to 0.25 ton ha^{-1} (that is, 12% of error) (Kouadio et al, 2015).

The long-term median (or average) yield forecast for a given coffee-producing province is calculated using predicted performance over the 30-year period, and the set of simulated outcomes associated with the projected climate conditions from SCF is used to derive the coffee yield forecast distribution. Probabilistic Robusta coffee yield forecasts for the year of the forecast are provided using analog approaches based on categorical indicators of climate drivers (e.g., Oceanic Niño index, Southern Oscillation Index, Tropical Pacific sea surface temperatures, etc.) and simulated coffee yields (Hansen et al, 2004, Lorenz, 1969, Potgieter et al, 2003, Stone et al, 2000, Zhao and Giannakis, 2016). Conventional analog forecasting produces a forecast $\widehat{F}_t(y)$ of an observable f (i.e., climate driver index) of a dynamical sysetm (i.e., GCMs) at forecast lead time m given initial data y in the space X (Lorenz, 1969, Zhao and Giannakis, 2016). The distance function $D : X \times X \mapsto \mathbb{R}$ is set to the Euclidean distance $D(x, y) = \|y - x\|$, when $X = \mathbb{R}^n$ (Zhao and Giannakis, 2016). A cluster analysis method is used to select and assign probability weight to a subset of k analog years based on their rank Euclidean distance, in predictor state space, to a given predictor state (Lall and Sharma, 1996, Stone et al, 2000). The expected value of predictand y in year t of a series is estimated as follows:

$$\widehat{y}_m = \sum_{i=1, i \neq m}^{n} w_i y_i \qquad (16.1)$$

with

$$w_i = \frac{1/j}{\sum_{i=1}^{k}(1/j)}, \qquad (16.2)$$

where i is the index of the neighbor, sorted by distance (closest to furthest) from the predictor, and k is the number of nearest neighbors. For all $i > k$, w_i is set to 0.

The ICCFS-Robusta allows the examination of the probabilistic yield anomaly (likelihood of exceeding the long-term median or average) associated with the prevailing climate pattern in the year of forecast throughout the cropping season at the provincial scale. Simulated potential yields are used in this approach rather than actual yields because long time series of actual coffee yield data at the provincial scale are not available. An example output of the ICCFS-Robusta is depicted in Figure 16.2.

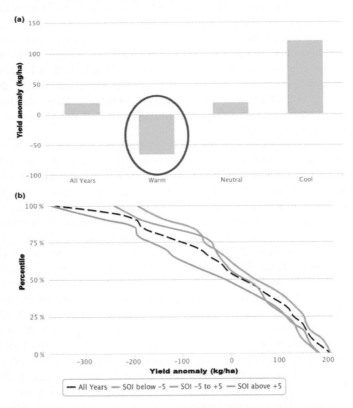

FIGURE 16.2: Example outputs of the ICCFS-Robusta for Gia Lai province, Vietnam. (a) Forecast of shift in Robusta coffee yield that would have been issued for harvest of 2015 based on the average Oceanic Niño index (ONI) in July–September. The climate pattern for 2015 is shown circled. (b) Probabilistic Robusta coffee yield forecast based on the Southern Oscillation Index (SOI) in April that would have been issued for harvest of 2015.

16.4 Challenges for operationalizing seasonal climate-crop modeling frameworks in Southeast Asia

Although various integrated SCF-crop models are used for operational purposes in several countries around the world, their adoption in the majority of Southeast Asian countries remains very limited. Challenges for moving toward the broader implementation of integrated SCF-crop modeling systems to support decision-making for climate risk management in Southeast Asia include addressing data scarcity for model calibration/validation, assessing fully SCF skills, communicating SCFs outputs to farmers, and extending the range of SCFs applications across Southeast Asian countries.

16.4.1 Data scarcity

Using SCFs for agricultural decisions depends on historic climate records that are sufficiently long to support downscaling, and assess the forecasting skill use of such SCFs at a spatial resolution that is consistent with the scale of decisions (Hansen et al, 2011, Meinke and Stone, 2005). There is a scarcity of reliable long-term climate data in the majority of Southeast Asian countries due to a lack of adequate infrastructures (e.g., constraints linked to complex topography, poor network of automatic weather stations, etc.). Satellite remote sensing provides a complementary source of climate variable estimates, but available satellite-based data sets are limited by their short duration or coarse spatial resolution. Nevertheless, they remain vital in regions where no climate data is available.

The robustness and reliability of crop models depend on the quality of data (e.g., crop variety, management practices) used for their calibration and validation. The availability of such data constitutes a key obstacle for using operationally crop models. For example, in CRAFT, gridded crop simulations can be conducted for any region for up to three scale levels, i.e., country, state/province, and district. But in the absence of information on crop varieties, irrigation, fertilizer input, and cultivated and irrigated area, the model runs are limited to the country level only (Shelia et al, 2019); thereby preventing the use of such an information for supporting agricultural decision at finer spatial scale (farm scale). It is noteworthy that some of the crop modeling systems have been designed for specific applications and, accordingly, have certain requirements and limitations that could restrict their use in operational SCF-crop modeling systems in developing countries. For example, depending on the time scale and spatial unit of simulation they may need to be run on clusters or on high performance computers (which might be costly due to associated implementation and maintenance issues).

16.4.2 Assessing the skills of seasonal climate forecasts

Inter-annual climate variations in Southeast Asia tend to be associated with the El Niño-Southern Oscillation, which is believed to influence monsoon behavior, resulting in drier and warmer than average conditions during El Niño years (Srinivas et al, 2019, Thirumalai et al, 2017). Forecasting monsoon precipitation across Southeast Asian countries remains a major challenge (Shin and Moon, 2018, Wang et al, 2009). Likewise, handling the occurrence of critical low temperatures and rain-induced chill damage on crops remain challenging in regions with complex topography, such as those in most Southeast Asia country (Promchote et al, 2018), highlighting a need to fully evaluate seasonal climate forecasts skill for enabling their broader use for operational purposes.

16.4.3 Communicating SCF outputs to farmers

Various forms of communication of SCF outputs need to be considered and tailored to the local context. Public or private extension systems are the most used channel of dissemination of agricultural advisory. Digital technology such as mobile phones are increasingly recognized and used as a potential advisory system. In Colombia, the CCAFS has implemented the Local Technical Agro-Climatic Committees with regular monthly meetings to bring together information from various sources, organize the ideas and thoughts, and disseminate the information (Loboguerrero et al, 2018). Another successful approach to deliver climate services to smallholder farmers is the Participatory Integrated Climate Services for Agriculture (PICSA) approach, developed by the University of Reading in partnership with CCAFS. PICSA is a structured process for evaluating farming and livelihood opportunities in light of historic climate risks, for identifying promising alternatives, and for adjusting management when seasonal forecasts shift relevant risks sufficiently. The idea is to integrate climate services into agricultural extension service by training staff, volunteer farmers, development NGO, and other intermediaries to integrate climate services into their work with farming communities (Dorward et al, 2015).

16.4.4 Extending the range of applications of integrated SCF-crop modeling systems

Managing climate-related risks in agricultural production implies synergies between the different levels of decision making (from farmers to institutional users). One way of extending the use of integrated SCF-crop modeling systems could be through incorporating their outcomes into the design of index-based insurance. This would offer a more robust approach to managing climate risk at different levels throughout the supply chain and would benefit to smallholder farmers particularly, who are dominant in Southeast Asia (Lowder et al, 2016, Samberg et al, 2016). Although they have to be tested in pilot implementations, factoring forecast information into the design of contract could increase the efficiency and livelihood benefits of index insurance, at least where it is designed to support access to credit and intensify market-oriented production (Hansen et al, 2011, Osgood et al, 2008).

16.5 Improved climate risk management in Southeast Asia—the way forward

As highlighted by (Sheinkman, 2015), several programmes and initiatives are underway across Southeast Asia, and likely to support seasonal forecast information services for agriculture, including SCFs use for climate-related risks management. However, there remains building and/or strengthening collaboration between research institutions, universities, national government agencies, industries and local stakeholders to mainstream climate information into effective and operational integrated forecasting systems for food security planning and policy formulation at regional, national, and sub-national local levels.

Recent investments in climate risk management systems for Southeast Asia (i.e., the De-RISK project) have been supported by the German Federal Ministry for the Environment, Nature Conservation and Nuclear Safety, targeting smallholder farmers and businesses engaged in the coffee, sugar, rice, cassava, rubber, maize, associated crops and fruits, and grazing industries in Vietnam, Cambodia, Lao PDR and Myanmar (https://deriskseasia.org/). The De-RISK project, promoted by the World Meteorological Organization (WMO), aims to develop resilient climate risk management systems that will shield stakeholders across the entire agricultural value chain in these countries from physical and financial disaster associated with climate variability and change. A description of the key comprehensive planned measures of the De-RISK project are presented in Figure 16.3. It is expected that the targeted seasonal climate forecasting system(s) developed for the needs of decision makers/agricultural sectors together with associated enhanced decision-support and delivery tools for each country will help adapting incrementally to climate change. This will be a good opportunity for developing and including integrated seasonal climate-crop forecasting systems in the region. Probabilistic forecasts of agricultural impacts (e.g., crop yields) based on SCF are most useful if they are timely, consistent and validated against other available or independent sources of information, and they meet the needs of the different agricultural stakeholders (Kouadio and Newlands, 2014). When updated through the growing season, they could serve multiple climate risk management interventions across the targeted agricultural value chains.

Climate change is threatening the livelihoods and food security of millions of poor smallholder farmers and agribusiness who depend on agriculture in Southeast Asia. Compared to countries such as the United States, Australia

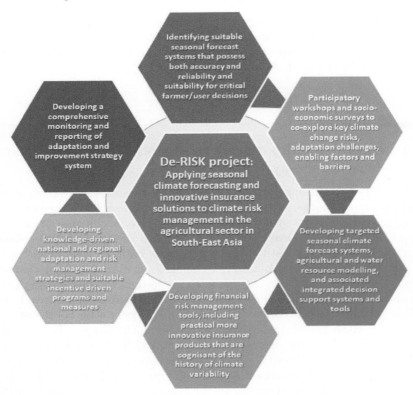

FIGURE 16.3: Comprehensive planned measures of the De-RISK project in four countries in Southeast Asia (Cambodia, Lao PDR, Myanmar, and Vietnam).

or India, effective seasonal climate modeling and forecasting for this region is dire in almost all circumstances, despite being vulnerable to impacts of extreme climate/climate change and major climate drivers such as ENSO. Such a vulnerability will increase under the changing climate if populations are not well prepared. Advances in the accuracy of climate information provide opportunities to increase lead times of early warnings. The ability to forecast extreme/unusual climate conditions months in advance is arguably one of the most potentially important developments in the environmental sciences of current times.

Acknowledgments

We gratefully acknowledge the funding received from the German Federal Ministry for the Environment, Nature Conservation, Building and Nuclear Safety (BMUB) and the World Meteorological Organization (WMO) through the De-RISK project.

References

Allan R (2000) ENSO and climate variability in the last 150 years, Cambridge University Press, Cambridge, UK, 3–56

Baron C, Bonnal V, Dingkuhn M, Maraux F, Sarr M (2003) SARRA-H : Système d'Analyse Régional des Risques Agroclimatiques-Habillé (System for Regional Analysis of Agro-Climatic Risks), IFDC, Muscle Shoals, Etats-Unis, 192–194

Cantelaube P, Terres JM (2005) Seasonal weather forecasts for crop yield modelling in Europe. Tellus A 57(3):476–487

Cirino PH, Féres JG, Braga MJ, Reis E (2015) Assessing the impacts of ENSO-related weather effects on the Brazilian agriculture. Procedia Economics and Finance 24:146–155

Coelho CAS, Costa SMS (2010) Challenges for integrating seasonal climate forecasts in user applications. Current Opinion in Environmental Sustainability 2(5):317–325

Crane TA, Roncoli C, Paz J, Breuer N, Broad K, Ingram KT, Hoogenboom G (2010) Forecast skill and farmers' skills: Seasonal climate forecasts and agricultural risk management in the Southeastern United States. Weather, Climate, and Society 2(1):44–59

Dorward P, Clarkson G, Stern R (2015) Participatory integrated climate services for agriculture (PICSA): Field manual. Walker Institute, University of Reading, Reading, UK

Gaydon DS, Balwinder S, Wang E, Poulton PL, Ahmad B, Ahmed F, Akhter S, Ali I, Amarasingha R, Chaki AK, Chen C, Choudhury BU, Darai R, Das A, Hochman Z, Horan H, Hosang EY, Kumar P, Khan ASMMR, Laing A, Liu L, Malaviachichi MAPWK, Mohapatra KP, Muttaleb MA, Power B, Radanielson AM, Rai GS, Rashid MH, Rathanayake WMUK, Sarker MMR, Sena DR, Shamim M, Subash N, Suriadi A, Suriyagoda LDB, Wang G, Wang J, Yadav RK, Roth CH (2017) Evaluation of the APSIM model in cropping systems of Asia. Field Crops Research 204:52–75

GSOV (2017) Statistical Yearbook of Vietnam 2017. Statistical documentation and service centre, General Statistics Office of Vietnam (GSOV), Hanoi, Vietnam. Available at $https://www.gso.gov.vn/default_en.aspx?tabid = 515\&idmid = 5\&ItemID = 18941$ (Accessed March 2019)

Hammer GL, Nicholls N, Mitchell C (2000) Applications of seasonal climate forecasting in agricultural and natural ecosystems. Atmospheric and Oceanographic Sciences Library, Springer, Dordrecht

Han E, Ines AVM (2017) Downscaling probabilistic seasonal climate forecasts for decision support in agriculture: A comparison of parametric and non-parametric approach. Climate Risk Management 18:51–65

Han E, Ines AVM, Baethgen WE (2017) Climate-agriculture-modeling and decision tool (camdt): A software framework for climate risk management in agriculture. Environmental Modelling & Software 95:102–114

Hansen JW, Indeje M (2004) Linking dynamic seasonal climate forecasts with crop simulation for maize yield prediction in semi-arid Kenya. Agricultural and Forest Meteorology 125(1):143–157

Hansen JW, Hodges AW, Jones JW (1998) ENSO influences on agriculture in the Southeastern United States. Journal of Climate 11(3):404–411

Hansen JW, Potgieter A, Tippett MK (2004) Using a general circulation model to forecast regional wheat yields in northeast Australia. Agricultural and Forest Meteorology 127(1):77–92

Hansen JW, Challinor A, Ines A, Wheeler T, Moron V (2006) Translating climate forecasts into agricultural terms: advances and challenges. Climate Research 33(1):27–41

Hansen JW, Mason SJ, Sun L, Tall A (2011) Review of seasonal climate forecasting for agriculture in Sub-Saharan Africa. Experimental Agriculture 47(2):205–240

Holzworth DP, Huth NI, deVoil PG, Zurcher EJ, Herrmann NI, McLean G, Chenu K, van Oosterom EJ, Snow V, Murphy C, Moore AD, Brown H, Whish JPM, Verrall S, Fainges J, Bell LW, Peake AS, Poulton PL, Hochman Z, Thorburn PJ, Gaydon DS, Dalgliesh NP, Rodriguez D, Cox H, Chapman S, Doherty A, Teixeira E, Sharp J, Cichota R, Vogeler I, Li FY, Wang E, Hammer GL, Robertson MJ, Dimes JP, Whitbread AM, Hunt J, van Rees H, McClelland T, Carberry PS, Hargreaves JNG, MacLeod N, McDonald C, Harsdorf J, Wedgwood S, Keating BA (2014) APSIM – Evolution towards a new generation of agricultural systems simulation. Environmental Modelling & Software 62(0):327–350

ICO (2019) Country coffee profile: Vietnam. International Coffee Council 124th Session, Paper ICC-124-9. International Coffee Organization (ICO), Nairobi, Kenya. Available at http://www.ico.org/documents/cy2018-19/icc-124-9e-profile-vietnam.pdf (Accessed on September 2019)

Iizumi T, Sakuma H, Yokozawa M, Luo JJ, Challinor AJ, Brown ME, Sakurai G, Yamagata T (2013) Prediction of seasonal climate-induced variations in global food production. Nature Climate Change 3(10):904–908

Iizumi T, Yokozawa M, Sakurai GEN, Sakuma H, Luo JJ, Challinor AJ, Yamagata T (2015) Characterizing the reliability of global crop prediction based on seasonal climate forecasts, World Scientific Series on Asia-Pacific Weather and Climate, vol Volume 7, World Scientific, 281–304

Iizumi T, Shin Y, Kim W, Kim M, Choi J (2018) Global crop yield forecasting using seasonal climate information from a multi-model ensemble. Climate Services 11:13–23

Jones JW, Hoogenboom G, Porter CH, Boote KJ, Batchelor WD, Hunt LA, Wilkens PW, Singh U, Gijsman AJ, Ritchie JT (2003) The DSSAT Cropping System Model. European Journal of Agronomy 18(3-4):235–265

Kontgis C, Schneider A, Ozdogan M, Kucharik C, Tri VPD, Duc NH, Schatz J (2019) Climate change impacts on rice productivity in the Mekong River delta. Applied Geography 102:71–83

Kouadio L, Newlands NK (2014) Data hungry models in a food hungry world—an interdisciplinary challenge bridged by statistics, CRC Press, Taylor & Francis Group, New York, book section 21, 371–385

Kouadio L, Tixier P, Stone R, Mushtaq S, Rapidel B, Marcussen T (2015) Robusta coffee model: An integrated model for coffee production at a regional scale. In: TropAg2015 "Meeting the Productivity Challenge in the Tropics"

Lall U, Sharma A (1996) A nearest neighbor bootstrap for resampling hydrologic time series. Water Resources Research 32(3):679–693

Liu Y, Yang X, Wang E, Xue C (2014) Climate and crop yields impacted by ENSO episodes on the North China Plain: 1956–2006. Regional Environmental Change 14(1):49–59

Loboguerrero AM, Boshell F, León G, Martinez-Baron D, Giraldo D, Recaman Mejía L, Díaz E, Cock J (2018) Bridging the gap between climate science and farmers in Colombia. Climate Risk Management 22:67–81

Lorenz EN (1969) Atmospheric predictability as revealed by naturally occurring analogues. Journal of the Atmospheric Sciences 26(4):636–646

Lowder SK, Skoet J, Raney T (2016) The number, size, and distribution of farms, smallholder farms, and family farms worldwide. World Development 87:16–29

Lyon B, Camargo SJ (2009) The seasonally-varying influence of enso on rainfall and tropical cyclone activity in the philippines. Climate Dynamics 32(1):125–141

Lyon B, Cristi H, Verceles ER, Hilario FD, Abastillas R (2006) Seasonal reversal of the enso rainfall signal in the philippines. Geophysical Research Letters 33(24)

Mason S, Tippett M (2016) Climate Predictability Tool Version 15.3. Columbia University Academic Commons, New York

Meinke H, Stone RC (2005) Seasonal and inter-annual climate forecasting: The new tool for increasing preparedness to climate variability and change in agricultural planning and operations. Climatic Change 70(1-2):221–253

Nguyen QK (2005) Evaluating drought situation and analysis drought events by drought indices. National Project Drought Research Forecast Centre South Central Highland Vietnam Constructing Prevent Solution

Osgood DE, Suarez P, Hansen JW, Carriquiry M, Mishra A (2008) Integrating seasonal forecasts and insurance for adaptation among subsistence farmers: the case of Malawi. World Bank Policy Research Working Paper No. 4651. World Bank, Washington, DC

Pasuquin JM, Pampolino MF, Witt C, Dobermann A, Oberthür T, Fisher MJ, Inubushi K (2014) Closing yield gaps in maize production in Southeast Asia through site-specific nutrient management. Field Crops Research 156:219–230

Potgieter AB, Everingham YL, Hammer GL (2003) On measuring quality of a probabilistic commodity forecast for a system that incorporates seasonal climate forecasts. International Journal of Climatology 23(10):1195–1210

Promchote P, Wang SYS, Shen Y, Johnson PG, Yao MH (2018) A seasonal prediction for the wet–cold spells leading to winter crop damage in northwestern Taiwan with a combined empirical–dynamical approach. International Journal of Climatology 38(2):571–583

Samberg LH, Gerber JS, Ramankutty N, Herrero M, West PC (2016) Subnational distribution of average farm size and smallholder contributions to global food production. Environmental Research Letters 11(12):124010

Sheinkman M (2015) Integrated Modeling of Climate Change Impacts on Agricultural Productivity and Socio-Economic Status (IMCASE) in the Philippines. CCAFS Workshop Report. Copenhagen, Denmark: CGIAR Research Program on Climate Change, Agriculture and Food Security (CCAFS)

Shelia V, Hansen J, Sharda V, Porter C, Aggarwal P, Wilkerson CJ, Hoogenboom G (2019) A multi-scale and multi-model gridded framework for forecasting crop production, risk analysis, and climate change impact studies. Environmental Modelling & Software 115:144–154

Shin SH, Moon JY (2018) Prediction skill for the east Asian winter monsoon based on apcc multi-models. Atmosphere 9(8): 300

Srinivas G, Chowdary JS, Gnanaseelan C, Parekh A, Dandi R, Prasad KVSR, Naidu CV (2019) Impact of differences in the decaying phase of El Niño on South and East Asia summer monsoon in CMIP5 models. International Journal of Climatology 39(14):5503–5521

Stephens D, Butler D, Hammer G (2000) Using seasonal climate forecasts in forecasting the Australian wheat crop, Atmospheric and Oceanographic Sciences Library, vol 21, Springer Netherlands, book section 21, 351–366

Stone R, Smith I, McIntosh P (2000) Statistical methods for deriving seasonal climate forecasts from GCM'S, Springer Netherlands, Dordrecht, 135–147

Thirumalai K, DiNezio PN, Okumura Y, Deser C (2017) Extreme temperatures in Southeast Asia caused by El Niño and worsened by global warming. Nature Communications 8(1):15531

Wang B, Lee JY, Kang IS, Shukla J, Park CK, Kumar A, Schemm J, Cocke S, Kug JS, Luo JJ, Zhou T, Wang B, Fu X, Yun WT, Alves O, Jin EK, Kinter J, Kirtman B, Krishnamurti T, Lau NC, Lau W, Liu P, Pegion P, Rosati T, Schubert S, Stern W, Suarez M, Yamagata T (2009) Advance and prospectus of seasonal prediction: assessment of the APCC/CliPAS 14-model ensemble retrospective seasonal prediction (1980–2004). Climate Dynamics 33(1):93–117

Zhao Z, Giannakis D (2016) Analog forecasting with dynamics-adapted kernels. Nonlinearity 29(9):2888–2939

17

Poppy Cultivation and Eradication in Mexico, 2000–2018: The Effects of Climate

S. Marcelo Olivera-Villarroel
Metropolitan Autonomous University Cuajimalpa, Mexico City, Mexico

Maria del Pilar Fuerte Celis
Research Center for Geospatial Information Sciences, Aguascalientes, Mexico

CONTENTS

17.1	Introduction	363
17.2	Context	365
17.3	Methodology	366
	17.3.1 Overview of index construction	367
	17.3.2 Statistical weighting of the index components, using the Shapley decomposition	367
	17.3.3 Components of the poppy eradication index	368
17.4	Results	370
17.5	Discussion	375
17.6	Conclusions	376
References		377

17.1 Introduction

Climate change and its effects are closely linked to farming activities, and may result in the loss of crops and the abandonment of agricultural regions, especially due to extreme droughts and floods (Chavas, 2019, Crost et al, 2018, De la Fuente and Olivera-Villarroel, 2013, Gümüşçü and Gümüşçü, 2015). Since opium poppy (*Papaver somniferum*) does not require a lot of water and gives high agricultural yield (Bauer, 2019, Collet, 2005), many farmers in Mexico have decided to stop cultivating legal crops and have started cultivating poppy (Dube et al, 2016, Herrera, 2019, Santacruz-De León and Palacio-Muñoz, 2014).

As reported by the United Nations Office on Drugs and Crime (UNODC, 2018), the area used for poppy in Mexico in 2016–2017 was the third-largest in the world (behind Afghanistan and Myanmar)—about 30,600 cultivated hectares (UNODC, 2018, Villa y Caña, 2017). Moreover, according to the data from the Ministry of National Defense (UNODC, 2018), the areas taken by poppy in Mexico have been increasing. This growth has invigorated violence near those areas and the competition among multiple criminal structures fighting over the control of the drug business (Calderón et al, 2015, Dube et al, 2016).

The phenomenon of illicit crops is complex; hence, its analysis requires an approach capable of managing economic, geographical, political, social, and environmental factors. In the conditions of increasing poppy cultivation, the concern is often directed to a public security debate (Mattiace et al, 2019), ignoring the causes that push farmers toward illicit cultivation. In this study, we focus on the relationships between climate change and poppy cultivation which has been poorly explored in the literature (Dube et al, 2016, Gümüşçü and Gümüşçü, 2015). How does climate affect the production of illicit crops? Our research is based on the hypothesis that if climate of a region discourages the production of legal crops, poppy's production increases, therefore, the amount of effort for its eradication by the state grows. Our objective is to systematically study the change in weather conditions in Mexico and the effects of the decline in agricultural productivity caused by droughts and floods, added to social conflicts and the low production of foodstuffs, which has pushed farmers to abandon traditional agriculture, especially seasonal corn (Dube et al, 2016, Gümüşçü and Gümüşçü, 2015, Olivera-Villarroel et al, 2011).

Opium poppy production is an illegal activity in Mexico. Government agencies report eradication, surveillance, and control activities in the cultivation areas. The information is reported at the municipal level and by month, hence, our minimum unit of analysis is municipality.

We add to the literature on illicit crops and drug trafficking by emphasizing the importance of climate impacts on illicit crops. Rain and temperature are important variables to consider in the analysis of the territorial patterns of poppy cultivation, what can be demonstrated through an exploratory analysis of areas with high concentration of eradicated crops.

Finally, in this study we emphasize that by using the suggested perspective to address the role of climate change on illicit crop cultivation, we transcend visions, which are usually divided by different political points of view that tend to simplify the problem and limit the implementation of efficient and sustainable solutions. The foregoing can play a crucial role in guaranteeing public safety in Mexico. By providing public policy tools and arguments, it is possible to implement alternative development programs and viable licit activities in areas affected by climate change, and to support those affected in rural areas, guaranteeing the sustainability of the local communities and the reduction of illicit crops (UNODC, 2016).

17.2 Context

Millions of people, mainly in the Global South, take part in illegal crop cultivation (coca, opium poppy, and cannabis) used to make narcotics (Chouvy, 2019, Chouvy and Laniel, 2007, Lincoln, 2019, Miltenburg, 2018, Musto, 1991, Thoumi, 2002). The Single Convention on Narcotic Drugs of 1961—the first and most influential of the three United Nations conventions on drugs—forced states to uproot all cultivation of coca, poppy, and cannabis not for medical or scientific needs (Boister, 2018, Buxton, 2016).

The "war on drugs," initiated by the United States in the early 1970s, was based on strategies to try to contain drug trafficking and reduce high levels of drug use (Chabat, 2009, Nadelmann, 1998, Sharp, 1994). The strategy followed by the United States towards the Latin American countries directed all efforts towards expansion of the justice system and to strengthening of the prison and justice procuring infrastructure. The greatest effort was directed to the eradication of plantations and prohibition, with an emphasis on countries such as Peru, Bolivia, and Colombia (Belenko, 2000, Rodríguez Luna, 2010, Rosen and Zepeda Martínez, 2015).

The cooperation with Mexico under these action lines was inaugurated with the signature Agreement between Mexico and the United States for Cooperation in the Fight against Drug Trafficking, in 1989. This document accepted the join responsibility of the two countries in dealing with the problem of drug trafficking and addictions (Chabat, 2009, Velázquez Flores, 2011). Also, an emphasis was placed on the development of programs for the prevention, reduction of the demand for recreational drugs (Nadelmann, 1998), and the eradication of illegal drug crops (Rodríguez Luna, 2010).

In view of drug prohibition and eradication of illicit crops, a large poppy production market in Mexico began to consolidate, desired by drug trafficking groups to develop a thriving business of banned substances. In addition to the intensification of illegal drug trade, recent climate change in Mexico has also favored the expansion of poppy (Bucardo et al, 2005, Dube et al, 2016, Medel and Lu, 2015).

The geographical pattern of precipitation and temperature in Mexico has generated regions known for the production of illicit poppy and cannabis crops. Among those renowned areas are the "Golden Triangle" in the Sierra Madre Occidental mountains, specifically, in the border area of Chihuahua, Durango, and Sinaloa; and "Tierra Caliente" in the Sierra de Guerrero, which include more than 1280 towns that are engaged in this illegal activity (Peacock et al, 2018, UNODC, 2016).

The total area under poppy cultivation in Mexico was estimated at 25,200 hectares between July 2015 and June 2016 (UNODC, 2016), which increased by 21% and reached 30,600 hectares of poppy between July 2016 and June 2017 (UNODC, 2018). Based on these two studies by UNODC

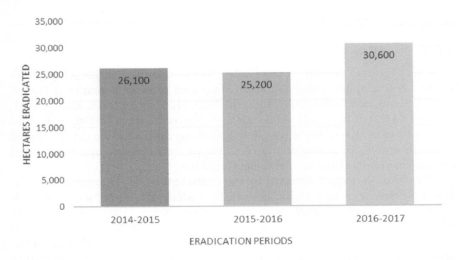

FIGURE 17.1: Areas of eradicated poppy cultivation in Mexico, 2014–2017. Source: UNODC (2018).

(2015–2016 and 2016–2017), poppy crops were mainly concentrated in the Golden Triangle, north of Nayarit, and in the states of Guerrero and Oaxaca in the Sierra Madre del Sur. The Mexican government reported that 26,426 hectares of poppy were eradicated in 2015; 22,436 hectares in 2016, and 29,692 hectares in 2017 (see UNODC, 2018, and Figure 17.1).

Mexican government efforts to eradicate illegal cultivation follow a complex state policy that came about in the 1990s and involves different sectors of the federal government, the army, and the navy. The strategy includes patrolling the territory; manual eradication and fumigation of illegal crops; securing areas; land, air, and sea money-laundering interception; providing help for addicts, and the development of rural activities (Gudiño-Chong, 2016).

The eradication strategies and the related patrolling activities have led to crops all over the territory, since producers attempt to cultivate and avoid elimination, while authorities try even harder to eradicate. Crops are moved between regions where they are the most prominent and where they are less likely to be eradicated, leading to complex interrelations, which is one of the reasons for this study.

17.3 Methodology

We propose a new poppy cultivation eradication index (PEI) representing the likelihood of poppy crop eradication in a municipality. This likelihood is based on the number of state patrols and on other geographic, sociodemographic,

Methodology

and climatic characteristics of the municipality. The index is used to visualize cultivation patterns in Mexico and to quantify the impact of climate and social factors, as well as the influence of the eradication strategy undertaken by the Mexico's three most recent governments (Vicente Fox, 2000–2006; Felipe Calderón, 2006–2012, and Enrique Peña-Nieto, 2012–2018). The premise is that the greater the number of crops eradicated, the more illegal activities move to regions where they are less likely to be eradicated, but where adequate climatic conditions for the cultivation exist.

17.3.1 Overview of index construction

The process of building an index entails several steps, including choosing, normalizing, weighting, and aggregating index components, represented by various indicators, into a final index (OECD, 2008). Weighting the indicators is the most complex step and can be based on statistical assessments (such as principal components analysis [PCA] or factor analysis), participatory approaches (such as analytic hierarchy process, Delphi De Loe, 1995), or budget allocation process (OECD, 2008). The main objectives of weighting the indicators are to: 1) detect variables with high correlations, and 2) choose an optimal weighting and aggregation approach for calculating the final index.

A comparison of 106 studies for building indices to assess risks showed that the most-often used approach (46 of all the studies) was the "equal weights" method (Beccari, 2016), where different indicators contribute to the final index in the same proportion (Barnett et al, 2008, Cutter et al, 2003, Nguefack-Tsague et al, 2011). Some studies (13) used weights defined by the authors, and some studies (19) used participatory methods, where the weights were based on opinions of experts or local agents, decision makers or government authorities. The rest of the studies (28) used different types of statistical methods. When there are a considerable number of variables, participatory approaches can be subjective, but the expert judgment is often based on many years of experience, which can be beneficial (Simpson and Katirai, 2006).

The choice of the weighting technique affects the index directly. Such effects stand out in the study by Becker et al (2017), where three indices were calculated (Resource Governance, Good Country, and Water Retention) using original and optimized weights, and the final classification results differed substantially between the two approaches. Optimization of the weighting in the Good Country Index showed improved results for up to 86 out of 125 countries (Becker et al, 2017). In other words, modifications of the weighting imply important changes in the estimated index. Therefore, the weighting method for index calculations should be well-justified.

17.3.2 Statistical weighting of the index components, using the Shapley decomposition

We propose a two-step procedure for calculation of the PEI. In the first step, all the indicators included in the index have the same weight. In the second step, a statistical re-weighting of the components is applied, which allows us to identify components with the highest weight, rank the components by their importance, and, based on that, prioritize certain public policy decisions.

Let Θ be the index with k components x_i and respective weights β_i ($i = 1, \ldots, k$):

$$\Theta = \beta_1 x_1 + \beta_2 x_2 + \ldots + \beta_k x_k, \tag{17.1}$$

where at the first step of our procedure $\beta_1 = \beta_2 = \ldots = \beta_k = 1$ (Shorrocks, 1999).

The index form (17.1) can be viewed as a multivariate linear regression. Determination of statistical significance and contribution of each explanatory variable to the variance of a dependent variable in regression is an important topic in applied economics. A systematic way of quantifying the different contributions of explanatory variables is quantifying their contribution to the regression's goodness-of-fit (Israeli, 2007). Hence, we propose to weight the index components using the Shapley–Owen decomposition, which provides partial coefficients of determination, R_i^2 ($i = 1, \ldots, k$), for each variable x_i (Sastre and Trannoy, 2002, Zaiontz, 2017):

$$R_i^2 = \sum_{T \subseteq V \setminus \{x_i\}} \frac{R^2(T \cup \{x_i\}) - R^2(T)}{k \cdot C(k-1, |T|)}, \tag{17.2}$$

where $V = \{x_1, x_2, \ldots, x_k\}$ is the set of components of the index, T is a subset of V, $|T|$ denotes cardinality (number of elements) of the set, and $C(a, b)$ is the number of possible combinations of b elements taken from the set of a elements ("a choose b"). We assume that $R^2(\varnothing) = 0$.

To calculate R_i^2 when $k = 16$, we need to compute R^2 for $2^{16} = 65,536$ regression models; this number goes up to 1,048,576 if $k = 20$. Thus, the approach is practical only for a relatively small number of independent variables (Zaiontz, 2017). The Shapley decomposition is available in statistical software, such as R and Stata (Shorrocks, 1999, Zaiontz, 2017).

17.3.3 Components of the poppy eradication index

The poppy cultivation eradication index (PEI) consists of five components, which include climatic variations, sociodemographic factors, geographic characteristics, patrol efforts, and eradication efforts. The five components come from the literature, which specifies links between different socioeconomic and environmental processes that are key to understanding the territorial patterns of illegal crops (Rocha García, 2015).

The components are carefully chosen groups of indicators that capture a specific aspect within the PEI and meet the "3 R" criteria: relevant, representative, and robust. At the intermediate stages of the analysis, a factorial test was applied to avoid data redundancy.

Methodology

Climatic variability

The first component of the PEI is the climate variability. Based on monthly average records of temperature and precipitation in each Mexican municipality, we create an indicator comparing the baseline behavior of climate variables in 1980–2000 to the behavior in three 6-year presidential administrations from 2000 to 2018.

Methodologically, it is necessary and reasonable to assume that seasonal crops are grown in places with predictable weather. From this point of view, there is an optimal crop yield as a function of meteorological conditions (rainfall and temperature). There are many climatic zones in Mexico that over the long period of agricultural development have been supporting certain kinds of agricultural practices and population living in those areas, including indigenous communities of many different ethnic groups. Hence, the recent climate perturbations in any direction (i.e., leading to suboptimal crop yields or leading to changes in agricultural practices) can be considered as unfavorable (IMCO, 2012, Olivera-Villarroel and Heard, 2019). Therefore, the analysis focuses on how much the climate variables differ from their average.

To quantify variability of temperature and precipitation in i-th municipality, we calculate relative deviation, d ($0 \leqslant d \leqslant 1$), from the average of the corresponding variable in the baseline period. The pairs of deviations calculated for each municipality and time step t (month),

$$\{d(temp)_{i,t}, d(precip)_{i,t}\} \qquad (17.3)$$

represent the municipality's location in the data cloud and serve as an index of climate volatility, with $\{0,0\}$ being the optimum value. Since the coordinates (17.3) are relative, they can be used to compare climate volatility across municipalities.

This approach of quantifying climate impacts, however, has some limitations. The distances (17.3) do not quantify trends in the local climate, in particular, the index does not show if a municipality is warmer or colder, more dry or more rainy when compared to previous years. Hence, it is necessary to assign categorical labels describing the climate traits of the municipalities.

The climate labels were assigned as follows. Based on the temperature dynamics, *warm municipality* is the area with a temperature increase in more than six months out of a year and *cold municipality* is the area with a temperature decrease in more than six months out of a year. Based on the precipitation dynamics, we call the area a *rainy municipality* if it is experiencing higher rainfall during at least 6 months of the year compared to previous years and *dry municipality* if precipitation has decreased in more than 6 months. These tags are aggregated in 6-year periods of the Mexico's administrations and used as qualitative variables in our analysis.

Sociodemographic indicators

Some of the sociodemographic indicators included in the index are the municipality's population density and the total population. It is assumed that the areas with lower population density and smaller population are more likely to have remote and secluded places for illicit activities. Hence, such territories are more susceptible to illegal poppy cultivation. Another variable in this group of indicators is the municipality's social gap index, which is a summary of the standard of living, unmet basic needs, and poverty level (Rocha García, 2015).

Geographic characteristics

Several geographic indicators were selected for the PEI based on their theoretical relationship with the presence of illegal crops in municipalities and the ease of moving narcotics to consumer markets or drug-processing regions. Thus, distances from the municipality to Mexico's northern and southern borders, the existence of migratory routes to the United States, and the number of criminal organizations in the municipality were considered as the geographical indicators (Fuerte Celis et al, 2019).

Eradication efforts and the probability of eradication

The group of variables characterizing eradication efforts includes the number of patrols within the municipality, the number of times poppy crops were eradicated, the number of hectares eliminated, and the average size of the area being eradicated. Based on this information, the probability of eradication of poppy cultivation was calculated for each municipality. There were cases when patrols did not find the crops, and in some other cases the patrolling was done specifically to eradicate crops detected by other means. Such means included analysis of satellite imagery and use of reconnaissance planes and drones to detect illegal cultivation (Jia et al, 2011, UNODC, 2016).

Using a combination of the described indicators, the index was calculated, the Shapley decomposition was carried out, and contributions of the indicators to the total variance of the index were estimated. The index itself and each of its components are measured on the scale from 0 to 1, hence, a similar approach can be used to analyze each of the components.

17.4 Results

The results are presented in two stages. The first stage is the visualization of the distribution of illegal cultivation patches, which shows that during the Vicente Fox and Felipe Calderón administrations (2000–2012) the crops were spread out, whereas with Enrique Peña-Nieto (2012–2018), the opposite is true (Figure 17.2). The most recent map shows plots in fewer municipalities,

Results 371

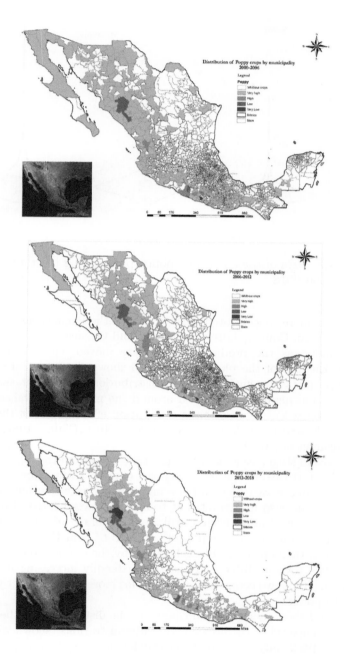

FIGURE 17.2: Distribution of poppy by municipality during each of the three recent Mexico's administrations.

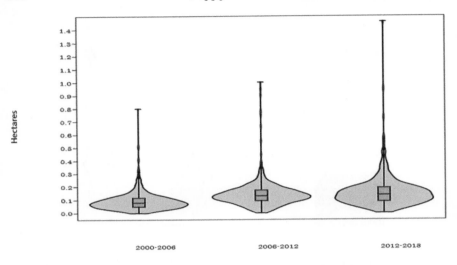

FIGURE 17.3: Sizes of the eradicated poppy plots during the three administrations in 2000–2018.

which are now more concentrated in the states on the Pacific coast, especially Sinaloa, Durango, Colima, Jalisco, Guerrero, and Oaxaca.

Furthermore, as the production zones are moved, there has been an increase in the size of the plots. Figure 17.3 shows that most of the eradicated poppy plots are small, with the distribution of the plot sizes being right-skewed and highly concentrated around the median. It is also possible to see that the recent more efficient eradication efforts warrant that larger plots are eradicated in the latter period of 2012–2018 (Chung, 1987, Kapoor, 1995, Yıldırım et al, 2016).

In the second stage, we look at the general results from the index analysis. Based on the statistical weighting, the impact of eradication efforts is the most substantial. Climate variables and the municipality's geographic and social characteristics are also important, but to a much lower degree (Table 17.1). The number of eradication events explains an average of 70% of the PEI, however, the weight of this component drops to 65% in the last period. At the same time, the percentage of explanation by the eradication effects (sum of the last two rows in Table 17.1) has been steadily increasing in the analyzed period. These two components account for more than 90% of the index's explanatory power.

Figure 17.4 shows a substantial change in the distribution of the index in 2012–2018, compared to the previous two administrations (shown with violin plots). More specifically, the median of the index increased from approximately 0.20–0.25 during the first two analyzed administrations to more than 0.70 in the 2012–2018 administration. Table 17.1 and Figure 17.4 show that the eradication efforts have become more efficient. For example, the investments by

Results

TABLE 17.1: Structure of the poppy crop eradication index in each period

Variables	2000–2006	2006–2012	2012–2018
Climate index	0.49%	0.36%	0.45%
Social index	0.64%	0.65%	0.69%
Geographic characteristics	6.66%	4.15%	2.26%
Prob. of finding poppy crops	14.02%	17.69%	29.17%
Eradication events	74.13%	73.70%	65.10%

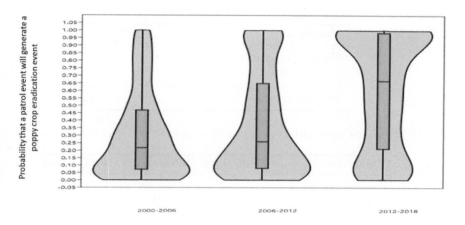

FIGURE 17.4: Poppy crop eradication index during the three administrations in 2000–2018.

Mexican navy and the army into infrastructure and use of satellite imaging (UNODC, 2016) lead to more directed efforts in fewer municipalities with illegal crops, which increases the probability that a poppy field can be effectively eradicated.

Climate variability and the qualitative representation of having a warm-cold or wet-dry climate show a slight but statistically significant effect on the crop eradication process. Collet (2005) explains that farming opium poppy in warm dry climates is not favorable to its growth during the first stages, so moving the crops to wetter regions is a strategy to raise production levels (Figure 17.1). However, during the Peña administration (2012–2018), some of the production moved to municipalities with dry climate (Table 17.2). The intensified poppy eradication practices force the choice of regions further from the traditional areas of eradication, but with less favorable weather conditions.

Note that the climate index focuses on the variability of climate conditions, so it leaves aside more homogeneous aspects of climate.

The explanatory power of the considered geographic characteristics decreased from 6.66% in 2000–2006 to 2.26% in 2012–2018 (Table 17.1),

TABLE 17.2: Structure of the weather index in each period

Variables	2000–2006	2006–2012	2012–2018
Climate variability	22.77%	21.02%	25.54%
Areas with dry months	24.79%	38.82%	48.55%
Areas with warm months	52.35%	40.04%	25.81%

TABLE 17.3: Poppy cultivation eradication index by geographic characteristics

Variables	2000–2018
Number of criminal organizations	37.5%
Distance from northern border	5.4%
Distance from southern border	4.5%
Migration route	52.6%

TABLE 17.4: Poppy cultivation eradication index by social indicators

Variables	2000–2006	2006–2012	2012–2018
Population density	11.03%	10.67%	14.28%
Population	9.52%	10.32%	14.46%
Social gap index	79.14%	78.75%	70.94%

whereas the characteristics themselves stayed the same over the whole period of 2000–2018. The existence of a migratory route within the municipality plays a key role in the geographic component of the index (Table 17.3). Migratory routes allow for temporary labor when agricultural demand is high and allow the illegal product to be distributed more efficiently. The number of criminal organizations has a lower explanatory power, while the distances to the borders are ranked as the least important (Table 17.3).

The weights of the variables constituting the social dimension of the index (Table 17.4) show a certain similarity of the types of poppy-producing municipalities in the first two administrations analyzed, while there was a considerable surge in more densely populated municipalities during the Peña-Nieto's administration (2012–2018), with the weight increasing from about 11% to 14.28%. Population size also showed a progressive increase of its relative weight (Table 17.4). The social gap index showed dynamics opposite to the population variables. Farming thus moved from highly marginalized areas to areas with larger population, greater population density, and better living standards.

Since the modern poppy eradication techniques include satellite imagery, there is now more certainty about the location of poppy fields (UNODC, 2016). There are now fewer eradication events in the region, with a drop from more

Discussion

TABLE 17.5: Crop eradication efforts

Variables	2000–2006	2006–2012	2012–2018
Number of municipalities with eradication events	1090	1016	700
Min number of eradication events made in a year	1	1	1
Max number of eradication events made in a year	398,633	162,180	193,290
Total number of eradication events per year	2,465,948	1,183,661	1,138,848
Average number of municipalities with eradication events per year	2262	1165	1627

TABLE 17.6: Poppy crop eradication index for eradication efforts

Variables	2000–2006	2006–2012	2012–2018
Hectares eradicated	6.15%	8.56%	5.75%
Number of plantations	6.71%	8.92%	5.48%
Number of excursions	5.52%	4.99%	5.12%
Probability of finding poppy plantations in the area	81.61%	77.52%	83.64%

than 2 million during the Fox administration to slightly more than 1 million during the Calderón and Peña administrations (Table 17.5).

The change in the number of eradication events and the spread of the crops over the territory has modified the weights of the variables within the component of eradication efforts and their final effect on the index. During the Calderón's administration (2006–2012), it becomes evident that production spreads to more municipalities, the weight of the odds of eradicating crops decreases, and the number and size of fields found increases, stabilizing with the concentration of poppy farming in fewer municipalities in the later period (see Tables 17.5 and 17.6).

17.5 Discussion

The eradication patterns of poppy show the importance of climate. Growers choose the best land, climate, and locations to develop this illegal activity. It is important to understand these effects to approach the study of the causes of violence based on the factors of production of the illegal drugs (Herrera, 2019).

The importance of the weather factor in the illegal poppy cultivation eradication index at first glance seems marginal. During the analyzed 18 years, more than 300 municipalities participated in the production of the illegal crop, however, only municipalities with traditional narcotics farming and processing networks remain prominent, and new municipalities-producers are those with weather conditions beneficial for poppy farming. Our study shows, municipalities with the least favorable weather conditions for poppy production discontinue the illegal farming. In other words, climate is significant and marginal, but it has a high weight when decisions are made regarding moving crops motivated by other factors.

In Mexico, the territorial concentration seen in the poppy cultivation during 2012–2018 increases the risks to the drug business, one that would hardly seem strategic. We highlight two central points: 1) cultivation has been moved to areas with a larger population and greater social visibility, and 2) price rises constantly on the export market, and producers can accept greater risks of loss compensated by higher relative profits (Kapoor, 1995, Yıldırım et al, 2016). Eradications of poppy crops are moving toward peri-urban municipalities that have strategic value for controlling the drug market. This is a new scenario for organized crime groups, which have expanded and evolved to maintain their structure and territorial dominance (Ryder, 2015).

This concentration pattern of poppy cultivation seen in the last administration could lead to struggles over territories with the best weather conditions to maintain poppy crop farming. The strategic movement of the crops is focused on more weather-based factors and on where there is a lower probability of being eradicated rather than on geographic and location factors (Dell, 2015).

Meanwhile, it is necessary to consider that there are several criminal groups specialized in the production of narcotics. The relationships between the state and criminal actions are complicated. Despite the improvements in detecting land areas used for poppy cultivation, poppy farming business has grown stronger. Additional analysis is needed to assess whether these actions have led to an increase in confrontations between public forces and criminal organizations. We believe we can answer this question with further research and with data collected for this study.

17.6 Conclusions

The climate factors are relevant for the study of illegal crops in Mexico. To develop a comprehensive strategy against organized crime, it is necessary to assess the specific patterns of regional traits sought after by producers of illicit crops. This strategy must include offering the growers—whose involvement into the illegal activity is motivated by financial considerations, social or criminal pressure—other paths to develop. The strategy also must take into account the social, environmental, and climate characteristics of the regions where illicit crops have become a viable economic option.

Despite its limitations, this study allows us to consider the phenomenon of illicit drug crops, specifically opium poppy in Mexico, from new perspectives. The migration of poppy crops from one region to another is partially motivated by the search for better climatic conditions. One of the main results of this study is the recognition of the importance of climatic factors in understanding the territorial pattern of poppy cultivation. With the analysis of 18 years of data, our model showed part of the production has been moving into areas with dry climate.

The illicit cultivation in Mexico is not happening just by chance; the empirical evidence shows patterns in the change of the crops that are strongly related to the climatic characteristics, the number of events of eradication, sociodemographic, and geographical aspects of the municipalities.

References

Barnett J, Lambert S, Fry I (2008) The hazards of indicators: insights from the environmental vulnerability index. Annals of the Association of American Geographers 98(1):102–119

Bauer R (2019) The costs and benefits of poppy cultivation. In: The Peasant Production of Opium in Nineteenth-Century India, Brill, 132–162

Beccari B (2016) A comparative analysis of disaster risk, vulnerability and resilience composite indicators. PLoS Currents 8

Becker W, Saisana M, Paruolo P, Vandecasteele I (2017) Weights and importance in composite indicators: Closing the gap. Ecological Indicators 80:12–22

Belenko SR (2000) Drugs and Drug Policy in America: A Documentary History. Greenwood Press, Westport, CT

Boister N (2018) Inter se modification of the UN drug control conventions. Law Review 20:456–492

Bucardo J, Brouwer KC, Magis-Rodríguez C, Ramos R, Fraga M, Perez SG, Patterson TL, Strathdee SA (2005) Historical trends in the production and consumption of illicit drugs in Mexico: implications for the prevention of blood borne infections. Drug and Alcohol Dependence 79(3):281–293

Buxton J (2016) Drug Crop Production, Poverty, and Development. Open Society Foundations, Washington, DC

Calderón G, Robles G, Díaz-Cayeros A, Magaloni B (2015) The beheading of criminal organizations and the dynamics of violence in Mexico. Journal of Conflict Resolution 59(8):1455–1485

Chabat J (2009) El narcotráfico en las relaciones México-Estados Unidos: Las fuentes del conflicto. Centro de Investigación y Docencia Económicas, Mexico City, Mexico

Chavas JP (2019) Adverse shocks in agriculture: The assessment and management of downside risk. Journal of Agricultural Economics 70(3):731–748

Chouvy PA (2019) Territorial control and the scope and resilience of cannabis and other illegal drug crop cultivation. EchoGéo 48

Chouvy PA, Laniel LR (2007) Agricultural drug economies: cause or alternative to intra-state conflicts? Crime, Law and Social Change 48(3–5):133–150

Chung B (1987) The effect of irrigation on the growth and yield components of poppies (*Papaver somniferum L.*). The Journal of Agricultural Science 108(2):389–394

Collet K (2005) Los factores favorables al desarrollo del cultivo de la adormidera: provincia de Albacete (España). Investigaciones Geográficas (Esp) 36:157–164

Crost B, Duquennois C, Felter JH, Rees DI (2018) Climate change, agricultural production and civil conflict: Evidence from the Philippines. Journal of Environmental Economics and Management 88:379–395

Cutter SL, Boruff BJ, Shirley WL (2003) Social vulnerability to environmental hazards. Social Science Quarterly 84(2):242–261

De Loe RC (1995) Exploring complex policy questions using the policy Delphi: A multi-round, interactive survey method. Applied Geography 15(1):53–68

Dell M (2015) Trafficking networks and the Mexican drug war. American Economic Review 105(6):1738–1779

Dube O, García-Ponce O, Thom K (2016) From maize to haze: agricultural shocks and the growth of the Mexican drug sector. Journal of the European Economic Association 14(5):1181–1224

De la Fuente A, Olivera-Villarroel SM (2013) The poverty impact of climate change in Mexico. The World Bank, Washington, DC

Fuerte Celis MdP, Lujan EP, Ponce RC (2019) Organized crime, violence, and territorial dispute in Mexico (2007–2011). Trends in Organized Crime 22(2):188–209

Gudiño-Chong E (2016) De las políticas públicas a las políticas castrenses en la erradicación de cultivos ilícitos en México, 1994–2015. ITESO, Tlaquepaque, Jalisco, Mexico

Gümüşçü A, Gümüşçü G (2015) Climate change and effect on yield components of opium poppy. Tarla Bitkileri Merkez Araştırma Enstitüsü Dergisi 24(1):79–84

Herrera JS (2019) Cultivating violence: trade liberalization, illicit labor, and the Mexican drug trade. Latin American Politics and Society 61(3):129–153

IMCO (2012) Índice de vulnerabilidad Climática. Instituto Mexicano de Competitividad, Mexico City, Mexico, URL http://imco.org.mx/images/pdf/Boletindeprensa_IVC_final.pdf

Israeli O (2007) A Shapley-based decomposition of the R-square of a linear regression. The Journal of Economic Inequality 5(2):199–212

Jia K, Wu B, Tian Y, Li Q, Du X (2011) Spectral discrimination of opium poppy using field spectrometry. IEEE Transactions on Geoscience and Remote Sensing 49(9):3414–3422

Kapoor L (1995) Opium Poppy: Botany, Chemistry, and Pharmacology. CRC Press, New York

Lincoln G (2019) An overview of the drug epidemic in the United States with a focus on opioids, cocaine, and marijuana. Integrated Studies 196

Mattiace S, Ley S, Trejo G (2019) Indigenous resistance to criminal governance: why regional ethnic autonomy institutions protect communities from narco rule in Mexico. Latin American Research Review 54(1):181

Medel M, Lu Y (2015) Illegal drug cultivation in Mexico: an examination of the environmental and human factors. Cartography and Geographic Information Science 42(2):190–204

Miltenburg J (2018) Supply chains for illicit products: case study of the global opiate production networks. Cogent Business & Management 5(1):1423871

Musto DF (1991) Opium, cocaine and marijuana in American history. Scientific American 265(1):40–47

Nadelmann E (1998) Challenging the global prohibition regime. International Journal of Drug Policy 2(9):85–93

Nguefack-Tsague G, Klasen S, Zucchini W (2011) On weighting the components of the human development index: a statistical justification. Journal of Human Development and Capabilities 12(2):183–202

OECD (2008) Handbook on Constructing Composite Indicators: Methodology and User Guide. OECD Publishing, Paris, France

Olivera-Villarroel SM, Heard C (2019) Increases in the extreme rainfall events: using the Weibull distribution. Environmetrics 30(4):e2532

Olivera-Villarroel SM, Binimelis Raga G, Orbe R (2011) The economic effects of intense rainfall in central states of the Pacific coast of Mexico: global warming impacts on agriculture. International Journal of Climate Change: Impacts and Responses 3(1):89–108

Peacock A, Leung J, Larney S, Colledge S, Hickman M, Rehm J, Giovino GA, West R, Hall W, Griffiths P, Robert Ali R, Gowing L, Marsden J, Ferrari AJ, Grebely J, Farrell M, Degenhardt L (2018) Global statistics on alcohol, tobacco and illicit drug use: 2017 status report. Addiction 113(10):1905–1926

Rocha García R (2015) Coca en Colombia: efecto balón, vulnerabilidad e integralidad de políticas. Archivos de Economía 431

Rodríguez Luna A (2010) La Iniciativa Mérida y la guerra contra las drogas. Pasado y presente. In: Benitez Manaut R (ed) Crimen Organizado e Iniciativa Mérida en las Relaciones México-Estados Unidos, Colectivo de Análisis de la Seguridad con Democracia México (CASEDE), Mexico City, Mexico, 31–68

Rosen JD, Zepeda Martínez R (2015) The war on drugs in Mexico: a lost war. Revista Reflexiones 94(1):153–168

Ryder N (2015) The Financial War on Terrorism: A Review of Counter-Terrorist Financing Strategies since 2001. Routledge, New York

Santacruz-De León EE, Palacio-Muñoz VH (2014) Campesinos mexicanos: entre la subsistencia, el mercado y los cultivos ilícitos. Quivera Revista de Estudios Territoriales 16(2014-2):11–25

Sastre M, Trannoy A (2002) Shapley inequality decomposition by factor components: some methodological issues. Journal of Economics 77(1):51–89

Sharp EB (1994) The Dilemma of Drug Policy in the United States. HarperCollins College Publishers, New York, NY

Shorrocks AF (1999) Decomposition procedures for distributional analysis: a unified framework based on the Shapley value. Tech. rep., University of Essex

Simpson DM, Katirai M (2006) Indicator Issues And Proposed Framework for a Disaster Preparedness index (DPi). University of Louisville, Louisville, KY, USA

Thoumi FE (2002) Illegal drugs in Colombia: From illegal economic boom to social crisis. The Annals of the American Academy of Political and Social Science 582(1):102–116

UNODC (2016) México: Monitoreo de cultivos de amapola 2014–2015. URL https://www.unodc.org/documents/crop-monitoring/Mexico/Mexico-Monitoreo-Cultivos-Amapola-2014-2015-LowR.pdf

UNODC (2018) México: Monitoreo de cultivos de amapola 2015–2016 y 2016–2017. URL https://www.unodc.org/documents/crop-monitoring/Mexico/Mexico-Monitoreo-Cultivos-Amapola-2015-2017.pdf

Velázquez Flores R (2011) La política exterior de Estados Unidos hacia México bajo la administración de Barack Obama: cambios y continuidades. Norteamérica 6(2):85–113

Villa y Caña P (2017) México, tercer productor mundial de amapola. URL https://www.eluniversal.com.mx/articulo/nacion/sociedad/2017/06/23/mexico-tercer-productor-mundial-de-amapola

Yıldırım U, Demircan M, Özdemir A, Sarıhan E (2016) Effect of climate change on poppy (*Papaver somniferum L.*) production area. Journal of Central Research Institute for Field Crops

Zaiontz C (2017) Shapley–Owen decomposition. URL https://www.real-statistics.com/multiple-regression/shapley-owen-decomposition/

Index

agriculture, 325, 348, 363
    coffee, 352
    illicit crop, 363
    poppy, 363
area
    Arctic, 152
    Canada, 325
        British Columbia, 48
    Mexico, 310, 363
        Mexico City, 310
    midlatitude, 152
    North Atlantic Basin, 27
    Norway, 259
        Bergen, 268
        Oslo, 268
    Southeast Asia, 349
    USA, 165, 201, 277
        Annapolis, 71
        Baltimore, 71
        California, 155, 203
        Chesapeake Bay, 71, 89, 123
        Dorchester County, 71
        Gulf Coast, 294
        Maryland, 71
        Midwest, 203
        New York, 290
        South Carolina, 201, 238
    Venezuela, 245
        Vargas, 245

benthos, 87
biodiversity, 88, 123
bootstrap, 11, 315

car accident, *see* traffic accident
causality, 132, 140
    causal graphical model, 145

convergent cross mapping
    (CCM), 144
    Granger, 141
changepoint, 28
climate model, 4
coastal inundation, *see* sea level rise
cyclone energy, 28

distribution
    Bernoulli, 269
    beta, 177
    binomial, 266
    gamma, 41, 93, 267
    Gaussian, 10, 32, 93, 244, 248
    generalized extreme value
        (GEV), 49, 183
    generalized Pareto, 169
    inverse Wishart, 249
    lognormal, 170
    negative binomial, 93, 249
    Poisson, 31, 93, 179, 249, 267
    Student's, 249
    unit Fréchet, 49
    zero-inflated negative binomial, 249
diversity, *see* biodiversity
drought, 46, 188, 203, 239, 277, 286, 363

ecosystem, 87, 123, 220, 328

fishery, 87, 155
flood, 65, 203, 363
forest fire, 45, 204, 287

greenhouse gas, 326

heat wave, 188, 239, 277, 284

hurricane, 27, 165, 201, 218, 239, 282
hypoxia, 87

index
    fire weather, 45
    poppy eradication, 366
    Shannon–Wiener, 93
    Simpson's, 93
    species richness, 93
infrastructure, 206, 259, 321
    electricity, 277
    transport, 218, 307

Jensen's inequality, 176
jet stream, 152

loss (economic), 165, 237, 259, 277

machine learning, 10, 260, 308
    classification and regression
        trees (CART), 314
    random forest, 314
minimum description length (MDL),
    30
model (climate)
    atmosphere-ocean general
        circulation model
        (AOGCM), 4
    earth system model (ESM), 4
    ensemble, 7
    general circulation model
        (GCM), 4, 140
    regional ocean model, 69
    representative concentration
        pathway (RCP), 66, 217,
        285
model (statistical)
    autoregressive moving average
        (ARMA), 32
    causal graphical model, 145
    conditional autoregressive
        (CAR), 241
    generalized additive model
        (GAM), 92, 313
    generalized linear model (GLM),
        266, 269

kriging, 247, 251, 265
    Bayesian, 251
    logistic regression, 266
    state space model, 143
    vector autoregressive (VAR),
        142

network (graph), 125
    alignment, 126
    causal, 140

organized crime, 363

principal component analysis (PCA),
    132
Python package
    skccm, 145
    statsmodels, 143
    TIGRAMITE, 149

R package
    extRemes, 49
    GA, 34
    ggplot2, 135
    Hmisc, 133
    indicspecies, 96
    ismev, 183
    lmtest, 143
    mgcv, 314
    MTS, 143
    netcom, 127, 132, 133
    pcalg, 149
    plotmo, 315
    randomForest, 315
    ranger, 315
    rEDM, 145, 149
    Rfast, 133
    SpatialExtremes, 52
    vegan, 96, 134

sea level rise, 65, 204, 239, 283
sea surface temperature, 155
Shapley decomposition, 367

traffic accident, 307

wildfire, 203, 204, 287

For Product Safety Concerns and Information please contact our EU representative GPSR@taylorandfrancis.com Taylor & Francis Verlag GmbH, Kaufingerstraße 24, 80331 München, Germany

Printed and bound by CPI Group (UK) Ltd, Croydon, CR0 4YY
08/06/2025
01896985-0007